The National Childbirth Trust
Book of
PREGNANCY, BIRTH, AND PARENTHOOD

The National Childbirth Trust,
*formed more than thirty years ago, is Britain's
foremost charity concerned with education for
parenthood. The Trust aims to help parents experience
greater confidence in, and enjoyment of, pregnancy,
childbirth, and the early days of parenthood. These
objectives are carried out through its antenatal
classes, counselling, and postnatal support
network. The NCT also extends its work into
schools and other organizations
for young people.*

Glynnis Tucker, *the editor of this book,
is an NCT antenatal teacher and counsellor.*

Contributors to this book
Elaine Antcliffe, Pauline Armstrong, Sheila Damon,
Hilary English, Gillian Fletcher, Alison Heffernan, Eileen Hutton,
Barbara Kott, Jeanne Langford, Helen Lewison, Anne Loader, Deirdre
Mackay, Mary Nolan, Jo O'Farrell, Gwen Rankin, Shirleyanne Seel,
Louise Simmonds, Mary Smale,
Glynnis Tucker.

Other contributors include all the members of the
National Childbirth Trust who have been involved in writing NCT
leaflets and booklets.

The National Childbirth Trust Book of

PREGNANCY, BIRTH, AND PARENTHOOD

Second Edition

*EDITED FOR THE NATIONAL CHILDBIRTH TRUST BY
GLYNNIS TUCKER*

Oxford Melbourne

OXFORD UNIVERSITY PRESS

1996

Oxford University Press, Walton Street, Oxford OX2 6DP

Oxford New York
Athens Auckland Bangkok Bombay
Calcutta Cape Town Dar es Salaam Delhi
Florence Hong Kong Istanbul Karachi
Kuala Lumpur Madras Madrid Melbourne
Mexico City Nairobi Paris Singapore
Taipei Tokyo Toronto
and associated companies in
Berlin Ibadan

Oxford is a trade mark of Oxford University Press

First edition published 1992 as an Oxford University Press paperback
Reprinted 1993, 1994
Second edition published 1996

British Library Cataloguing in Publication Data
Data available

Library of Congress Cataloging in Publication Data
The National Childbirth Trust book of pregnancy, birth, and parenthood / edited
for the National Childbirth Trust by Glynnis Tucker.—2nd ed
p. cm. Includes bibliographical references and index.
1. Pregnancy. 2. Childbirth. 3. Infants—Care. 4. Parenthood.
I. Tucker, Glynnis. II. National Childbirth Trust (Great Britain)
618.2—dc20 RG525.P678 1995 95–37002
ISBN 0-19-286187-5

Designed and produced for Oxford University Press by Richard Garratt Design,
Le Moulin de la Pacaudière 49700 Les Verchers sur Layon, France
Picture Research by Jennifer Garratt
Illustrations by Taurus Graphics Limited

Printed in Hong Kong

Preface

The National Childbirth Trust aims to help parents achieve greater enjoyment and satisfaction during pregnancy, birth, and early parenthood; this is the aim of this book, which contains a distillation of the wisdom, experience, and expertise of the NCT, which has been helping parents for more than thirty years.

The book will provide you with the essential information you will need to guide you through your pregnancy, birth, and the early stages of your baby's life. It will not tell you what to do — any decisions will be yours. What it will do is offer the information to help you make your own choices. There are no right or wrong ways of giving birth or being a parent; there may, however, be ways that are better for individuals, and this book will suggest some of the options open to you. Because the NCT is a consumer organization, of and for parents, any ideas, tips, and suggestions have come from parents, have worked for other parents, and may work for you.

The book will also offer you an opportunity to reappraise much of what you already know or assume, and suggests

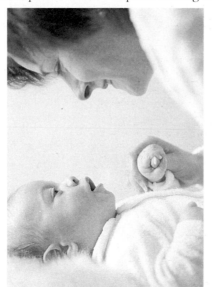

some ways of meeting the challenges of birth sensitively and intelligently. When it comes to understanding about your own body, your baby, your feelings, and your parenting skills, you, the parents, are the experts. Finding out as much as you can about all aspects of pregnancy, birth, and parenthood will help you gain the confidence to do what you want to do in the right way for you.

This book is written for fathers as well as for mothers. Read it and share your thoughts and feelings about it — use it as a stimulus to start you thinking about the questions you want to ask; the sort of birth you would like to have; how you are going to achieve the birth you are hoping for; how you will feel if pregnancy, birth, or parenthood do not always live up to your expectations; how you can help yourselves become the sort of parents you would like to be.

Although reading a book is a good beginning, it is no substitute for finding things out for yourselves: by attending antenatal classes, meeting other people, especially other parents, and having the chance to discuss all sorts of issues, concerns, and feelings at length with them. If you want to find out about pregnancy and birth, NCT antenatal classes will offer you the best opportunity of doing so. If you would like to breastfeed, NCT breastfeeding counsellors are there to help you. If you would like support and friendship once your baby has been born, the NCT offers opportunities for mothers and fathers to get together with other parents to share some of the delights and drawbacks of being a parent. You will find more about the NCT's approach and what it can offer as you read this book.

If you would like to contact the National Childbirth Trust for further information or help, you should write or phone NCT Headquarters. You will find the address listed at the back of this book.

For the purpose of clarity, the baby and older children are referred to as 'she'. Whilst appreciating that by no means all doctors are male, nor all midwives female, doctors are referred to throughout as 'he' and midwives as 'she'.

CONTENTS

Part 3: PARENTHOOD

Part 1
PREGNANCY

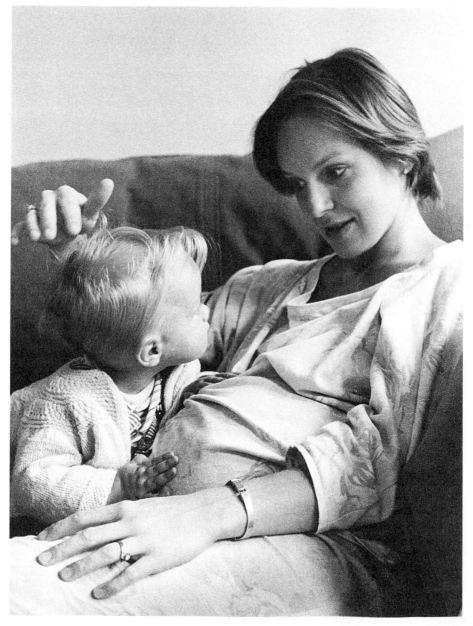

1 Beginning a Pregnancy

Whilst many women find themselves pregnant with little or no previous forethought, or indeed intention, and others choose a time that feels about right to go ahead with trying for a baby, many plan a pregnancy well in advance and alter their life-styles accordingly.

This first chapter is aimed at anyone who is considering becoming pregnant sometime in the near future, or who is in the very early stages of a pregnancy, either with a first or a subsequent baby. If you are hoping to conceive and would like the child you conceive to have the best possible start you can offer it, this chapter may help you decide what, if anything, you could usefully do to prepare for your pregnancy.

If, as is more than likely, you are reading this book because you are already pregnant, you do not have to skip this chapter; there may well be information or suggestions which could be of use or interest to you for this or a future pregnancy. If you happen to be pregnant unintentionally, or did not think to prepare for it, it is possible you will come across something which may make you feel worried or even guilty. If this is the case and you are concerned about the welfare of the child you are carrying, you could perhaps discuss your fears with your doctor or midwife, who can either reassure you or suggest appropriate action you might take. It may also be that there are things you could do now which could alleviate your worry, such as cutting out smoking or making sensible changes to your diet. It is also worth remembering that the vast majority of babies born in the United Kingdom are perfectly strong and healthy. Most women and men are sufficiently well-nourished, housed, and educated, having received good health care all their lives, to be fit and ready to conceive a healthy baby, and, in a woman's case, to enjoy a healthy pregnancy. This does not mean that, as a society, we should be complacent about conditions throughout the community, but it does put some of the worst fears into a different perspective.

Although this chapter will be looking at ways in which you can prepare for your pregnancy, and take care of your baby from the beginning, this will not, in itself, ever guarantee you a perfect baby. Parents of babies who are born with handicaps or other problems may feel guilty, or that they have failed their child in some way. But parenthood is not something you can swot up for then pass or fail, like an exam. There are no right or wrong answers, no absolute guarantees of perfection. Bearing this in mind, it is worth giving some thought to the best time for you to have a baby, in order to maximize your chances of conceiving a healthy baby and enjoying a successful pregnancy.

TIMING YOUR PREGNANCY

YOUR AGE Physically, the best time for a woman to have a baby is when she is in her twenties. At this age her body is fully grown and sufficiently mature to cope with a pregnancy — there is no risk of damage to growing bones, yet she is supple and flexible with plenty of energy. The older a woman is, particularly once she is past her early thirties, the less supple her body becomes and the more likely she is to experience complications. An older mother also carries a greater risk of having a handicapped baby (Chapter 4, Antenatal Screening, will offer some information so that you can assess the relative risks for yourself).

There are, however, aspects other than the purely physical. Older mothers and fathers may feel more settled in themselves, having enjoyed interesting, developing careers as well as leisure opportunities, and may be better able to cope with the financial and emotional demands of parenthood. More and more couples are choosing to start their families later in life, feeling no desperate rush to have children until well into their thirties. Indeed, it is common for people to say that they had never intended to have children, but they realized that soon the time would come when it really would be too late, and then they felt an overwhelming need to have children before it became impossible. Parents who have their children in their thirties and after can enjoy a maturity of outlook and experience rarely matched by their younger counterparts. The adjustment to parenthood may, of course, be harder for people who have become more used to doing things their own way!

SPACING YOUR FAMILY There is no right answer as to how to space your family. While a short gap between babies may suit some families better, others feel happier leaving several years between children. Often, the experience with one child will help to make the decision — you might originally intend having your family very close together, but find that a poor sleeper means you postpone the next baby until you are getting more manageable nights!

From the physical viewpoint, it is probably advisable to allow your body about eighteen months to recover before getting pregnant again, but you may feel that the advantages of a small gap outweigh the potential drain on your body. Only you will know how fit you feel, how well able to cope with the challenges of another pregnancy and baby. It can be useful to talk to friends who already have more than one child to hear the relative pros and cons of various age differences. Friends and relatives are often free with their advice about what the perfect answer is, but only you can decide what your family's needs and capabilities are, and therefore what would be most appropriate for you all.

PREPARING FOR PREGNANCY

Whereas some experts believe three months to be a perfectly adequate length of time to prepare for a pregnancy, others advise waiting six months or a year. How long you take may depend on your own situation: you may currently be taking medication which you would prefer to be free of first; you may have a health problem which needs clearing up; there may be other aspects of your life and health which it might be advisable to sort out now, while you have the chance.

Once you have decided when you would ideally like to become pregnant, it is a good idea to visit your GP both for advice and help with your general health, and also for specific tests he can carry out, at least three months before you hope to conceive.

RUBELLA Rubella, or German Measles, is a common, mild infection under normal circumstances, but if contracted by a pregnant woman in the first four months of pregnancy, it can have disastrous effects on the development of the baby's vital organs. You may be immune to the virus already through having had the disease or the immunization, but it is possible that you are unprotected, as neither is a guaranteed protection for life. A blood test will tell if you are immune. If you are not, your GP can immunize you, but you must be very careful not to get pregnant for the following three months, and you may wish to have a blood test to check that immunity has now developed.

You will be given a blood test for immunity to Rubella at your first antenatal appointment, but if you are worried that you may have been in contact with Rubella since becoming pregnant, do talk to your GP, who will be able to advise you.

ANAEMIA It is worth checking that you are not deficient in iron before beginning a pregnancy, so that you do not begin your pregnancy suffering the debilitating effects of anaemia. If you are of African, West Indian, Asian, or Southern Mediterranean origin, you can also be tested for sickle-cell anaemia and thalassaemia, both genetic disorders, which cause potentially very serious problems in pregnancy.

THE CONTRACEPTIVE PILL If you are taking the Pill and have decided to become pregnant, it is suggested you leave at least three months after coming off the Pill before trying to conceive. This will not only allow your body to begin adjusting its hormone levels; it will also mean that you stand a better chance of resuming a normal menstrual cycle. Getting pregnant before your periods have become regular again (if they ever were!) means you will not find it easy to work out when your baby was conceived. Many doctors advocate leaving a much longer gap between coming off the Pill and conceiving to be quite sure all the Pill's hormones have passed out of your system. Since the Pill also destroys vitamins, you will need to eat a particularly nourishing diet with plenty of fresh, raw fruit and vegetables (see Chapter 6, Looking After Yourself).

GENERAL HEALTH Since the health of both partners affects the baby you conceive, and since pregnancy imposes a strain on the woman's body, it is worth making sure any specific health problems either of you has are cleared up before you do conceive. If you, the woman, have long-term health problems, your GP or specialist will be able to advise you about how a pregnancy could affect your health, and vice versa. If your GP has insufficient information about your condition in relation to pregnancy, you can be referred to a specialist who should provide you with the information you need to make your decisions.

It is important that both partners consider their general health, as both eggs and sperm are affected by your physical well-being. It takes at least eight weeks for eggs and sperm to develop to the stage of being ready to be released, so you should consider waiting several months after a serious illness before conceiving a baby, particularly if you have been prescribed drugs to treat the illness.

SEXUALLY TRANSMITTED DISEASES Although all women are tested for VD antenatally, you might prefer to be tested beforehand if you think there is a chance you have contracted some form of sexually transmitted disease. Apart from the threat to your own health, babies can contract these infections in the uterus. Likewise, if you are in a risk category for contracting AIDS, you can be tested to discover whether or not you are HIV positive, in order to help you decide whether to risk becoming pregnant at all. You might well prefer any testing for sexually transmitted diseases to be done at a local clinic rather than by your GP.

GENETIC COUNSELLING If a relative of yours or of your partner has had a baby with a defect, you can be referred for genetic counselling, when a specialist will help you understand the nature of the problem and can offer advice about the likelihood of a child of yours being similarly affected, as well as advising you on any steps you could take to help yourselves.

DRUGS AND MEDICATION All chemical substances affect the production and growth of cells in our bodies, so, if you are used to taking drugs or medicines for any reason, now is a good time to reassess your use of them. If you are seeing your GP about other pre-pregnancy matters, you could ask him about this too. Even sleeping-pills and pain-killers are better avoided at this stage, so you may like to discuss with your GP alternative means of dealing with the problem. This may prove to be an ideal opportunity for looking at the cause of your problem rather than tackling the symptoms. Once you think you are pregnant, it is safest to avoid drugs of all kinds, even common remedies you might take for an upset stomach or a headache. If you do have to be prescribed drugs by your doctor, remind him that you are, or may be, pregnant, as there may be distinct choices between a drug which could harm the fetus and one which will not. If you are taking drugs for an existing condition such as diabetes or a heart problem, the most important thing is that you continue taking them unless advised otherwise. You and your specialist or GP can discuss between you the relative risks and benefits of any drugs you are taking.

ALCOHOL Alcohol contains chemicals which can damage both the developing sperm itself and also a man's fertility levels. If you bear in mind the fact that it takes a minimum of eight weeks for the sperm to get from production line to its intended egg, you will need to think about your alcohol consumption for at least three months in advance.

Alcohol intake will also affect a growing baby once a pregnancy is established, as any substance present in the mother's blood, whether beneficial or harmful, will pass to the baby. Nobody yet knows what a safe amount of alcohol during pregnancy might be, if indeed there is any safe level. Alcohol crosses the placenta, the organ which nourishes your baby during pregnancy (see Chapter 5, How You and Your Baby Grow), reducing the flow of nutrients and oxygen. Regular serious drinking can lead to both physical and mental retardation in a baby, but a bout of really heavy drinking, particularly in the early stages of pregnancy, is also potentially dangerous. Moderate social drinking, however, is unlikely to cause any problems.

SMOKING Apart from the adverse effects smoking has on the fetus, not to mention on the smoker him- or herself, it does not do a lot for your chances of conception. Smoking affects fertility as well as damaging the developing sperm. Smoking by a pregnant woman increases the risk of miscarriage and, by reducing the flow of nutrients and oxygen to the baby, also reduces its size and slows brain development. Smaller babies tend to have more problems than larger ones during their early months of life. Smoking also increases the chance of your baby being born pre-term, with all the inherent problems that brings. If you decide to continue smoking through your pregnancy, you may like to ask advice about supplements of vitamins B and C and zinc, as smoking interferes with your absorption of these elements. You and your partner may decide that the beginning of a pregnancy is a prime opportunity for giving up smoking altogether, so that your baby can be born into a non-smoking household without the risks of passive smoking. Many women do go off cigarettes while pregnant and you may, therefore, find it relatively easy to give up smoking now. If you would like to give up or cut down, but find the flesh less willing than the spirit, do ask your GP or midwife for help and support.

DIET AND NUTRITION Again, both partners need to consider their diets, checking that the overall nutritional balance is good, preferably for at least three months before trying to conceive, whilst sperm and eggs are maturing. Your nutritional intake will not only help ensure your sperm and eggs are well formed; it will also protect them against other harmful substances with which you come into contact (see below, Pollutants).You will find information to help you maintain a well-balanced, nourishing diet in Chapter 6, Looking After Yourself.

Some people are convinced that problems of congenital malformation or conceptual and pregnancy problems are caused by vitamin and mineral insufficiency in some women. Folic acid, a vitamin in the B group, has been found to be especially important in the prevention of neural-tube defects such as spina bifida or anencephaly. The Department of Health has recommended that a folic acid supplement of 0.4 mg. per day be taken both before pregnancy and for the first 12 weeks of pregnancy. Some studies suggest taking a supplement of 0.8 mg. a day to reduce the risk. Women who have previously had a baby with neural-tube defects are recommended to take a supplement of 5 mg. a day. (These recommendations do not apply to any woman who suffers from epilepsy, or to those taking the anti-convulsant drug valproic acid, or to women who have a vitamin B12 deficiency.) You may also like to make sure that your diet is rich in folic acid—good sources include wholegrain cereals, yeast extracts, and fruit and vegetables. Dark-green, leafy vegetables such as spinach and broccoli are excellent sources of this vitamin, and if you can eat them raw, or very lightly cooked, so much the better. Folic acid is quickly destroyed by cooking processes, particularly boiling.

If you are at all worried about your nutritional intake, contacting your GP or a dietician will provide you with further information.

POLLUTANTS It is not reasonably feasible to avoid all of the unpleasant, harmful substances we encounter in everyday life, but you could reconsider your life-style and become aware of what you are actually in contact with, thus minimizing your intake. Any form of X-ray or radiation is best avoided completely in this period, and the less you are exposed to traffic fumes, chemicals, pesticides, and sprays of all descriptions, the better. You can determine what you take in in the way of food to a large extent; less easy to control is what you inhale or take in through your skin. Try to be conscious of the substances you are exposed to. Now is not the time to use paint-stripper on your furniture or to sit in the garden while the farmer sprays his crops in the next-door field. You may also need to consider the jobs you or your partner do, in case either of you works with potentially damaging substances. You may be pregnant already and decorating your house, in which case you will need to make sure the rooms are well ventilated, and you should stop if you feel at all nauseous.

KNOWING YOUR MENSTRUAL CYCLE One advantage of preparing yourself for a pregnancy is that you are giving yourself time to get to know your own body: its rhythms, its likes and dislikes, its needs and capabilities. You may not have stopped to think much about the way your body works until now, so, by preparing yourself, you are pre-empting a natural desire to take care of your body, to listen to it, and to nourish it effectively.

You might like to start keeping a record of your menstrual cycle during this preparation period, noting how long it lasts, when you think you are ovulating (see below), and how regular your cycle seems to be. It is amazing how many women making their first antenatal appointments do not know when their last period started or how long their normal cycle lasts. Taking note of your body's rhythms in advance will help you decide when is your best chance of conceiving and when your baby is likely to be due. It is also excellent practice for listening to your body ready for pregnancy and labour.

BECOMING PREGNANT

Conception   A baby is conceived when a sperm from the male partner fuses with an egg from the female partner to form a single cell. This single cell then begins to divide, eventually implanting itself in the lining on the uterus, or womb, to start a pregnancy. Each contribution to this single cell, both egg and sperm, carries all the genetic material necessary to make your baby the person she will become — thus, in this tiny, fused cell, invisible to the naked eye, is a complete mixture of both parents which is, at the same time, utterly unique.

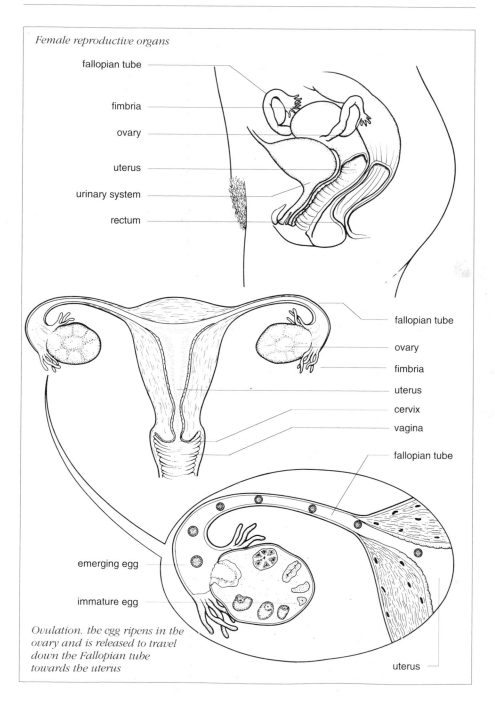

Female reproductive organs

fallopian tube

fimbria

ovary

uterus

urinary system

rectum

fallopian tube

ovary

fimbria

uterus

cervix

vagina

fallopian tube

emerging egg

immature egg

uterus

Ovulation. the egg ripens in the ovary and is released to travel down the Fallopian tube towards the uterus

One of the most exciting aspects of being a parent is in enjoying the knowledge that your children have physical and mental character- istics from both sides of the family; not just from the previous generation, but from all their ancestors. Your child will not only be a blend of the two parents; she will be entirely herself from the moment of conception — her obvious individuality and personality even in the earliest days of life is one of the great surprises and delights of parenthood.

Although you probably have a very clear idea about how the reproductive system works already, the information in this section can help you plan things for yourself more accurately, which is an important first step towards an active involvement with your baby.

THE FEMALE REPRODUCTIVE SYSTEM Normally every woman releases a ripened egg from one or other of her ovaries each month throughout her child-bearing years. On leaving the ovary, the egg is gently guided along the Fallopian tube towards the uterus. If it happens to meet a healthy sperm travelling along the Fallopian tube from the opposite direction, the two may become fused to create a single cell, which will develop into a baby. If it does not meet a healthy sperm *en route* for the uterus, then it will be swept away during your period with the endometrium, or lining of the uterus.

THE MENSTRUAL CYCLE The day a period starts is counted as Day 1 of the menstrual cycle. When the two-to-seven days of your period are over, the ovary begins ripening another egg ready for release during the next ovulation. Meanwhile the uterus begins to build up another inner lining ready to receive a fertilized egg. Ovulation normally occurs fourteen days before the beginning of the next

Normal menstual cycle

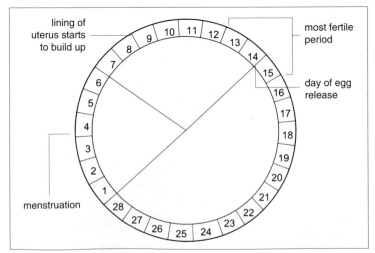

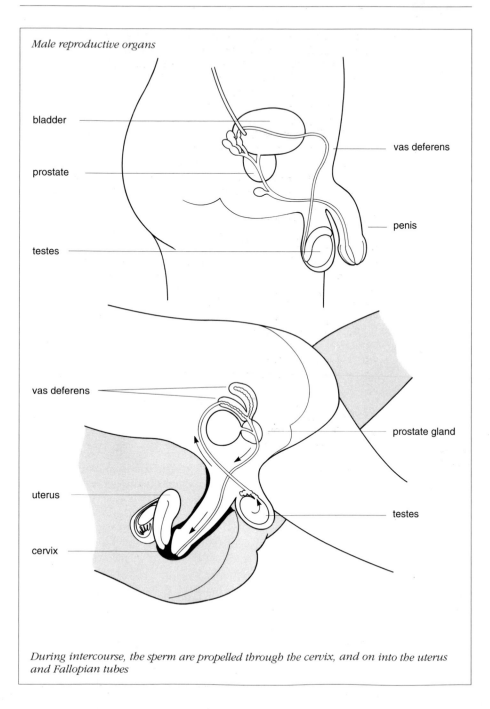

Male reproductive organs

bladder

prostate

testes

vas deferens

penis

vas deferens

prostate gland

uterus

testes

cervix

During intercourse, the sperm are propelled through the cervix, and on into the uterus and Fallopian tubes

period, regardless of the length of the cycle; this is why it is useful to build up a picture of your own menstrual cycle, so that you can work out when you might be likely to ovulate. Some women have a standard twenty-eight day menstrual cycle, starting a period on Day 1, ovulating around Day 14, then starting a period again two weeks later. As with most things in life, however, there are wide variations in what is considered normal, and menstrual cycles may be almost any length, though they will most commonly vary between twenty-three and thirty-six days.

An egg has a very brief life on its own, and, if unfertilized, will disintegrate rapidly after one-to-three days in the Fallopian tube. The more you know about when your body is ovulating the better you will be able to judge how to get the sperm to a good fresh egg.

THE MALE REPRODUCTIVE SYSTEM The sperm, the male cells, are produced in the testicles, being released during ejaculation. Millions of sperm are wasted, as anything from 20 to 500 million sperm may be released during an orgasm. When a man ejaculates, the muscle contractions propel the sperm into the vagina towards the uterus. Very few of the original sperm ever make it as far as the uterus. It is possible for sperm to remain alive and healthy for up to forty-eight hours, waiting at the top of the vagina for the mucus plug in the cervix to become sufficiently welcoming for them to get through the cervical opening. When conditions are right, it can take as little as thirty minutes for sperm to get up into the Fallopian tubes after orgasm.

FERTILIZATION If an egg is waiting in the tube, the surviving sperm cluster around it until one manages to break through first the outer, then the inner, membranes of the egg to reach the maternal cell nucleus. Immediately, a coating forms round the egg to prevent other sperm breaking through. Once the sperm and egg cells fuse to form a single new cell, this cell begins dividing rapidly, again and again, until it forms a cluster of cells which continues to travel down towards the uterus.

On reaching the uterus, about a week after fertilization, the cluster of cells buries itself in the endometrium. Once this implantation has occurred, another important step towards a successful pregnancy has taken place.

Maximizing your chances of conception

It is interesting that, until now, much of your reproductive life will probably have been spent attempting to avoid pregnancy, and here you are, trying very hard to do the opposite. In view of the fact that you actually have a rather precariously brief fertile period in your menstrual cycle — possibly only three or four days at most — you may like to know exactly when is your best opportunity for love-making to lead to pregnancy.

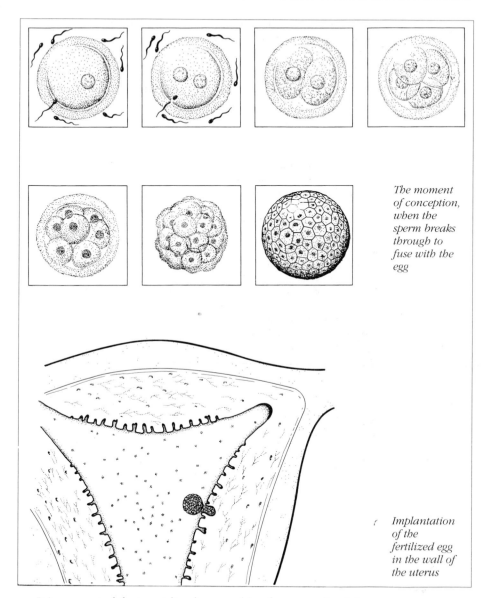

The moment of conception, when the sperm breaks through to fuse with the egg

Implantation of the fertilized egg in the wall of the uterus

It is suggested that avoiding love-making for a couple of days before your anticipated fertile time increases the number of sperm in the semen, enhancing your chances of conception. Once you have settled on the best time to have sex for conception to occur, the most effective way of making love is in the conventional 'Missionary' position, with the man on top. You could also put a pillow under your bottom, tilting your pelvis to allow full penetration, giving the sperm a head start into the top of the vagina. If you remain lying down for at least thirty minutes after making love, your chances of conception are increased still further.

If you are not one of the women who have a regular accountable menstrual cycle, you may be looking for a less hit-and-miss method. There are, fortunately, other signs that you may be approaching your peak of fertility.

OVULATION PAIN Some women experience a pain or ache low in the abdomen when about to ovulate. The pain is the result of a slight leakage of fluid as the egg ripens and bursts from the ovary. Whereas in the past you may have found this ache a mildly debilitating nuisance, you may now find yourself welcoming it as a useful sign from your body.

TEMPERATURE METHOD Another sign to watch for is a change in temperature. Immediately after ovulation your body temperature will rise sharply. It is possible, though rather fiddly, to test your temperature for yourself and assess your fertile days. You will need an ovulation thermometer (ordinary ones are rarely precise enough for such minute degrees of change) and some graph paper. You can then plot your own temperature graph every day, taking your temperature before you do *anything* else in the morning — before getting out of bed or having a cup of tea!

Normal fluctuations of body temperature during the menstrual cycle

Immediately before you ovulate, your temperature will drop slightly, a little further than the usual fluctuations, then there will be a sudden, steeper rise in temperature the follow-

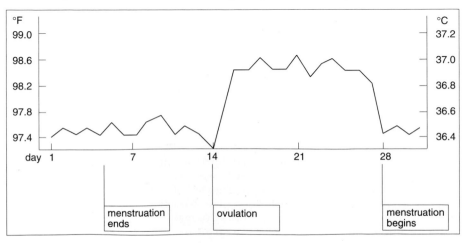

ing day. After this, the temperature will remain high until your period begins. Your most fertile day is the one immediately before the rise in temperature, so you need to have a very predictable cycle to be sure of your most fertile period. This can be a useful method to employ if you are wanting to find out if you are ovulating or not.

However, you may not feel like bothering to do this — indeed if you already have a child, it may be quite impossible to be so organized first thing in the morning!

MUCUS METHOD There is another method, which is to observe your vaginal mucus. Looking carefully at your vaginal mucus may not be something you had ever imagined yourself doing, and you may feel rather odd about doing it now. You may, however, find yourself increasingly fascinated by the way your body works once you start to take an interest. You may well find that your desire to find out about your body or to become pregnant overcomes any initial feelings of distaste. The mucus in the vagina and cervix, or neck of the uterus, is only actively receptive towards the sperm during your fertile period. It changes consistency throughout the menstrual cycle, and when you are at your most fertile it will alter in such a way as to enable the sperm to swim through into your uterus and beyond, to the Fallopian tubes.

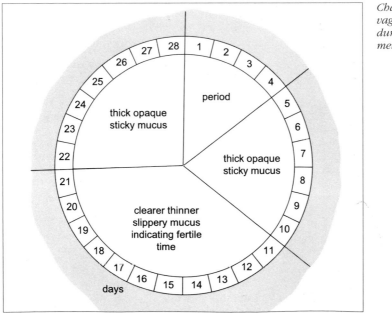

Changes in vaginal mucus during the menstrual cycle

As with the temperature method, it is better to keep a chart, noting the mucus changes from day to day. You can check your mucus each time you go to the lavatory, using either your fingers or a piece of tissue. Once your period has finished, in the pre-fertile stage, the vaginal mucus is cloudy, rather sticky, dryish, and relatively little is produced. If you pull it between your fingers, it will break and not stretch at all. As ovulation and fertility approach, the mucus alters to become wet and slippery, is often profuse enough to be noticeable some of the time, and, if you pull this type of mucus between your fingers, it will be quite clear and stretchy, resembling white of egg. This is the mucus which will enable the sperm to swim rapidly through the cervix. Things can happen extremely swiftly, so you do need to check your mucus several times a day to be sure of catching the right time when the mucus is most plentiful and stretchy, indicating fertility. Whether your partner is available on the right days is, of course, another matter! Once your fertile time is past, your mucus will quickly become cloudier and stickier again until your period starts — or not, if you have successfully become pregnant.

When conception does not occur

Although 80 per cent of couples manage to become pregnant in the first few months of trying, this still leaves 20 per cent who do not find it so easy. Of this 20 per cent, 10 per cent will be pregnant within a year; others may have longer-term fertility problems. If you have made the decision that you do want to have a baby, and have decided when you would ideally like that baby to be born, failure to conceive can be quite devastatingly disappointing. Many women find that, even if they began trying to conceive in a rather haphazard alright-if-it-happens-but-I-won't-mind-if-it-doesn't approach, they discover, once they start trying, that they become desperate to conceive. This may be the first time you feel your body has 'let you down', or you may suddenly realize there are aspects of your life you cannot control. You may be aware that the years are slipping past fast, so feel that every lost month counts. Each month you find your period has started seems more and more confidence-shattering — you begin to wonder why things are not going according to plan.

Couples can find that what began as a rather enjoyable new challenge has turned into a more clinical, calculated exercise, seemingly remote from the previous spontaneously loving relationship. Making love because you both wanted to rather than because the time of the month dictated it may appear to be a thing of the past, which can impose a strain on even the very best relationship. Other people too may make unfeeling, inconsiderate remarks about when you are going to start a family, which can be particularly hurtful at this time. However fulfilling your life is, you may feel as though all your emotional energy is being channelled into this attempt to become pregnant.

Most couples do become pregnant within the first six months of trying, and it is quite normal for it to take four to six months. Even six months can seem an eternity when you want a baby; every month comes to represent another lost opportunity. If, however, you have been having unprotected sex for a year, or if you have been taking accurate tests for ovulation for six months, you should consider going to see your GP for referral to a specialist. Some GPs are reluctant to refer someone after 'only' a year, but, if you are concerned, the sooner you are referred, the sooner your problem, if there is one, can be dealt with.

Doing something positive about not conceiving can help alleviate some of the frustration and depression of seeing month after month slip by with no pregnancy in sight. Just talking things over with your GP may help to lessen some of the intensity of feelings which can surround you both, may help you to look at the issue with a wider, better-informed perspective. You do not need to feel foolish for worrying so early, or a nuisance for bothering your GP when you are not ill; you are right to be looking for help at what can be a very miserable time indeed.

There are a number of books written about fertility problems which can help you understand what is happening and what the various forms of treatment may entail. There are also a number of support groups which you may find helpful and which are listed at the back of this book.

A TIME OF UNCERTAINTY

It may be obvious to you from the very morning after you have conceived that you are indeed pregnant — many women do report feeling 'strange' or 'different' immediately. There may be nothing as tangible as this, merely a sense that something has occurred which is new and different. There may be a more definite response in that you go off tea or coffee, or notice certain smells very distinctly. One woman found that she could not bear to go into her greenhouse because the smell of the tomato plants suddenly seemed so unpleasant. It may well be, of course, that you only recognize these differences in retrospect, once a pregnancy has been confirmed, or at the beginning of a second pregnancy.

If you do not have the benefit of knowing you are pregnant straightaway, there are a rather uncertain few weeks ahead, waiting and watching your body for any sign that you might be pregnant. Missing a period is the most obvious indication, but there are others which you may, or may not, experience. Many women do find they have a rather heavy, aching, cramp-like feeling, just as though they were about to start a period, but which may continue for several days, or longer. This is quite normal, and nothing to be concerned about, though it can feel both confusing and worrying if you are keen to be pregnant.

EARLY SIGNS The early signs of pregnancy include:

- ○ A MISSED PERIOD, OR A RATHER SCANTY ONE
- ○ TENDER, HEAVY BREASTS WHICH MAY ALSO TINGLE A LITTLE
- ○ DARKENED NIPPLES AND AREOLAE
- ○ NAUSEA AND SICKNESS, OR CHANGING TASTES
- ○ A HEIGHTENED OR ALTERED SENSE OF SMELL
- ○ A NEED TO EMPTY YOUR BLADDER MORE FREQUENTLY
- ○ AN ALMOST UNBELIEVABLE FEELING OF TIREDNESS
- ○ CONSTIPATION

PREGNANCY-TESTING You may prefer not to wait until you visit your GP round about the time of the second missed period and decide to buy a pregnancy-testing kit. Most of these are only effective once the first period is missed. Some family planning clinics will do a test for you, but this is becoming increasingly rare as it is expensive to carry out. Some GPs will also do tests, but, again, cost is a limiting factor. A number of chemists' shops will do a test for you, but for a price, of course. Beware of using old kits left over from your last pregnancy or a friend's test from some time ago, as the chemicals will not give a true reading if they are stale.

YOUR FEELINGS These early weeks, when you either suspect you may be pregnant or have just had your pregnancy confirmed, are very special. You may find yourself feeling excited, apprehensive, happy, resentful, proud, and incredulous all at the same time. It may be a time of very mixed emotions for you: you may have been looking forward eagerly to becoming pregnant and may be surprised by the ambivalence of feeling — resentment and fear alongside the pleasure and excitement. You may have been unpleasantly surprised to find yourself pregnant in the first place but may still feel clever and enjoy hugging your special secret inside yourself. Changing hormone levels as well as a natural delight and fear about what you may have let yourselves in for are all part of the normal processes of pregnancy. It may be particularly difficult for your partner at this stage, who has no tangible evidence of pregnancy, yet is also caught up in the heightened emotional responses. You may want to tell everyone how clever you have been, yet wish to hold on to your secret; you want everyone to share your happiness and excitement yet are aware that you may still be mistaken, that some pregnancies do miscarry, and not wish to be too definite too soon.

* *I didn't want to tell too many people to begin with, just in case, but I was desperate to shout out to everyone that I was going to have a baby.* **'**

* *Although we knew that thousands of babies are conceived every day, we still felt immensely proud, as though we were the only ones ever to have been so clever.* **'**

* *In the early weeks it was rather nice, sort of hugging my special secret inside myself.* **'**

* *After all those months when I'd burst into tears every time my period started, I could hardly dare believe I really was pregnant this time.* **'**

LOOKING AFTER YOUR PREGNANCY

Even though you may be uncertain as to whether or not you are pregnant, though there is nothing to see or feel as yet, this is a good time to begin being aware of your developing fetus. By the time your period is two weeks overdue, you are actually six weeks pregnant and your embryo is roughly pea-sized, with spine, arms, and legs all visibly forming. By the time you are three months pregnant, all your baby's vital organs will have been formed and she will be a recognizable human being, complete with fingers, toes, and ears. Until your baby is born, you are providing her whole environment for growth and development, so the way you care for yourself inevitably affects your baby.

By making some positive choices about your life-style and avoiding certain things, you can help create a good environment for your baby's growth, though it may not be possible to eliminate all potentially harmful aspects of your life while continuing to lead a normal social and working life. Some of these choices have already been considered earlier in the chapter, but there are others which you may wish to take into account once your pregnancy is suspected or confirmed.

X-RAYS X-rays should be completely avoided during the first three months of a pregnancy, so tell any doctor, dentist, or X-ray technician that there is a chance you may be pregnant, even if you are not sure. In a situation where an X-ray becomes truly essential for your safety, lead aprons can be used to protect the baby, but this would be for emergencies only.

EMPLOYMENT If you are in an occupation which involves extremely fatiguing or hazardous work (such as lifting heavy goods or dealing with strong chemicals), and you feel this may affect your own or your baby's health now that you are pregnant, you can ask your doctor or midwife for support in getting your job altered. Those women not in paid employment, but who nevertheless have an extremely demanding and fatiguing job looking after small children, will unfortunately find it hard to get their occupation changed. Asking for some extra help and support from your partner, if you have one, is useful, but the most important thing may simply be to be aware that being pregnant may impose limitations.

VDUs There has been much discussion about the effects of VDUs on pregnant women, particularly the risk of causing miscarriage. As yet, there is no firm evidence to substantiate their safety or lack of it. If you do work with VDUs and are concerned, discuss your fears with your employer and your union representative. It may be possible for your job to be altered to minimize the time you need to spend in front of a screen, and for you to take frequent breaks. Make sure your chair is comfortable, enabling you to maintain a good posture, and that you stop if or whenever you begin to feel strained or unwell.

CHICKEN-POX Although normally considered a fairly innocuous childhood infection, chicken-pox can pose a real threat should it be caught during pregnancy. There is a danger of the fetus suffering malformations, similar to those caused by German measles, if it is contracted during weeks 13–20 of a pregnancy. A further potential danger for the baby arises if the mother catches the infection seven days before she gives birth, when there is a risk of the baby contracting neonatal chicken-pox, which can lead to very serious consequences. Chicken-pox contracted during pregnancy also carries a risk for the mother, regardless of the stage at which it is caught. This infection is often much more serious for adults, and may cause respiratory complications for a pregnant woman. If you contract the infection whilst pregnant, you should ask your doctor to prescribe Acyclovar immediately to minimize the risk of respiratory problems occurring. As yet there is no chicken-pox immunization available, so if you know that you are not naturally immune, it may be as well to try to keep away from children who are known to have the infection. This may be rather difficult if you have older children who are at school or playgroup, but it may be worth asking to be made aware of any outbreak of chicken-pox as soon as possible. You could then decide what would be a sensible course of action for you to take in order to reduce your exposure to infection.

LISTERIA Though you may have felt prepared to take risks in eating certain foods up to now, you may feel less happy to do so now that you are responsible for another's welfare. Listeria in a pregnant woman causes miscarriage and still birth. Babies who are born, having caught the illness in the uterus, rarely survive. Cook-chill foods and the ready-made dishes found in cold cabinets in food stores are a recognized source of the listeria bacteria, but Government guidelines suggest you should also avoid eating soft cheeses or unpasteurized dairy products. Ice-cream stalls of the scoop variety are other possible sources of listeria and are better avoided unless you are certain of the hygiene precautions. You may also decide that eating any form of processed meat product, such as pâté, is to be avoided. If you are reheating foods of any description, make sure they are very well heated right through.

TOXOPLASMOSIS In a healthy adult, the toxoplasmosis infection is virtually unnoticeable, producing mild flu-like symptoms, but a pregnant woman catching it may pass it on to the baby. The earlier in pregnancy it is caught, the less likely it is to cross the placenta, but the greater the risk to the baby. There is no routine antenatal testing for immunity from this virus in the United Kingdom, but, if you are particularly concerned, you could ask your GP about the possibility of testing before conception. It is perfectly possible to avoid infection with toxoplasmosis by taking a few basic precautions.

Toxoplasmosis is most commonly caught from cat faeces and undercooked meat. Undercooked or raw meat is easily avoided. Cats can pose more of a problem, especially if they are hunters who will pick up the organism from the animals and birds they catch. If you make sure you keep away from your cat litter tray or wear rubber gloves when handling it, and wear gloves while gardening, you should be reasonably safe. If you grow your own vegetables, you should also wash them thoroughly — even if you do not own a cat, the chances are that another neighbourhood cat will have chosen your nicely dug vegetable patch as a comfortable lavatory. With strict attention to hygiene there should be no problem, and stroking your pet is fine as long as you remember to wash your hands well afterwards.

SALMONELLA Salmonella is a food-poisoning organism which contaminates food such as poultry and eggs. It is destroyed by thorough cooking. Although not directly dangerous to the fetus, it is a most unpleasant infection for the pregnant mother, and it is better to avoid any food which might cause the illness. If you avoid eating raw eggs, and make sure all food you cook is heated right through until piping hot, you should not have any problems.

LIVER Animal liver contains very high concentrations of vitamin A because of the vitamin supplements added to animal feed. The liver of a live animal acts as a filter, absorbing and storing much of the circulating vitamin A, which is then passed on to the person eating the liver. Very high doses of vitamin A have been implicated in some fetal abnormalities, and therefore the Department of Health has recommended that pregnant women should avoid eating liver.

This may all seem rather a bleak picture of abstinence — of a pregnancy fraught with potentially lethal mines under every step. Given that you are probably feeling concerned to take good care of your child in the uterus, most of these are not unreasonable restrictions to place on yourself. There is more information about looking after yourself and therefore your baby in Chapter 5, How You and Your Baby Grow.

Changing Perspectives 2

The knowledge that a baby is indeed on the way will inevitably have a profound impact on a woman and her family. The effect may be most acutely felt with a first baby, because everything is so new: physical signs and symptoms; the reactions of the father, parents, friends, and work colleagues. Each succeeding pregnancy will have its own impact as each new baby alters relationships within the family and provides the outside world with a different perspective on the family. Much will depend on the state of mind of both parents. If this baby has long been wanted and planned, then the mother and father may react with relief and exultation to the news of the pregnancy. The feelings of a woman whose relationship with the father is not secure or who did not wish or expect to become pregnant in the first place will inevitably be very different. The decisions to be faced will be unique and different for each couple and each pregnancy.

YOUR REACTIONS

The mother

If you listen to many women talking about their initial feelings on discovering they were pregnant, the wide range of emotions expressed seems quite staggering — shock, surprise, delight, panic, fear, elation, relief, interest, anxiety, happiness, and excitement may all be there, jumbled together in an almost overwhelming glut of feelings. Most women find they need to sit down and take stock of the new situation, realizing that they have embarked on a course which will lead them inexorably towards the birth of a baby for whom they will be responsible, and whose arrival will irrevocably alter their lives.

You may feel that your life will no longer be your own in quite the same way any more, as other people will have to be consulted during your pregnancy, and midwives, doctors, and hospitals will have their views on the best course to be taken for the safe arrival of your child. You may feel excited but apprehensive at the prospect of moving into a different phase of your life. If this is your first baby, you may feel rather sad at leaving behind your former life as a non-parent, as well as excitement about what is in store. In common with many women, you may find the pregnancy does not seem real for a long while, despite physical responses to it such as sickness or tender breasts. You may feel the first twinge of reality with the first movements you notice inside your abdomen. It may be an ultrasound scan which heralds the recognition that this baby is for real — it is often a scan which brings the reality of the pregnancy home to the father as well. If you are unhappy about being pregnant, you may manage to deny the baby's existence for much of the pregnancy. Many parents, especially those expecting a first baby, say they do understand intellectually that there is a baby waiting to be born, but cannot actually imagine the reality of it until the moment of birth, and, even then, reality may dawn slowly, or by fits and starts.

The father   Your reactions as a father may be equally wide and variable. Many men find it hard to express their innermost feelings, but those who can say that disbelief and shock were often the initial reactions,

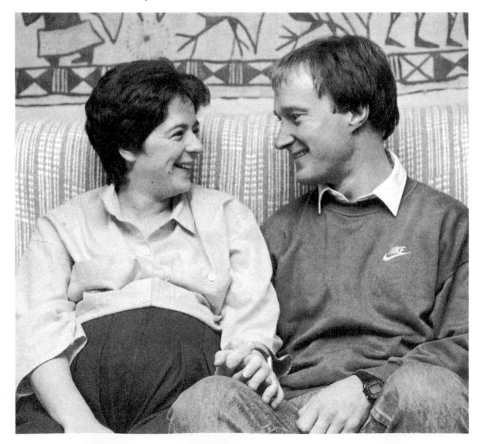

along with a pride in this proof of their virility and their partner's fertility. These feelings may be swiftly followed by anxiety and apprehension about the commitment with which they are now faced, and some fear for the woman during the ordeal of birth. Few men have had very much in the way of helpful or reliable education for parenthood during their upbringing, taking their only cues from their own parents or half understood conversations at school, work, or during social activities. So you may be taken aback by the immediate effects of pregnancy on your partner, whom you thought you knew well. It can come as a great surprise to find that the same person who enjoyed driving miles to a party, or was happy to stay up talking late into the night, suddenly prefers to stay at home and go to bed early. If your efficient, capable partner, who has been holding down a responsible and demanding job, now forgets important dates or meetings, and feels too tired or sick to bother about much besides dragging herself through work each day, sinking into bed at 8.00 every evening, you may well wonder what you have let yourself in for. If your partner feels sick during the early months of pregnancy or beyond, the lack of interest in cooking or eating meals may seem incomprehensible or even, eventually, irritating. The very fluctuation of her emotions during pregnancy may be hard for you to come to grips with — you may wish to be understanding and supportive but find it hard to strike the right balance between helpful concern and over-protective mollycoddling. Most women like the feeling of being a bit 'special' during pregnancy, but also want to remain as normal and independent as possible. There may well be occasions when you wonder if you will ever manage to hit the right note!

Your need for adjustment is as great as hers, even in the most contented and uncomplicated relationship. The need to cope with new and bewildering feelings during pregnancy is the beginning of the subtly altering relationship which characterizes the advent of parenthood. Whatever worries, frightens, delights, or confuses you now, this is a good time to start talking openly and honestly about all your feelings, even the more negative ones, so that you will have a strong basis of trust and understanding to cope with the differences you will encounter once your baby is born.

CHANGES IN OUTLOOK

SECURITY Many women say that, if they are honest, they would prefer to be in a stable relationship with some security when they become pregnant. Parents' relationships come in many varieties, and the need to have a secure base may not become apparent until the reality of children asserts itself. A woman may suddenly feel very vulnerable, realizing that for several years someone will be dependent on her. If she has more than one child, this vulnerability will be prolonged; she may see the advantages of some degree of financial protection as well as emotional security. Her partner, if she has one, may be the most obvious source of protection, but the society into which her child will be born also has some responsibility for the safety and well-being of each child.

FINANCE For both parents, the first major anxiety is usually money. Children are expensive: governments and institutions have published surveys of the estimated overall cost of raising a child to maturity, with the result reckoned in many thousands of pounds. For most couples, this amount seems initially as remote and daunting as Mount Everest, and the more immediate impact is going to be the loss of a second income, for a short while or for many years. This may be a heavy worry for the father, who may be, for a time, the sole wage-earner. Most people hate financial stringency. One problem for some couples is that the mother, who also hates financial stringency, may be made to feel guilty for being pregnant and staying at home to care for her very young baby. There is nothing that spoils happiness and threatens the enjoyment of parenthood more than feeling guilty. Resentments about money are a constant threat to satisfying parenthood, so it is as well to talk over all feelings and plans on financial matters, so that you each understand the strains on each other. Your baby may well prefer to have parents who are bright and smiling, enjoying each other's company and her, rather than the best new baby equipment but glum, strained parents.

THE BIRTH The next most obvious anxiety is the approaching birth. Most parents now know a good deal about the dangers of pregnancy and birth, with newspapers and magazines supplying information about research into safety for the new-born and her mother. At the same time, belief in the essential straightforwardness of pregnancy and birth is undermined. Sorting out the true from the false or misleading is vital, as is keeping a sense of proportion about the ghastly stories of pain and drama with which so many expectant parents are regaled by friends and relatives.

It is worth searching for really good childbirth education classes, preferably ones which are offered to both parents. Men often cannot see how they could benefit from going to a series of antenatal classes, but, since they are more than likely to be present during long hours of labour, it is valuable for them to find out what happens, what to expect and how they can best support their partners. Most men see the sense in being an informed participant at the birth rather than an observer, possibly scared or embarrassed. The benefits of going to such classes locally do not stop at the birth either — many good friendships have been initiated through antenatal classes and the reunions and postnatal support which follow on. It is hard to understand the potential value of peer-group support before you become a parent; impossible to imagine sane life without it once you are. The NCT specializes in providing excellent antenatal classes so that parents can make informed choices when faced with a variety of decisions. NCT classes will also provide a chance to think about the changing nature of your relationships and life-styles once the baby is here.

RESPONSIBILITY Although money worries loom so large in parents' minds during pregnancy, there are plenty of other factors to be taken into consideration, which are equally important but which may easily be overlooked. The confirmation of a first pregnancy marks a point of no return for the parents. From now on there is a third person to be considered, and, even if they decide on a termination for powerful reasons, they have still made a decision for someone other than themselves. It is the realization of this inevitable fact which often induces a feeling of panic. Parents may ask themselves if they were really quite ready for this, saying, 'If only we could have a little more time to ourselves, just a bit longer to prepare ourselves for all this.' Once you are pregnant it is too late; planning is in the past, and life will be different from now on. Many parents nowadays have grown up in smallish families and therefore have little or no experience of young children or babies in their own homes as they grew up; you may find yourselves thinking of a baby as an episode in your lives which will last a few months, maybe a few years, possibly up to school age. But babies grow into children, into teenagers, into adults, and are a lifelong source of interest. For much of this time, their welfare will be your responsibility — an awesome yet fascinating prospect. The most important thing is for the gloomy notion of a 'life sentence' to be balanced by the excitement and interest of the child you have made, and the fun you and she will have over the years to come.

SINGLE MOTHERS

Single women have special problems in pregnancy. They may have to deal with attitudes from those around them which are particularly unhelpful. Whether you have chosen single parenthood, whether the pregnancy has been the reason for your single status because the baby's father has moved out, or whether your pregnancy is the result of an unwanted experience, which in itself is hard to endure, you may feel acutely lonely. However supportive and understanding your family may be, you may be aware that this is something you will have to cope with all by yourself in the long run, and you may at times doubt your confidence to achieve all that will be required of you.

Your financial situation will be an almost inevitable anxiety, especially if you have no supportive family to turn to and will be dependent on working throughout your pregnancy to gain maximum state benefit. You may be worried about the possibility of losing your present accommodation once the baby arrives. You may feel you dare not be ill or take time off work, and this in itself is a stress that can cause illness. Decisions must be made alone and it is easy to view your coming baby more as a series of problems than a fulfilling and enjoyable event.

Attending warm and welcoming antenatal classes with other mothers and couples can be a source of relief and help for you as well. The fears and feelings of pregnancy are the same whoever you are, whether you are wealthy or destitute, younger or older, married or single, able-bodied or disabled, and the differences fade into insignificance when everyone is approaching labour. Support and friendship can develop across all sorts of barriers at such a time, which can ease any loneliness you feel.

WORKING MOTHERS

Mothers who are working outside the home and expecting a second or subsequent child also have particular stresses in pregnancy. You may have managed to solve the difficulty of continuing in employment after having one child, with family help or a reliable child-minding service, but be worried that the extra cost and effort of more children cannot be met in the same way. If you are in mid-career and have a professional future which will be difficult to interrupt with a gap for raising children, then you may be preoccupied with the need to find a carer for your children who will be both wise and kind. Good child-care facilities are not easy to find, and come very expensive in our society, so the parents' dilemma is often acute. It may be especially so if a woman's partner would actually prefer her to give up her job and stay at home to look after the children, while she would prefer to maintain her career. It may be worth sorting out your relative expectations during your pregnancy, so that some degree of harmony and compromise can be agreed upon. Children prefer their parents to be happy, and, hard though it may be to juggle everyone's needs all the time, there may be occasions when a child's needs must take preference. Individual babies react very differently once they are born, and it might be that an arrangement which has suited one child turns out to be totally inappropriate for another of a different temperament. It is worth being as flexible as is practically possible when considering arrangements for your children in order to achieve peace of mind for both parents in the long term.

Adults, after all, are able to adapt and modify their behaviour and ideas, can develop and change for good reasons, but babies and children remain at the mercy of the adults to whom they have been born.

RELATIONSHIPS WITH OTHERS

GRANDPARENTS Your new baby will have an impact on every member of your family. The approaching change of status for the parents often dominates their own thinking, so that they do not see what is happening in their wider circle; their own parents are going to be grandparents, which confers a new status upon them too. It will usually make them feel extremely proud, with a sense of continuity for the future. But it will also make them feel older — the senior generation — and that much closer to death, which may be frightening for some. The current emphasis on young grand-mothers in popular culture often covers a fear of growing old and can lead to unpredictable behaviour, including some resentment of their children for forcing recognition of a possibly painful fact.

Relationships with in-laws may be affected too, especially if the sex of the baby is important to grandparents on either side for whatever reasons, and all these attitudes tend to focus on the mother and the birth. Grandparents can be wholly supportive or very unhelpful. You may find it useful as a couple to discuss what each of you is expecting of your parents in their new roles as grandparents. There may be some discrepancy between what you would ideally like and what you realistically can expect. If you sense that there may be some tension within the family as everyone moves into a different stage of life, it may be worthwhile discussing your feelings with your parents. You may not feel brave enough to broach a potentially difficult subject, but, if you are able to, some later stresses and resentment could be avoided. On the whole, people prefer to know what is expected of them in any job, and being a grandparent is no exception. They may have no intention of conforming precisely to your expectations, but at least they will know what you are asking of them.

SIBLINGS If this baby is a second child, then her arrival will turn your first child into an older sister or brother. Many parents feel particularly ambivalent about a second pregnancy; you may feel you have committed an act which will change for ever the wonderful relationship you are enjoying with your first child. You may worry about how you will ever be able to love another baby as intensely as the one you already know, and may find it hard to focus on this pregnancy and this baby, because you do not want to lose what you have with your older child. Much has been written and expressed about sibling rivalry and the anticipated jealousy of the ex-baby, whether it is an eldest child or one of a larger family.

It is not always the very youngest child in a large family who shows the most resentment and jealousy when a new baby is expected or arrives, and parents are sometimes surprised by the reactions of children they had not anticipated would be so deeply affected. Sorting out and dissipating any harmful reactions is in the parents' hands, and they can usually be avoided with skill and kindness. It is important to be aware that every new baby causes a rearrangement among the family members, rather like a shuffling of the pack, and you will need to allow time for new positions to be worked out and accepted.

FRIENDS A first baby also changes relationships with friends. If you have been a couple with a wide circle of friends with whom you spend time and share interests, the relationships may be dramatically altered by pregnancy. A whole new world of interests and concerns opens up for the couple expecting a baby, which non-pregnant friends cannot be expected to share. As a newly pregnant woman you may not enjoy food or outings as you used to, and, as the months pass, your thoughts and those of your partner will increasingly turn towards the birth and the baby. Plans for holidays and weekends will change once the baby is born, and priorities for sleep and companionship will be different. Friends may find it hard to understand your altered way of thinking and may even feel rejected as the gap between you widens, but it is amazing how quickly these friends will catch up on new priorities if they too embark on a pregnancy.

At the same time, pregnancy can cause you to lose touch with friends and acquaintances with whom you may have had little in common. The same thing happens to each of us all through life, as we move on towards any new landmark: starting secondary school; going to college; leaving home; getting a new job; getting married. At each landmark, happy or sad, there is a new group of people with whom you share experiences, whom you understand and by whom you are understood. Pregnancy widens your horizons, and both parents can find themselves looking into the future with new eyes and new interests, and also with more friends.

THINKING AHEAD

It is worth using these months of pregnancy to think at least a little towards life after the birth, if you can. This can be difficult, as labour seems to loom ever larger on the horizon as the pregnancy progresses; but labour, though the end of pregnancy, is really only the beginning of your life with your baby, and it is incredible how much this small person will change your days and nights, whatever preconceptions you may have had. New parents often have strong views on the way that babies should be treated, and these may be both sensible and good, but it is wise to be prepared for shocks, and prepared also to change your mind and adapt if ideas do not quite fit the child you have, as opposed to the one you had imagined. If you are both willing to be flexible and ready to watch and learn from your baby, to help her cope with the enormous changes she will have to go through, you will make few mistakes. Breathing, seeing, hearing, feeding, responding are all new and strange for the new-born, and it is a hard life for several weeks. If a baby is cared for by adults who are prepared to help her get settled into living with compassion and common sense, she will be quick to respond as the months pass, and will learn confidence and independence safely.

One point worth remembering is that pregnancy is actually a very short part of a couple's or woman's time, though this may not be so apparent until you look back later: it may seem endless at the time, and so may the first few weeks after the baby is born. Short though it is, the foundations can be well laid and many difficulties smoothed away by recognizing and adjusting to your changing perspectives.

❛ I always wanted to have a baby, but at the right time, in a secure relationship — I never imagined life without a child, and I wish it had happened a bit earlier, but I hadn't met the man I wanted to marry and have a baby with. ❜

❛ Instead of feeling irritable and grumpy during my pregnancy, like all my friends said, I've felt particularly close to my husband. Suddenly there's this extra bond between us. ❜

❛ I hate the way everyone seems to think they've got a right to tell you how to run your life once you're pregnant, and the way even virtual strangers come up and touch your abdomen, as though it's not part of you any more. ❜

❛ We tried making this list of all the things we thought might be different once the baby's here, but we couldn't really imagine that there really is going to be a baby, so we couldn't plan much at all. ❜

3   ANTENATAL MEDICAL CARE

Once your pregnancy has been confirmed by your GP, you will be booked in for your antenatal care, your labour, and your postnatal care. The aim of antenatal care is to confirm that all is well with you, your pregnancy, and your baby, and to provide appropriate medical care should a problem arise. It should work as a two-way process, offering you an opportunity to ask questions, to discuss any worries or concerns you may have, and to build up a relationship with those who will be attending you during the birth and the postnatal period whenever possible.

Precisely how your antenatal care is organized will largely depend on the local arrangements your hospital, GP, or midwives usually make. It will also depend on what options you have taken up — whether hospital, home birth, GP unit, or domino scheme.

THE OPTIONS FOR ANTENATAL CARE

At your first appointment your GP will probably examine you briefly to check that you are in fact pregnant and that everything is progressing well, and will discuss with you the sort of antenatal care you would prefer and your choice of place for labour and delivery. This may seem rather early to be making definitive decisions about where you would like your baby to be born, and you might prefer to wait until you have found out more before coming to a firm conclusion. Some GPs do not make all the choices clear at this first visit, so you may not realize until later that you do have any choice. If you do discover later in pregnancy that you wish you had chosen a different option, it is possible to change as late as you wish. Occasionally women do have a problem moving to a different hospital or unit, but in general there is no reason why you should not.

If a particular type of care appeals to you but you find your GP has automatically booked you in for a consultant delivery at the local hospital, do ask your GP to go through all the options available locally. If your GP is unhelpful, you could try asking the Community Health Council, your community midwife, or your local NCT branch. Many people find it hard to talk to doctors or other medical personnel, and some medical professionals do not find it easy to encourage those who are uncomfortable when faced by professionals. There are some suggestions for helping yourself cope when meeting medical staff in Chapter 11, Communicating with Health Professionals.

If you feel unsure about what you would like in these early weeks, you could postpone making your decision until you have made some further investigations, then you could take your partner or a friend along with you for your next appointment. There may be more information than you feel one person can sensibly take in, and you may find the moral support of another person gives you the confidence to speak up for what you would prefer. In any case, it is quite common for fathers to attend many, if not all, of the antenatal checks, which can increase your joint involvement in this baby.

If you have questions to ask, then go ahead, even if your doctor seems dismissive — the questions are important to you and you should be treated with common courtesy. Antenatal care can easily become rather frustrating and feel like a waste of time if you are not getting all that you need out of it. Making sure you are getting answers sufficient for your needs and are having all the options placed before you so you make the decisions you want is important. If you are concerned that you may have made the wrong choice, do not feel afraid to ask to change — it is not silly to change your mind about something as important as the medical care for you and your baby. On the contrary, it shows a mature responsibility for knowing what is right in your individual circumstances.

CHOOSING A GP FOR PREGNANCY It may be that your own GP does not do obstetric work, in which case you can go to a different GP for your maternity care whilst remaining with your usual GP for medical purposes. You might decide that your usual GP is not someone you want to remain with during a pregnancy and wish to choose a different GP for your maternity care. Some women feel that a GP who was fine while they were working women is not someone they feel will care for their children sensitively. Your local Family Health Services Authority will provide you with an up-to-date list of GPs who do obstetric work so that you can ask to be put on another's list. Copies of this list will also be kept at most larger Post Offices.

SHARED CARE The most common option for women who are choosing to have their babies in hospital is a shared-care scheme, whereby you visit the hospital two or three times during your pregnancy while your GP and/or your community midwife undertake the rest of your antenatal care. You would normally visit the hospital for a booking appointment at around 10–12 weeks (though community midwives arrange this in many areas now); at 16 weeks for an ultrasound scan (if you are having one); again at 34 or 36 weeks; and possibly once more when your baby is due.

DOMINO DELIVERY If you have chosen a GP or midwife domino (see below) for your delivery, all your antenatal care may be undertaken by these people rather than the hospital. Community midwives will often visit your home for antenatal appointments as well, as they do for a home birth.

MIDWIFE DELIVERY   If you have chosen a midwife delivery, community midwives will care for you throughout the ante- and postnatal periods, and you will be delivered by hospital midwives, thus possibly never seeing a doctor at all.

THE OPTIONS FOR THE BIRTH

There is not a straight choice between birth at home and birth in hospital; there are various schemes available in most areas, and even, for many women, a choice of hospital. The choice for women in urban areas tends to be greater than for those in rural districts. There are, however, usually alternatives to having your baby in hospital under consultant care.

CHOOSING A HOSPITAL If there is a choice of hospitals in your area, you will need to find out which might suit you best. Visiting a hospital even at this early stage can give you a fair idea of the atmosphere of the place and can start you thinking about the sort of delivery you would like. There may be certain criteria about which you feel particularly strongly and wish to ask.

Important criteria about the hospital might include:

○   **ITS RATES OF CAESAREAN SECTION**
○   **ITS RATES FOR INDUCTION**
○   **ITS RATES FOR EPISIOTOMY**
○   **ITS RATES OF INTERVENTION IN NORMAL LABOURS**
○   **ITS POLICY ON ROOMING-IN**
○   **ITS POLICY ON AND ATTITUDES TOWARDS BREASTFEEDING**
○   **ITS POLICY ON AND ATTITUDES TOWARDS ACTIVE BIRTH**

You might also feel that the quality of the food plays a part too, if there is little else to choose between them. Asking friends who have used the different local hospitals can be very informative, as can contacting your local NCT branch or the Community Health Council.

CHOOSING CONSULTANT CARE Should you decide to have your baby in hospital under consultant care, you will be seen by your consultant's team of doctors during your antenatal visits and your overall care will be supervised by the consultant's team. When you go into hospital for delivery, you will be attended by the hospital midwives on the labour ward, and, should any problem arise during either pregnancy or labour, it will be referred to the consultant's team of senior house officers and registrars. You may be surprised to find at the end of pregnancy, labour, delivery, and your postnatal stay that you have never met your consultant. Consultants lead the team and set the policies but usually only attend when there are problems. Some consultants do like to meet the women in their care at some point during the pregnancy, but, as not all introduce themselves, it may be hard to know if you have just met the consultant or another registrar. A few consultants also hold their antenatal clinics locally rather than expecting the women to go into the hospital, particularly where travelling is difficult, and this is very much more convenient for many mothers.

Your hospital will possibly have two or three consultants working in obstetrics — individual GPs tend to favour one particular consultant, so do make it clear if there is a different one you would prefer. Again, the local NCT is a useful source of information about what sort of care and service the different consultants provide.

TEAM MIDWIFERY SCHEMES Certain hospitals are now setting up schemes whereby teams of about five midwives work together to care for the woman and her baby throughout pregnancy, delivery, and the postnatal period. Under such a scheme, you would get to know your team of midwives well over the months, building up a rapport with them, and feeling able to ask about any worries at any time. You will also be able to discuss in detail the plans you have for the actual labour and delivery, knowing that these are the midwives with whom you will be in contact throughout. This scheme, which is a relatively recent and very welcome addition to the maternity services on offer, has great advantages both for mothers and for midwives, who gain a great deal of job satisfaction from caring for women and their families right through the maternity period.

GP-UNIT DELIVERY Under a GP-unit delivery scheme, you would see either your GP or a community midwife for the majority of your antenatal care, and when you go into labour your GP or midwife will come into hospital to look after you. Your GP will be informed that you are in labour but will not necessarily come out unless he particularly wants to be there for the delivery. Should a problem arise during pregnancy or labour you will be transferred to the hospital team under consultant care. This can be rather distressing and disappointing, especially if you have to travel some distance from the unit to the hospital during labour, though in some areas GP units are situated in the hospital itself. For many women, being delivered by their GP in a small familiar unit closer to home is an excellent choice and a pleasant, safe alternative to the more institutional atmosphere of a larger hospital. Women who are delivered in small units have statistically less likelihood of being delivered by forceps, vacuum extraction, or Caesarean section compared with low-risk women delivering in larger hospitals, and are less likely to need any pain relief in the form of drugs during labour. The outcomes for both women and babies are extremely good, so this is a safe and positive alternative to delivery in a consultant unit.

DOMINO SCHEMES Domino stands for DOMiciliary-IN-Out. In this scheme a community midwife will share your antenatal care with the hospital and GP, often coming to your home to do your antenatal checks. When you think you are in labour, you call your midwife, or her relief, and she will either come out to visit you at home to assess how things are going or meet you in hospital if that seems more appropriate. If she comes out to your home, she may well stay with you at home for several hours until you both decide it is time to go into hospital. Providing all goes well, she will then deliver your baby and will look after you once you have gone home. Your stay on the hospital postnatal ward may be very brief, as women choosing this option often choose to go home very soon after the birth — a stay of between six and forty-eight hours is usual. You can, of course, stay longer in hospital if you wish or if there is a medical reason to, but many women choosing this scheme are keen to get back home as soon as they feel ready.

BIRTH AT HOME Many women believe that the right place to have a baby is at home, in their own surroundings, where they will feel relaxed and comfortable and where the medical attendants are invited guests. If you decide to have your baby at home, it is your statutory right, though it will not be advisable in all cases for medical reasons. It may be that you like the idea of giving birth at home but lack the confidence to ask for a home birth or are worried about the safety aspect. Chapter 19, Birth at Home, explores many of the issues surrounding home births in detail, as well as offering advice on how to get one if you wish it. Home birth is not going to feel right for everyone, but, if you want one, there is plenty of help and support available to enable you to achieve what you have chosen.

INDEPENDENT MIDWIVES There are a few midwives who have decided, for various reasons, that they cannot provide the sort of service for women and babies they would wish while working within the NHS, and have decided to become independent practitioners. These midwives usually look after women having their babies at home. You do have to pay for the services of an independent midwife, who will then attend you during your pregnancy, labour, and the postnatal period. Occasionally an independent midwife may agree to attend for the labour and birth as long as the local community midwives will provide antenatal and postnatal care.

PRIVATE CARE Some women prefer to have their maternity care privately; they will be provided either with a private bed in a local NHS hospital, or with a bed in a private maternity home. If you choose private care, you can usually guarantee that your consultant will be there should any complications arise, but you will, of course, have to pay for the privilege. You will also need to make sure you know precisely what items of care you will be billed for at the end of your maternity care.

THE POSTNATAL OPTIONS

You will be asked at your booking appointment how long you will want to stay in hospital. The reaction of most first-time mothers is: 'I don't know; you tell me what's normal.' Many women feel they want to get back home as quickly as possible to be in familiar surroundings, to get to know their baby in their own way and in their own time. Other women prefer their initial confidence in handling a new-born baby to be built up while staying in hospital with constant help to hand. Women are not left entirely alone at home. The community midwife can visit at least once a day for a minimum of ten days and possibly for up to twenty-eight days. Mothers and midwives now usually negotiate a visiting schedule which is felt to be most appropriate for the individual mother and her baby. The average stay in hospital seems to be between two and five days for a first baby; many mothers having second or subsequent babies also choose a few days' stay in hospital, where they might have a chance of some relative peace and quiet, particularly if there is a bouncy, talkative toddler at home. Many mothers find home infinitely more restful than hospital.

Postnatal units Some districts have small postnatal units attached to local cottage hospitals to which a mother and baby can be transferred after a day or so; these usually have homely, friendly atmospheres without the bustle and noise of a larger hospital, and, for many, the added advantage of being much closer to home for relatives and friends to visit. (The food is often better too, as the catering is not on such a vast scale.)

Amenity beds Many hospitals also have private rooms off the ward for mothers who would prefer not to be on the main postnatal ward. These cost varying amounts per day according to what your hospital decides, and there may not always be one available. If you are interested, it may be worth discussing the possibility with a midwife at an antenatal appointment.

WHO'S WHO

Unless you have a medical background, you may find it hard to comprehend the precise role of everyone you meet during the maternity period. This brief guide should help you understand where everyone fits in.

MIDWIFE A midwife is a specialist in the management of normal pregnancy and labour. You will be cared for by midwives antenatally, during labour, and postnatally. They are independent practitioners in their own right, calling in a doctor only when problems arise.

COMMUNITY MIDWIFE A community midwife is one who is working out in the community, usually responsible for a certain area or attached to a GP practice.

OBSTETRICIAN An obstetrician is a doctor specializing and trained in the management of abnormal labour.

CONSULTANT OBSTETRICIAN A consultant obstetrician is the senior obstetrician in the team caring for you. (Consultants are referred to as Mr, Mrs, or Miss; all other doctors as Dr.)

REGISTRAR A registrar is an obstetrician immediately junior to a consultant.

SENIOR HOUSE OFFICER (SHO) A senior house officer is a junior doctor doing his obstetric training.

PAEDIATRICIAN A paediatrician is a doctor specializing in the care of babies and children.

RADIOGRAPHER A radiographer is a technician who will perform and explain an ultrasound scan.

HEALTH VISITOR A health visitor is attached to a health centre or GP practice, and will visit you from the time the midwife care finishes, at about ten days postnatally. Her role is to help and advise you in the care of your baby. Your health visitor should introduce herself to you sometime in the antenatal period. She will have been a trained nurse and may have been a midwife as well.

SOCIAL WORKER A social worker's role is to find ways of supporting a mother or family with particular needs. This may be important if you have a disability or a specific problem and think you may need extra support, or help with housing, or money for help and equipment. You can ask your doctor or hospital to put you in touch with a social worker.

ANTENATAL APPOINTMENTS

A common pattern of visits for antenatal care is as follows:-

- A BOOKING APPOINTMENT AT AROUND 8–12 WEEKS EITHER WITH YOUR COMMUNITY MIDWIFE OR AT THE HOSPITAL
- APPOINTMENTS EVERY FOUR WEEKS UNTIL 28 WEEKS
- APPOINTMENTS EVERY TWO WEEKS UNTIL 36 WEEKS
- APPOINTMENTS EVERY WEEK UNTIL YOUR BABY IS BORN

The booking appointment

You might also visit the hospital for an ultrasound scan at 16–18 weeks; some hospitals also offer an alpha-feto-protein (AFP) blood test at this time (see Chapter 4, Antenatal Screening, for further information about these tests).

Assuming your pregnancy has already been confirmed, the booking appointment will be to check on your general medical history and in particular your obstetric history.

GENERAL QUERIES Questions you will be asked might include information on:

- ANY PREVIOUS PREGNANCIES, INCLUDING MISCARRIAGES AND TERMINATIONS
- ANY PREVIOUS BIRTHS AND THEIR OUTCOME
- ANY SPECIAL FAMILY OCCURRENCES SUCH AS TWINS OR ABNORMALITIES
- YOUR GENERAL STATE OF HEALTH
- PAST ILLNESSES AND OPERATIONS YOU MAY HAVE HAD
- YOUR IMMEDIATE FAMILY'S MEDICAL HISTORY
- ANY MEDICINES OR DRUGS YOU MAY BE TAKING
- THE DATE OF YOUR LAST MENSTRUAL PERIOD
- DETAILS OF YOUR USUAL MENSTRUAL CYCLE
- WHAT KIND OF CONTRACEPTION YOU HAVE BEEN USING UNTIL NOW
- WHETHER OR NOT YOU BREASTFED YOUR OTHER BABIES
- HOW YOU PLAN TO FEED THIS BABY

EXAMINATION Your doctor will probably also make a general medical examination. Your breasts will be examined for lumps, and you should also be taught how to check your breasts yourself if you do not already know. Your abdomen will be examined (palpated) to assess the progress of your pregnancy. You may already be more than 12 weeks pregnant, in which case your doctor will be able to feel your uterus just above the pubic bone at the front of your pelvis. Your pregnancy may not be as far advanced as this, in which case your doctor will only be able to assess the uterus by doing a bimanual examination — that is, with one hand on your abdomen, and one or two fingers of the other hand feeling your cervix and the lower part of your uterus through your vagina.

This examination will also give the doctor an idea as to the shape and size of your pelvis and whether or not you have any fibroids (common, benign tumours of the uterus) or ovarian cysts that might cause problems. You may also have a cervical smear taken now, though some doctors prefer to wait until the postnatal check to do this. If you do have a smear at this stage, your doctor will be able to have a close look at your cervix through the speculum and detect any signs of thrush or other vaginal infection. You will find some suggestions for coping with vaginal examinations further on in this chapter.

CHECKS During this first appointment you will also have checks made on:

○ **YOUR HEIGHT**
○ **YOUR BLOOD PRESSURE**
○ **YOUR URINE**
○ **YOUR HEART AND LUNGS**
○ **YOUR BLOOD**
○ **YOUR WEIGHT**

BLOOD TESTS Blood tests will be carried out to discover the following information:

○ **YOUR IMMUNITY OR OTHERWISE TO RUBELLA**
○ **YOUR HAEMOGLOBIN LEVELS, TO TEST FOR ANAEMIA**
○ **YOUR BLOOD GROUP, IN PARTICULAR TO DISCOVER WHETHER YOU HAVE RHESUS-NEGATIVE BLOOD**
○ **WHETHER YOUR BLOOD CONTAINS ANY ANTIBODIES WHICH COULD AFFECT THE BABY**
○ **WHETHER YOUR BLOOD CONTAINS ANY UNUSUAL HAEMO- GLOBIN, WHICH CAUSES ANAEMIA (SICKLE-CELL TEST), IF YOU COME FROM AFRICA, ASIA, THE WEST INDIES, OR A MEDITERRANEAN COUNTRY**
○ **WHETHER YOU HAVE ANY FORM OF VD**

AIDS Although the test is not yet routinely carried out in all areas, it looks increasingly probable that pregnant women's blood will also be tested for the HIV virus, which causes AIDS. This will be done anonymously, as an indication of the spread of the disease rather than as a test for the individual.

If you are concerned that you may have been in contact with the HIV virus, you may ask to have your blood tested for this. Otherwise you will not be informed of the result. (For further information, see Chapter 4, Antenatal Screening.)

Blood tests to check haemoglobin levels and detect any

antibody formation are also carried out later in pregnancy, at 28 weeks and 36 weeks. Rhesus-negative mothers may find they have blood tests at other times as well.

MEDICAL NOTES You will either be given your medical notes or a co-op (co-operation) card at your first visit. You then take these along to each appointment for them to be filled in. The idea is that you carry your notes with you always, so that all the necessary information about your pregnancy is to hand should you need to visit a doctor or hospital anywhere, at any time.

However your antenatal care is arranged, the checks are pretty well standard, and you can expect the following procedures to be gone through at each visit.

Subsequent visits

URINE Your urine will be tested for the presence of sugar, ketones, and protein.

The presence of sugar may be only a trace, in which case it could mean you ate rather a lot the previous evening. It could also signal the onset of diabetes.

Ketones may also indicate diabetes, though they may simply be showing up the fact that you forgot to eat any breakfast or have suffered from sickness during your pregnancy. They are produced when your body is burning up fats for energy.

Protein in your urine may be the result of contamination in your sample, or it may indicate a urine infection (unfortunately and painfully common in pregnancy). A third possibility is that you may have pre-eclampsia, an illness of pregnancy where blood pressure rises and your body retains fluid, creating potentially extremely serious problems for you and your baby.

MID-STREAM URINE SAMPLE You may be asked to produce a mid-stream urine sample to rule out the possibility of contamination. Precisely how to do this will be carefully explained to you at the time. You will first need to clean your vulva very thoroughly, carefully rinsing away any soap which might contaminate your sample. You will also need to make sure that your hands are scrupulously clean. You then sit on the lavatory and begin to empty your bladder. After a few seconds, when a little urine has been passed, you stop emptying your bladder, by pulling up your pelvic-floor muscles (see Chapter 6, Looking After Yourself), and then catch the required amount of urine in the container provided. The container will have been sterilized. You can then put the top on the container and finish emptying your bladder. Any urine collected in this way will be unlikely to have been contaminated from outside, and medical staff can check more accurately for any signs of infection or other problems.

WEIGHT You may have expected to have your weight checked, but in fact very few hospitals or midwives now weigh women routinely, as no useful information about the mother's or baby's well-being is obtained. If you are concerned about putting on weight that will be hard to lose once your baby is born, cutting down on foods containing fat or sugar is usually all that is necessary. You will find a breakdown of the usual weight-gain in pregnancy in Chapter 5, How You and Your Baby Grow.

BLOOD PRESSURE Your blood pressure will be taken, as raised blood pressure is another sign of pre-eclampsia. It is the lower reading on your blood pressure which is significant. Although it is not possible to prevent pre-eclampsia, you can help to keep your blood pressure down whilst waiting in the clinic by relaxing as much as possible.

OEDEMA You will be asked if your rings seem tight, or your feet or hands are swollen with fluid, and you may have your legs checked for signs of oedema or fluid retention causing swelling.

ABDOMINAL PALPATION Your abdomen will be felt at each visit (abdominal palpation) to determine the size of the uterus, the height of the fundus (the top of the uterus), which way your baby is lying, which way it is facing, and whether your baby is growing as would be expected.

FETAL HEART From about 18 weeks your baby's heart may be listened to. The heartbeat is very fast, about 120–40 beats per minute (twice as fast as an adult's). If your doctor or midwife has listened to the heartbeat with a Sonicaid or Doptone device, a form of portable ultrasound, you will be able to listen as well.

Recent evidence suggests that listening for the fetal heart has little, if any, clinical significance, and is used mainly to reassure the woman that her baby is alive. If you are not sure about the safety of ultrasound, you may find it helpful to consider whether or not any useful information will be gathered from this practice. You may feel happy about a fetal stethoscope being used, but prefer not to have your baby subjected to unnecessary levels of ultrasound. You will find further information on ultrasound in Chapter 4, Antenatal Screening.

BLOOD If it is appropriate, a blood sample may be taken.

ASKING QUESTIONS Once all the routine procedures have been gone through, you should have your opportunity to discuss anything that is bothering you. Many midwives and doctors happily explain everything as they go along; others leave you to do the asking afterwards. Some seem surprised to be asked anything at all and may start to walk off before you have had a chance to sit up and collect your thoughts. Do feel entitled to call your doctor back to answer your queries; it is better for you to be reassured about your pregnancy now, than to worry about something for several weeks. Likewise, it is sensible to read your notes or co-op card before leaving the clinic, so that you can ask to have any hieroglyphics translated before you go home. The midwife may be able to answer your queries about what the doctor meant.

You may come away from an antenatal visit puzzled or upset by some comment from a doctor or midwife. These are usually kindly, if thoughtlessly, meant and indicate no abnormality, but, because they are made by a medical professional, you may assume they have some significance which is not in fact the case. They often refer to the size of your abdomen or other personal characteristics. Common remarks are:

The throwaway remark

- THIS IS A *BIG* BABY.
- YOU'VE GOT A LOT OF WATER IN THERE.
- YOU'VE GOT SUCH A LITTLE BUMP.
- YOUR BREASTS ARE RATHER SMALL/LARGE FOR BREASTFEEDING.
- PLENTY OF ROOM IN THIS PELVIS.
- BIT OF A TIGHT SQUEEZE IN HERE, ISN'T IT!

Unless a medical explanation is given, such comments can safely be ignored as meaningless small talk. If you are worried about what is meant, then do ask, to save yourself worrying about it until your next visit.

Many women find vaginal examinations unpleasant, uncomfortable, or even painful, and become anxious at the prospect of having one. It helps to make an examination less unpleasant if you consciously relax yourself, and especially your pelvic floor. The more tense you are, the harder the doctor or midwife will have to work to be able to put his or her fingers into your vagina and the more uncomfortable it will be for you. Breathing out and relaxing into the examination rather than tensing up against it is a useful skill to learn — it works well for all sorts of other examinations too, including dental check-ups and work. (See Chapter 6, Looking After Yourself, for suggestions about how to relax yourself.)

Coping with vaginal examinations

Vaginal examinations carried out gently in early pregnancy will not provoke a miscarriage, but, if you are worried about the possibility, do explain this to your doctor before the examination, so that extra care can be taken or the internal examination postponed until the pregnancy is further advanced.

Under-standing your medical notes

The best way to understand your notes is to ask your midwife to go through them with you. If you can remember to look at your notes while you are still at the surgery or clinic, this is the best time to pick up anything you do not understand or of which you are unsure. The person who has written your notes is the best one to decipher and explain what has been written, but the explanations below will help you translate your notes:

Weeks	The figure gives the number of weeks since your last period (therefore the number of weeks into your pregnancy).
Weight	Weight is usually measured in kilos; not all scales are the same, so you may need to take account of the discrepancy between one set of scales and another if your weight is checked at all.
Urine	Urine is tested for albumen (the protein which may be present in your urine), sugar, and ketones; a small amount found is termed a trace. Urine is also checked for any trace of blood, usually the result of a urine infection.

ALB	albumen
tr.	trace
+,++,+++	an indication of the amount found
NAD	no abnormality detected
NIL	none found, so the same as NAD

BP	Blood Pressure. The lower figure is the significant one. A rise in this figure can be one of the indications of pre-eclampsia.
Height fundus	The fundus, or top of the uterus, becomes higher in the abdomen as your pregnancy progresses and your uterus grows. This is measured as a comparison between your fundal height and the average height for that number of weeks. A difference between the figures could mean:

○   **YOUR DATES ARE WRONG.**

○   **YOUR BLADDER IS VERY FULL, PUSHING YOUR UTERUS UP.**

○   **YOUR BABY'S GROWTH IS SLOWER OR FASTER THAN AVERAGE.**

36
32
40
28
24
20
16
12
weeks

The growth of the uterus in pregnancy

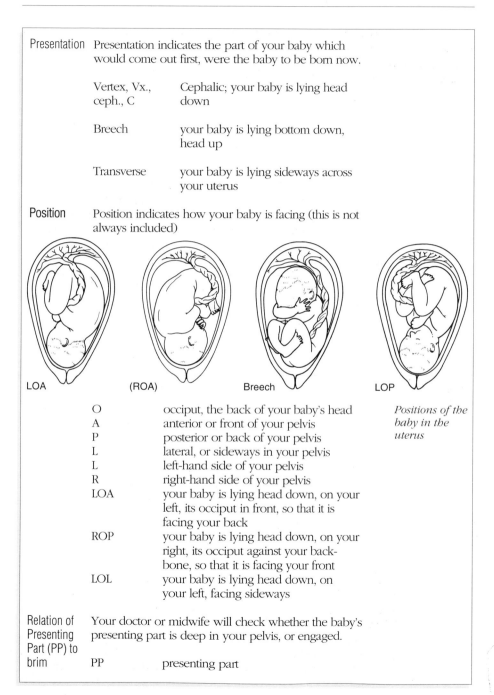

Presentation   Presentation indicates the part of your baby which would come out first, were the baby to be born now.

Vertex, Vx., ceph., C   Cephalic; your baby is lying head down

Breech   your baby is lying bottom down, head up

Transverse   your baby is lying sideways across your uterus

Position   Position indicates how your baby is facing (this is not always included)

LOA   (ROA)   Breech   LOP

O   occiput, the back of your baby's head
A   anterior or front of your pelvis
P   posterior or back of your pelvis
L   lateral, or sideways in your pelvis
L   left-hand side of your pelvis
R   right-hand side of your pelvis
LOA   your baby is lying head down, on your left, its occiput in front, so that it is facing your back
ROP   your baby is lying head down, on your right, its occiput against your backbone, so that it is facing your front
LOL   your baby is lying head down, on your left, facing sideways

Positions of the baby in the uterus

Relation of Presenting Part (PP) to brim   Your doctor or midwife will check whether the baby's presenting part is deep in your pelvis, or engaged.

PP   presenting part

Eng	engaged
NE, Not Eng	not engaged

Your doctor or midwife will check how much of the baby's head has descended into the pelvis, and how much can be felt above the brim of the pelvis. Some hospitals indicate how much remains above the brim, others how much has descended into the pelvis. Thus ⅕ could mean that:

○ **ONE-FIFTH REMAINS ABOVE THE BRIM, AND FOUR-FIFTHS HAVE DESCENDED INTO THE PELVIS**

○ **ONE-FIFTH HAS DESCENDED INTO THE PELVIS, AND FOUR-FIFTHS REMAIN ABOVE THE BRIM**

You might like to check which method your hospital uses.

Fetal heart

Fetal heartbeats and fetal movements are checked.

FH	fetal heart
FHH	fetal heart heard
FHNH	fetal heart not heard
FMF	fetal movements felt
FMNF	fetal movements not felt

Oedema

You will be checked for oedema or swelling. Oedema is another of the indications of pre-eclampsia.

NIL	no swelling
+, ++, +++	degrees of swelling

HB

Haemoglobin. Average readings in pregnancy are around 11–12; a drop could indicate anaemia.

Notes

An opportunity to record any comments that the person examining you thinks important; do ask if anything puzzles or concerns you.

COPING WITH ANTENATAL CLINICS

Antenatal checks ought to be positive experiences, reaffirming your confidence in your body to nourish your baby and make it grow, leaving you feeling reassured and delighted with yourself and your pregnancy. All too often, however, women leave clinics feeling hot and irritated, aware of all the questions they really wanted to ask, frustrated by the time wasted having to wait so long, and disappointed at having been treated as nothing more than another part of that day's production line.

Many hospital clinics have a poor appointments system, resulting in long waits. You might turn up for a 9.30 a.m. appointment, to find you are one of the twenty-plus women block-booked for the same time. If a doctor on duty is then called to assist at a delivery or is late arriving, the queue will inevitably build up. If you are then seen by five or six different people during your visit, none of whom you have previously met, and whom you suspect you may never see again, the whole experience can be most dispiriting.

On the other hand, clinics where mothers and their companions are welcomed, where they are attended by midwives and doctors whom they recognize and know, who introduce themselves by name, and who take a real interest in them as people, troubling to put them at their ease and answer queries clearly, not in a patronizing way, can lift the spirits and give a positive glow. The antenatal check will then become an event to be looked forward to rather than a beastly chore to be survived.

Should you be finding your antenatal visits less than enjoyable, some of the following suggestions may help.

CHILDREN Some clinics are better equipped than others, physically and in their attitude, for dealing with small children. Some children are better equipped than others for dealing with waiting patiently and quietly in fairly confined spaces. Most children prefer not to. The best solution is to leave them at home with someone else during your visit. If you cannot arrange this, taking a varied supply of drinks, books, toys or games without small, losable bits, something for wiping sticky hands and faces, and a reasonable supply of non-messy food such as sandwiches, fruit, packets of raisins, etc., will help to keep the peace and preserve your sanity. Planning for the visit as for an expedition demands forethought, but is well worth the trouble.

TIME Allow plenty of this. You might be lucky and get through in under an hour, but a better bet is to anticipate that it might take at least an hour and possibly three. Expecting the worst will mean that you will not be on tenterhooks as time drags on and you are due elsewhere. If you are out fairly soon, then any 'extra' time can be regarded as a bonus.

PREVENTING BOREDOM Make an occasion of your visit. Take plenty of interesting things to do — a book you are enjoying and never have enough time to read; some knitting you would like to get on with; some letters you would like to write to old friends. If the clinic fails to provide a really good cup of tea or coffee, take your own, plus something interesting to nibble while you wait. Treating yourself, in however small a way, may also help you relax. Promise yourself a treat at the end of the visit — lunch out, or some time spent shopping or enjoying a quiet half-hour's walk if the surroundings are conducive to this; anything you do not normally have time to indulge in will make you feel better. Treat it as *your* special time.

TAKING A FRIEND If you do not find your visits at all sympathetic, take a companion along — your partner, friend, mother, or sister. Even if the companion chooses not to come in to see the doctor with you, you will have someone to talk to while you wait.

If your mind goes blank when faced with a doctor, your companion can be useful in nudging your memory about the questions you meant to ask, and writing down what the doctor actually said.

Making further appointments

If you feel dissatisfied with what you have been told and would like to find out more, or if you have something to discuss which you suspect may take a while, it may be wise to make a separate appointment, asking to see the consultant if you wish. This way, you will have plenty of time without having to worry about the other women waiting, and could arrange for your partner or other companion to be present. Nor will you be in the disadvantageous position of wearing nothing but your knickers and a dressing-gown, having just been through a medical examination.

Chapter 11, Communicating with Health Professionals, will help you think about ways of expressing yourself to your best advantage.

Improving the service

Once your antenatal visits are over and your baby is born, writing a letter to the Director of Midwifery Services explaining precisely what you found good and bad about the antenatal care provided will help improve the service for the future. The same applies to any of the maternity services — staff will not necessarily know what you find impressive or unpleasant unless you tell them. It is easy to drift into a routine without considering its effect on those at the receiving end: saying what you think and offering suggestions will perhaps provide some insight into a consumer's viewpoint, and help staff to reconsider the impact of the service they are providing.

• *I do like going to see my GP and the community midwife — they make me feel I matter. At the hospital it's just like I'm the next one in the line, not a real person.*

• *I used to look forward to my antenatal visits, as some kind of milestones in the pregnancy. What actually happened was a total anticlimax — we all sat around for two hours or more, to be whisked in and out of the consulting room in five minutes flat. Hardly worth taking your clothes off for that.*

ANTENATAL SCREENING
4

The outcome of pregnancy for both mother and baby is nowadays generally very good, and pregnancy is embarked upon with few anxieties for the mother's or the baby's health. It is rightly viewed as one of the normal functions a healthy body can perform. There are still, however, some serious problems that affect a small minority of babies and pregnancies, and you will come across tests during your pregnancy to screen for some of these.

You may already have thought about Down's syndrome or spina bifida, or you may have a hereditary disorder in your family, in which case such tests will be a welcome way of receiving reassurance or of preparing yourself to cope with a sick or disabled baby, or they will play a necessary part in making a difficult decision to terminate the pregnancy. On the other hand, you may have been blissfully free of anxieties until these tests cropped up, in which case you will probably have rather mixed feelings about their benefits.

It is at least helpful to know the significance of each of them, and those who feel strongly that they do not want to have them can discuss this with their doctors. There tends to be a common assumption that all pregnant women will have certain screening tests, but many choose not to and it is their right to refuse them. Some women have also said that, as well as some pressure from the medical profession to be screened if they are over a certain age, there has been a strong degree of censure from other people if they have decided not to have the tests. For those couples who know that they would not countenance a termination of pregnancy even if a handicap were discovered, or who believe that the risks to the fetus and the pregnancy outweigh any possible likelihood of abnormality, this pressure is most distressing and highly unwelcome. These are very personal choices to be made, and once you have decided what is right for you, any further pressure from others is simply interference in a private matter.

All screening tests are performed as early in pregnancy as they can be, to get the information to the parents and doctors as soon as possible. Some, however, cannot be done until 16 weeks, and, if there are specific anxieties, this can be a frustrating time to wait.

ULTRASOUND

Ultrasound scanning is a technique which underpins other screening procedures, but is an important and widely used device in itself. A routine scan is offered to most women at about 16 weeks.

What ultrasound scanning tests for

ASSESSING GESTATIONAL AGE One common justification for an ultrasound scan is to assess gestational age, but the most accurate measurement of that is obtained during the first trimester (the first fourteen weeks of a pregnancy). Warnings have however been issued not to use ultrasound routinely during the first trimester until there is more information on its safety. Between 14 and 20 weeks, measuring the bi-parietal diameter (the distance between the two bony prominences above the baby's ears) enables a due date to be calculated which is probably accurate to within a week.

DETECTION OF ABNORMALITIES Ultrasound will usually detect multiple pregnancies, an ectopic pregnancy (where the fetus lodges and is growing outside the uterus, usually in a Fallopian tube), and some fetal abnormalities. Many cases of neural-tube defect, such as spina bifida, will be shown up, as will some urinary-tract abnormalities. The development of high-resolution scanning, and trans-vaginal ultrasound, means that it is now possible to detect the majority of congenital abnormalities. This can only happen, however, if the scanning equipment is of a very high quality, the person interpreting the pictures is extremely skilled, and the time allocated for the scan is sufficient. Under normal, everyday circumstances, a woman would not expect to experience such a high level of technological and medical input at a routine scan.

ASSESSING GROWTH Ultrasound may also be used to assess how well a baby is growing when there is some doubt as to whether or not it is the right size for the given dates.

SITE OF PLACENTA A scan will also locate the placenta. If the placenta is found to be low-lying, so that it could possibly interfere with a normal vaginal delivery, there will be a follow-up scan at about 32 weeks, when, in most cases, the placenta will be seen to have moved as the uterus has expanded and to be in a favourable position higher up the uterus. If it is still covering the cervix (*placenta praevia*), then the baby will have to be born by Caesarean section.

(Opposite) A radiographer explains the ultrasound image to the mother

DETECTION OF HEARTBEAT With ultrasound a heartbeat can be detected as early as 6–7 weeks, so it is occasionally used to confirm a pregnancy or to determine whether or not a baby has died.

Another form of ultrasound, the Doptone or Sonicaid, is more commonly used to detect fetal heart sounds which can be heard at about 10 or 12 weeks. It is sometimes used at antenatal check-ups, and it can be very satisfying for the mother, father, or an older sibling to hear the baby's heartbeat. The scan too, showing the baby *in utero* on the screen, is often an exciting, moving experience — one which makes the baby seem a more real human entity. Women who have experienced a good deal of nausea and illness in the pregnancy so far often feel vastly encouraged once they have seen the baby on the screen. Unfortunately the uncommunicativeness of some ultrasonographers can serve to outweigh the benefits of the scan. Every woman should be able to see the monitor clearly, should have her baby's image pointed out, and be given all the information she requests. Some hospitals will offer parents a photograph or even a video of the recording — but at a price!

Ultrasound is the name given to sound waves which are of too high a frequency for the human ear to detect. The sound waves pass through a transducer and focus on the mother's abdomen just above where her baby is lying. They then bounce off the various different surfaces within the body and send back 'echoes' which are translated as a picture (albeit a fuzzy one) on to a television screen.

How ultra-sound is performed

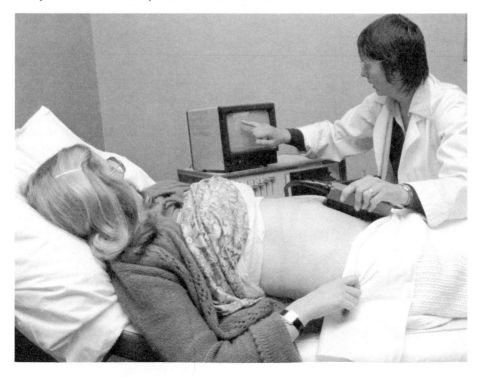

Before having the scan you will be asked to drink up to a pint of liquid, or not to empty your bladder, because a full bladder helps to push the intestines out of the way, and acts as a reference point during the examination. You then lie on a table and the doctor or radiographer applies mineral oil or gel liberally on to your abdomen. The oil helps conduct the sound waves. Gradually, the uterine contours, bladder, placenta and baby are revealed in a moving picture, but it takes a skilled and experienced operator to take measurements and interpret their meaning. The procedure is quite painless, although your full bladder may become increasingly uncomfortable as time progresses!

Question marks

Despite all the valuable information that ultrasound can give, there is still a question mark over its safety. It may take a long time to determine the effects of ultrasound, because exposure may have delayed effects which will show up later in life or in the next generation. Doctors who are keen on using ultrasound say that millions of babies have been scanned with no harmful effects, but others, less keen, point out that, unless or until the safety issue is proven, we cannot simply assume it must be safe. Much of the ultrasound scanning equipment now being used is relatively new, and babies are receiving higher resolution soundwaves for longer periods than was formerly the case. As yet no long-term biological effects of these scans have been determined, except for suggestions of an increase in the incidence of left-handedness.

Scans are mainly used to assess gestational age. They do not always give totally reliable information, however, and any reliability decreases with the length of the pregnancy. Some centres give routine scans in later pregnancy to assess the baby's growth. This practice is often accompanied by an increase both in the number of women admitted to hospital antenatally, and in induction of labour. There is, however, no beneficial effect on the condition of babies at birth, so there would seem to be little point in hospitals continuing to offer these late scans routinely when no real advantage is gained.

In the short term there is also the danger of misreadings of an ultrasound scan, because it is no simple matter to interpret the picture on the screen. Between 15 and 25 per cent of detectable abnormalities remain undetected. At worst, in some units, unacceptable numbers of false positives are being 'discovered'. The effectiveness of ultrasound scanning can vary widely from unit to unit, so if an abnormality is diagnosed from the scan, it is worth having a further scan or a second opinion before taking any further action.

You may be unsure about whether or not to have a scan; whether it is a routine one, or one specifically offered to you, asking the following questions may help you decide:

○ **WHAT ACTUAL INFORMATION WILL THE TEST PROVIDE?**
○ **ARE THE TEST RESULTS ESSENTIAL IN DETERMINING THE COURSE OF CARE?**

○ **IF THEY ARE ESSENTIAL, HOW?**
○ **HOW WOULD NOT DOING THE SCAN AFFECT THE COURSE OF CARE?**
○ **HOW ACCURATE IS THE TEST?**
○ **WILL ENOUGH BE LEARNED TO JUSTIFY EXPOSING THE BABY TO ULTRASOUND?**

Whatever decision you make regarding whether or not to have ultrasound, in whatever form, should be respected, and you should not need to feel pressurized into accepting something about which you feel unhappy. Both the Royal College of Midwives and the College of Radiographers say that scans should be carried out 'only after careful consideration of benefit versus risk, with emphasis on full information and choice for the patient'.

Whether you are being offered a routine scan, a scan for a particular purpose, or regular use of Sonicaid or Doptone to listen to your baby's heartbeat, you should be made aware of all the information you need beforehand, and your final choice should be a genuinely well-informed one.

An ultrasound image of a fetus at 19 weeks. The fetus is sucking its thumb

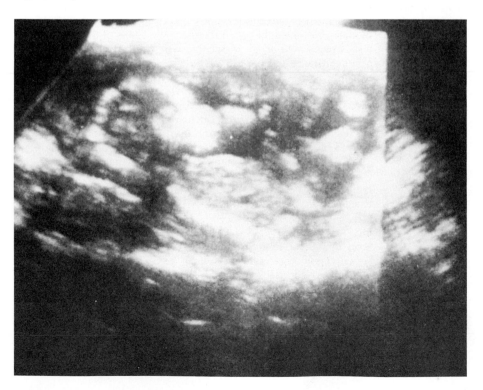

‘ *When I saw our baby on the ultrasound screen, I felt as though all those weeks of sickness and tiredness were worthwhile.* ’

‘ *I don't think Mike had believed in the pregnancy until he saw the baby on the screen.* ’

‘ *I didn't bother with a scan for any of my babies — I was certain my dates were correct and there was no apparent problem, so what would I have gained by it?* ’

ALPHA-FETO-PROTEIN (AFP) TEST

What alpha-feto-protein screening tests for

The AFP screening programme is intended to detect a fetus which has an abnormality of the central nervous system, where there is a failure of part of the neural tube to close. This leads to problems with the development of the spinal column, spinal cord, brain, or skull, as in spina bifida or anencephaly. These are jointly referred to as neural-tube defects.

How alpha-feto-protein screening is performed

AFP is a substance found in the blood of a baby before birth, a little of which leaks into the mother's bloodstream, so a sample of the mother's blood can be taken to assess the levels of the protein. The test is performed at 16–18 weeks, when the AFP levels can most accurately be assessed. Because the timing is crucial, the blood test is usually linked with an ultrasound scan to assess gestational age.

If the level of AFP is abnormally high or low, this can indicate the possibility of problems, but a measurement from this single blood sample is not, on its own, conclusive. If an abnormal reading is obtained, the normal procedure is for the mother to be recalled for a second blood test; if this also resulted in an abnormal reading, an amniocentesis would be offered as a more accurate indication.

The results of blood tests are usually available in about one week. If a hospital offers this test routinely and nothing further is heard, the usual assumption is that there is no apparent problem.

Question marks

On its own, the AFP blood test is not necessarily significant — a high level might, for instance, indicate that you are carrying twins or supertwins (not insignificant in itself, of course!), that the pregnancy is further advanced than was realized, or, sadly, that the baby has died. An ultrasound scan can check any of these factors.

There is no risk to mother or baby from a blood sample being taken, but if a decision is made to have an amniocentesis, there are specific risks attached to that test as we shall discuss later in this chapter. Because the information obtained from AFP testing alone is not particularly conclusive, many hospitals do not offer this test unless there is a history of neural-tube defects.

MATERNAL SERUM SCREENING TEST (BARTS' TEST)

The maternal serum screening test is used to assess the risk factor of any one mother for the following conditions:

What maternal serum screening tests for

O **DOWN'S SYNDROME**
O **ANENCEPHALY**
O **SPINA BIFIDA**

This is a test which has been developed at St Bartholomew's Hospital in London. It is offered routinely to all women in the London borough of Hackney, and there are other centres around the country which also offer this test, but as yet it is not freely available. It is, however, possible to arrange to have it done privately, either at St Bartholomew's or through your GP or local hospital.

A blood sample is taken from the mother, and levels of three substances in the blood are used in combination with the woman's age to estimate the risk of Down's syndrome.

How maternal serum screening is performed

ALPHA-FETO-PROTEIN LEVELS AFP levels are low in mothers carrying a Down's syndrome baby. The AFP level alone is used to determine the risk of neural-tube defects.

OESTRIOL LEVELS Oestriol levels also tend to be low in Down's syndrome.

HUMAN CHORIONIC GONADOTROPHIN (HCG) LEVELS The levels of human chorionic gonadotrophin (HCG, the 'pregnancy-hormone') tend to be high in Down's syndrome.

If the risk of Down's syndrome is assessed at less than 1 in 250, and the AFP level is not too high, a mother will be assessed as 'screen negative'. A woman may be 'screen positive' if her AFP level is greater than 2 times the normal level, or if she has an increased risk of Down's syndrome. More than nine out of ten women will have a negative result, and, whilst this is not in itself any form of guarantee, the test does detect:

O **2 OUT OF 3 CASES OF DOWN'S SYNDROME**
O **ALMOST ALL CASES OF ANENCEPHALY**
O **4 OUT OF 5 CASES OF SPINA BIFIDA**

If a woman is assessed as screen positive, she can then be offered an amniocentesis for more precise information.

The timing of the test is crucial. A woman must be at least 15 weeks and not more than 22 weeks for the levels of the three substances to be assessed as accurately as possible. It may be necessary to have an ultrasound scan to ensure that dates are exact.

Question marks

This test is non-invasive and may be considered a reasonable way of determining the risk factors for a woman who does not wish to go through the additional risks of an amniocentesis (see below). It does not, evidently, pick up every case of Down's syndrome or spina bifida, but many women will feel reassured knowing their risk is no greater than might be expected in the population as a whole.

The relative newness of this test does mean that there is still some evaluation to be done to assess its overall usefulness to women as a form of antenatal screening. Some midwives and doctors are reluctant to offer this test, as they feel that it only gives the woman another set of statistics, rather than any hard information. For many women, however, being able to judge whether they personally are more or less at risk than any other women of their age is a useful tool in helping them decide whether to undergo more invasive testing.

AMNIOCENTESIS

An amniocentesis tests a sample of amniotic fluid from the uterus.

What amniocentesis tests for

Because the baby drinks the amniotic fluid and passes it out again, the fluid contains cells from the baby's system which can provide a good deal of information.

An amniocentesis will thus test for neural-tube defects and chromosomal abnormalities. It can also detect the sex of your baby, though it would not be offered for this reason alone unless there is a family history of problems relating to the sex of a baby, such as haemophilia or muscular dystrophy.

Situations in which you might decide to have an amniocentesis:

○   YOUR AFP BLOOD TEST READING IS ABNORMALLY HIGH OR LOW AND YOU WOULD LIKE FURTHER, MORE ACCURATE INFORMATION.

○   YOU HAVE A FAMILY HISTORY OF GENETIC PROBLEMS, OR HAVE HAD A HANDICAPPED BABY ALREADY.

○   YOU ARE OVER 35 (OR 37 OR 38, DEPENDING ON YOUR HOSPITAL'S POLICY) AND ARE CONCERNED ABOUT THE INCREASING POSSIBILITY OF CHROMOSOMAL ABNORMALITIES, SUCH AS DOWN'S SYNDROME, RELATED TO INCREASING AGE.

Down's syndrome — the risks

Your age	Down's syndrome
25	1 in 1,500
30	1 in 800

Your age	Down's syndrome
35	1 in 300
38	1 in 180
40	1 in 100
45	1 in 30

If you decide to opt for an amniocentesis but do not wish to know your baby's sex before birth, make sure your doctor knows this so that you are not told and the information is not included in your notes.

How amniocentesis is performed

An amniocentesis is always carried out in hospital. It is usually carried out at about 14–16 weeks. It involves a sample of amniotic fluid being extracted from within the uterus through a hollow needle which is inserted very carefully so that it touches neither the placenta nor the baby. Ultrasound equipment is used to locate a safe place to insert the needle. A local anaesthetic may or may not be used to numb the tissues around the point of entry — this is something you might want to discuss with your doctor. Some women find the amniocentesis very uncomfortable; others report just a slight sensation. Most women, however, are surprised at how bruised and tired they feel afterwards, and you will be encouraged to rest for the remainder of the day, although you do not stay in hospital for long.

After an amniocentesis, a mother who has rhesus-negative blood must be given an injection of Anti-D to counteract any antibodies produced in her blood if some of the baby's blood escapes into her bloodstream during the procedure.

The results of the AFP test can be obtained in a few days, but, because the fetal cells have to be cultured for a chromosomal analysis, there is a delay of about four weeks. This waiting period can cause much anxiety and tension for the pregnant woman and her partner.

Question marks

Although amniocentesis is extremely accurate in detecting Down's syndrome, and detects nearly every case of neural-tube defect, there are risks to be considered. As with CVS, the young fetus may be exposed to prolonged doses of ultrasound. It is not thought to have any long-term effects on the baby (unless the needle damages it), but there has been shown to be an increase in the numbers of babies with very low birthweights, and in those suffering from respiratory problems after birth following amniocentesis. There is also a 0.5–1 per cent chance of miscarrying (this percentage is over and above those that would have miscarried anyway). Although the risk of miscarriage is very slight, you may decide not to have the test unless you feel that there is a strong indication that your baby may be affected in some way. It is perfectly reasonable for you to ask your doctor how many amniocenteses he has performed, and what his miscarriage rate is. The more experienced the operator, the less the risk of any complication arising becomes. You might decide that the overall risk is actually greater than the risk of having a handicapped baby. You might wish to think about finding an alternative consultant.

The long wait for results is difficult to live through, especially as, by the time they come through, you may well have felt your baby moving and kicking. A therapeutic termination performed at this relatively late stage is very distressing for the parents and may be a most uncomfortable procedure. If your baby does prove to have some abnormality, caring counselling should be available to help you decide what you want to do; whether or not you wish to have an abortion or would prefer to keep the baby. Not all hospitals offer as good a counselling service as parents would like, which is unfortunate when you may be making extremely difficult and important decisions.

It may help you to talk to parents who are bringing up a Down's syndrome child or those who have already been through this experience.

If your hospital does not offer these opportunities, you could contact the relevant support organizations listed at the back of this book.

* *It was very much more painful than I'd been led to believe.* *

* *Those weeks when we were waiting for the result of the amniocentesis to come through were the most nerve-racking I've ever lived through. All I could think about was how many more days before I'd hear something.* *

CHORIONIC VILLUS SAMPLING (CVS)

What chorionic villus sampling tests for

CVS is a relatively new procedure, not available in all areas, and its safety is still being assessed. CVS can be used to detect the same chromosomal abnormalities as an amniocentesis. It can detect genetic disorders such as thalassaemia and sickle-cell anaemia, as well as discover the sex of the baby. Developmental defects such as spina bifida cannot be detected by CVS.

CVS is carried out during the first trimester of pregnancy, at about 10 weeks. A narrow plastic tube is passed into the uterus through the cervix, and some cells from the developing placenta are drawn off by aspiration. Alternatively, it can be performed by piercing the abdominal wall with a hollow needle. Using ultrasound, the tube or needle is guided into place, and care has to be taken neither to rupture the amniotic membrane nor to injure the fetus in any way. The trans-abdominal method has a lower failure rate than the trans-cervical route, and results in less bleeding and fewer miscarriages. The procedure takes about five minutes and is described as uncomfortable to relatively painless. It has been likened to having a cervical smear taken, or an intra-uterine device fitted.

How chorionic villus sampling is performed

There has been some suggestion, as yet unproven, that early CVS (before 10 weeks) could be linked with a higher incidence of limb and facial deformities. Many centres, therefore, prefer not to perform CVS before 10 weeks, which does reduce some of its advantage over amniocentesis.

The results are obtainable after only 7–10 days, though some centres prefer to do tests which they feel are more accurate, which take three weeks. Either way, it does mean that parents know of a disorder in the baby much earlier than is usual with amniocentesis. If a termination of pregnancy is chosen, this can be performed before 12 weeks, when it is safer for the mother and less distressing for both parents. It also provides some measure of privacy, as a pregnancy at this stage may not yet be obvious to friends and family.

Although much of the long agonizing waiting is dispensed with in CVS, there are risks to be considered:

Question marks

- ○ THE RISK OF MISCARRIAGE IS HIGHER—UP TO 2 PER CENT.
- ○ THE AMNIOTIC SAC MAY BE ACCIDENTALLY PUNCTURED.
- ○ THERE IS A RISK OF INFECTION TO THE BABY.
- ○ THE YOUNG FETUS MAY BE EXPOSED TO VERY HIGH DOSES OF ULTRASOUND.
- ○ THERE IS A RISK OF RHESUS ISO-IMMUNIZATION, AS FETAL AND MATERNAL BLOOD CELLS MAY MINGLE (RHESUS-NEGATIVE MOTHERS MUST BE GIVEN ANTI-D FOLLOWING CVS, AS WITH AMNIOCENTESIS).
- ○ THERE IS A GREATER NEED FOR REPEAT TESTS THAN WITH AMNIOCENTESIS.
- ○ THERE ARE MORE FALSE POSITIVE DIAGNOSES.
- ○ THERE IS MORE BLEEDING FOLLOWING THE TEST.

As with amniocentesis, you and your partner will have to weigh up the potential risks against the information you would receive from a CVS and make what you believe to be the best decision, given what you know.

● *I decided the extra risk of miscarriage was worth it, given that the result would come earlier in the pregnancy and it might not feel quite so awful if something was wrong.* ●

❝ *When the results came through and they showed a problem, we were devastated. Although we were aware of the possibility, we hadn't really imagined we would be the ones. Fortunately we had very good counselling, for which I'm very grateful.* ❞

FETOSCOPY

What fetoscopy tests for

Fetoscopy, which involves a microscopic camera being inserted into the uterus, can detect some other fetal abnormalities, such as cleft palate.

Amazingly, some problems suffered by babies *in utero* can actually be surgically treated before birth, and fetoscopy can be a valuable aid in this. For a baby with an excess of fluid on the brain, a small shunt can be put in place to drain the fluid off into the amniotic cavity so that the brain is not damaged, nor the skull malformed. A urinary tract obstruction can be similarly treated by draining urine into the amniotic fluid. A baby can even have a complete blood transfusion whilst in the uterus. It is more usual, however, that the diagnoses reached by the various tests in pregnancy are used to alert the paediatricians to the need for swift treatment once the baby is born.

How fetoscopy is performed

The procedure is very similar to an amniocentesis, with the microscopic camera being passed through the hollow needle. More can be seen than with ultrasound, because it gives direct vision. It is not commonly used, however, because it is associated with a higher risk of miscarriage.

X-RAYS

What X-rays test for

X-rays used to be more widely used in obstetrics until it was discovered that they could damage the developing baby, particularly in the early stages of pregnancy when rapid formation is taking place. There is also the risk that the radiation might have a delayed effect on future generations. In obstetrics X-rays are mostly used to measure the size and shape of the pelvis (pelvimetry), shortly before the estimated due date, if there is any query about whether the baby will be able to pass through the pelvic bones. This is particularly important if the baby is in a breech position or another of the less favourable positions for labour. Usually only a single X-ray is taken to minimize the dose of radiation the baby receives.

AIDS

AIDS is now posing quite a problem in antenatal care. It is especially significant in pregnancy, because a mother who is a carrier of the disease can pass it on to her unborn baby. Also, for the mother herself, the pregnancy can cause the disease to pass from an asymptomatic HIV positive phase into full-blown AIDS. The current question is whether there should be a screening process which would routinely test all pregnant women (as they are checked for syphilis now), or whether the test should simply be available to all women as it is at present. The argument against routine screening is that it will present a mother with a problem which cannot be solved — there is as yet no treatment for the disease which would prevent the baby becoming infected or the mother seriously ill. Termination of pregnancy is offered to all mothers who are infected, but not all mothers want to take up this option. Many might feel pressurized to have an abortion, and the problem will inevitably involve much suffering for those identified as carriers. For a woman who knows she is HIV positive, and chooses to go ahead with the pregnancy, the knowledge can decrease the likelihood of the baby becoming infected, as measures can be taken to safeguard the baby against infection. The mother can be offered drugs which lessen the chances of infection crossing to the baby, a Caesarean section may be suggested for the delivery, and she may be very strongly advised against breastfeeding.

Ideally, if there is any cause for doubt, screening for AIDS should take place before conception, when the information derived can help women to make important decisions in their lives.

The availability of good counselling, both before the AIDS test and following a positive result, is imperative, and some authorities have trained midwives to provide this service.

COUNSELLING

It is not, of course, only AIDS and its related problems that necessitate counselling care. All antenatal screening, with its potential for producing painful information, should be accompanied by equally skilled care in helping people reach difficult decisions, or come to terms with the fact that their baby is in some way handicapped, whatever choice they eventually make. If you are on the receiving end of such screening, search out a sympathetic and helpful counsellor. This may be a particular midwife, or a doctor, an antenatal teacher, or a specialist counsellor.

The minute you decide to have any form of antenatal screening, you will need to start thinking about how you can best use the information you receive and how best you can make what may be extremely difficult and painful decisions. The following suggestions may help you consider how you will get the best from the services offered to you:

Suggestions which may help you make your decisions

○ ONCE YOU HAVE CHOSEN TO HAVE A SPECIFIC TEST, START ASKING QUESTIONS, AND DO NOT STOP UNTIL YOU ARE SATISFIED YOU HAVE ALL THE INFORMATION YOU THINK YOU NEED.

○ PRECISE INFORMATION ABOUT HOW TERMINATIONS ARE CARRIED OUT IS VERY HARD TO COME BY. YOU WILL NEED TO ASK WHAT THE PROCEDURE AT YOUR LOCAL HOSPITAL IS FOR TERMINATIONS AT DIFFERENT STAGES OF PREGNANCY.

○ ALTHOUGH SOME HOSPITALS SUGGEST YOU SHOULD ONLY HAVE CERTAIN TESTS IF YOU WOULD THEN TERMINATE THE PREGNANCY IF AN ABNORMALITY WERE DETECTED, YOU NEED NOT FEEL BOUND BY THIS. YOUR REASONS FOR WANTING SCREENING ARE VALID, WHATEVER YOU FEEL ABOUT THE OUTCOME. IF YOU ENCOUNTER PROBLEMS, EXPLAIN YOUR REASONS TO YOUR DOCTOR OR MIDWIFE, AND DO WHATEVER YOU KNOW IS BEST FOR YOU.

○ DISCUSS HOW YOU FEEL WITH YOUR PARTNER — ONE OF YOU MIGHT FEEL A TERMINATION WOULD BE BEST, THE OTHER MIGHT BE PREPARED TO BRING A HANDICAPPED CHILD INTO THE FAMILY. YOU NEED TO KNOW HOW THE OTHER FEELS BEFORE POTENTIALLY DIFFICULT DECISIONS HAVE TO BE MADE.

○ FIND SOMEBODY TO TALK TO WHO HAS BEEN THROUGH THE EXPERIENCE HERSELF; WHATEVER FINAL DECISION SHE TOOK, MANY OF THE PROBLEMS ENCOUNTERED WILL BE RELEVANT TO YOU.

○ TALK TO ANYONE WHO YOU THINK MAY BE HELPFUL, ESPECIALLY IF YOUR HOSPITAL DOES NOT OFFER A GOOD COUNSELLING SERVICE; TRY THE NCT, LOCAL COUNSELLING SERVICES, THE SAMARITANS, THE SUPPORT AROUND TERMINATION FOR ABNORMALITY ORGANIZATION (SATFA) — ANYONE WHO WILL LISTEN WITHOUT BEING JUDGEMENTAL.

○ TALK AND KEEP TALKING. THESE ARE EMOTIONAL AS WELL AS PHYSICAL DECISIONS YOU ARE MAKING. THE PEOPLE WHO COPE BEST IN THE END ARE THOSE WHO HAVE TALKED IT THROUGH AT EVERY STAGE: BEFORE, DURING, AND AFTER THE SCREENING PROCESS AND ITS AFTERMATH.

HOW YOU AND YOUR BABY GROW

5

The changes which enable your baby to grow and allow your body to change and grow to accommodate your baby are governed by hormones produced immediately conception has occurred. The age of your baby during pregnancy and your 'expected date of delivery' (EDD) are counted from the first day of your last period. Conception is assumed to have taken place around the fourteenth day of your menstrual cycle. For women with a cycle longer than twenty-eight days, this may result in a discrepancy in dates, but nowadays this can often be resolved with the help of ultrasound scans. If you are sure of your dates and know the normal length of your cycle, there should be little problem. Forty weeks is an average duration of pregnancy, but anything from thirty-eight weeks to forty-four weeks is considered a normal gestational length.

HOW YOUR BABY GROWS

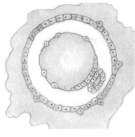

Within a week the fertilized ovum, or egg, now a cluster of over a hundred cells, has implanted itself into the inner lining of the uterus.

The first week

You may be aware that you are pregnant, but most women do not notice any obvious symptoms this early. According to the calculations, you are now 3 weeks pregnant.

The fertilized egg implants itself into the wall of the uterus during the first week of pregnancy

By 6 weeks a recognizable embryo has formed. It is the size of a pea and has a head with rudimentary eyes, ears, mouth, and a brain. It has simple kidneys, a liver, a digestive tract, a primitive umbilical cord, a beating heart, and a bloodstream already obtaining food from the rich lining of the uterus. It is surrounded by the bag of waters, or amniotic sac, which keeps it safe from infection and safely cushioned. The sac is composed of two membranes, the 'amnion' and the 'chorion', and is filled with amniotic fluid. At this stage, the groove which will form the backbone appears.

6 weeks

You may be aware of early pregnancy signs, such as tender

breasts or nausea, or be finding it difficult to keep tight jeans done up in the evenings!

The embryo at 6 weeks

12 weeks

Your baby is now fully formed and its spinal column developed, but it needs to grow and mature before being capable of independent existence. Its organs are fully functioning, co-ordinated by the brain, and it will begin to move about, developing and toning its muscles. Blood vessels in the umbilical cord carry food and oxygen from the placenta to the baby, and carbon dioxide back again.

The baby begins to swallow amniotic fluid continuously at this stage, helping its lungs develop ready for breathing at birth.

The baby passes urine into the amniotic fluid, which is continuously cleansed and changed by the uterus. The amniotic fluid is completely replaced every twenty-four hours until the baby is born. Any other waste products are stored in the baby's intestines and will be excreted as meconium after the birth. Meconium is the tar-like substance which plugs the baby's bowel before birth.

You will almost certainly be aware of your pregnancy. Though your uterus is still down in the pelvis, you may have a noticeable bulge above your pubic bone as the growing uterus displaces other organs. Many women find that any sickness or nausea they have been feeling begins to ease off now.

At 12 weeks, the baby is already fully formed

(Opposite) By 20 weeks your growing uterus will mean that your abdomen is beginning to swell visibly

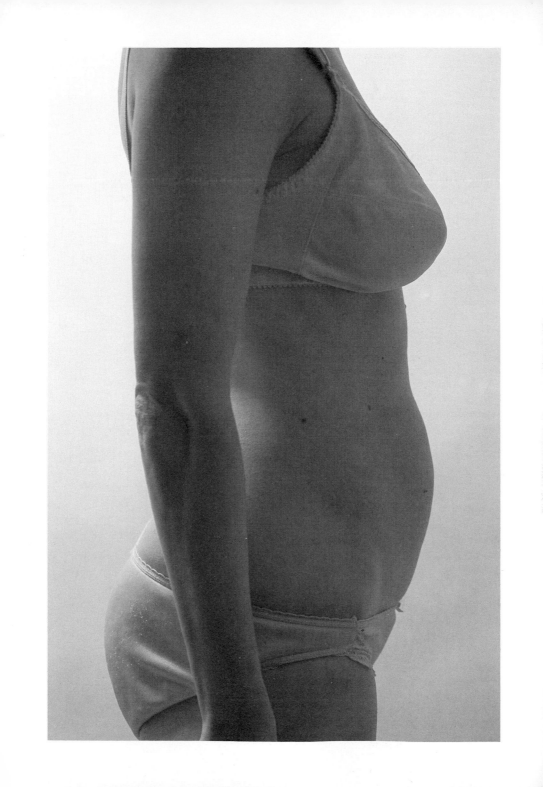

20 weeks

The baby is 25 cm. long — just half as tall as it will be at birth. The sense of touch is developed at 17 weeks so it is able to feel its surroundings.

Its sense of hearing is developed, so it can hear your heartbeat, along with the whooshings and gurglings of your digestive system. As it grows, it will hear sounds outside the uterus, enabling it to recognize your voice, and your partner's, at birth. It has a recognizably human face and a covering of soft hair or down, the lanugo.

You will start to notice your baby move about now, feeling first a series of fluttering sensations, as if bubbles were floating or gently popping inside you. Some women describe these early movements as being like butterflies fluttering in their abdomens; others find it hard to differentiate between the baby's movements and wind in these early stages. As your baby grows, you will feel definite kicks, punches, and squirms, including whole body movements, often surprisingly vigorous.

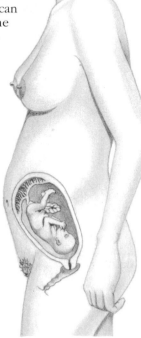

At 20 weeks, the baby may be large enough for you to feel the first movements

28 weeks

The baby might have a fair chance of survival in an incubator if born prematurely. It now weighs about 900 g. and is 37 cm. long. It will be covered in a white creamy substance called vernix, which prevents the skin becoming waterlogged.

You will be obviously pregnant, with a very definitely rounded abdomen, and may be beginning to find it hard to eat large meals as the uterus grows and takes up some of the room your stomach used to have!

The baby at 28 weeks

32 weeks

The baby's head and body are in proportion; it has begun to lay down a layer of subcutaneous fat, but is still rather thin. It will weigh roughly 1.6 kg. and be 40 cm. long. From now until birth it will gain about 250 g. a week. Some babies may suck their thumbs and some have hiccups.

You may be able to recognize a foot or elbow sticking out as well as the general heavings and lurchings which babies enjoy in the uterus. If the baby has hiccups, you will also notice these as regular rhythmical movements. The baby may bump its head uncomfortably into your bladder or stick its bottom under your ribs. Some babies make sudden bouncing movements with their heads which feel like 'buzzing' sensations at the top of your vagina, which may stop you in your tracks for a moment.

36 weeks

Most babies will have settled into a position with their head down, most of them facing towards their mother's back. At this stage many babies, especially first babies, 'engage'; that is, the baby's head descends well into the mother's pelvis ready for birth. Other babies wait until labour to move down into the pelvis. Your baby will still be active, but the scope of its movements will be restricted by its size: it now weighs about 2.5 kg. and is about 46 cm. long. It has a good covering of fat to keep it warm after birth and its lungs are probably almost fully mature.

You may feel very uncomfortable at times, with the heavy uterus a real weight to carry around all day. Your bladder may need emptying very frequently and you may find

By 34 weeks, the growing baby is beginning to have less space in which to move freely

The baby at full term — 40 weeks

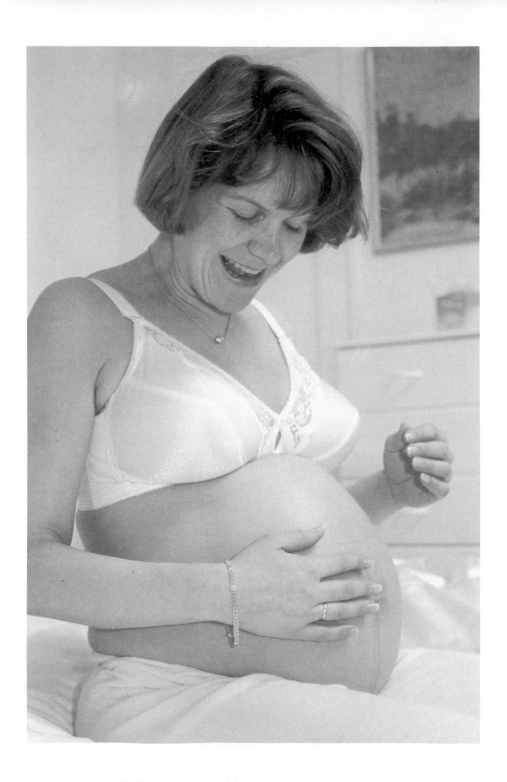

your legs swelling by the end of the day. Your feet may ache if you have to stand for any length of time, particularly if the weather is hot.

40 weeks

This is the average time for a baby to be ready to be born; however, most babies are born either earlier or later than this; partly because they take different times to mature, and partly because women vary in the time it takes for their bodies to be ready to go into labour. Some vernix will usually be left on your baby, and it may still have some lanugo on its shoulders or back.

You may feel ready to give birth to your baby and look forward to greeting him or her. You may find you have rather ambivalent feelings as the end of your pregnancy approaches and the next phase is in sight.

The placenta

The placenta is the organ which grows with your baby on the inside of the uterus at the site where the embryo first embedded itself. It has direct contact with your bloodstream: this is how nicotine, drugs, and alcohol, as well as food, oxygen, and immunities, are passed from you to the baby.

The umbilical cord

The umbilical cord is about 50 cm. long and is surrounded by a substance known as Wharton's jelly, which acts as a buffer and prevents the cord from kinking, which could interfere with circulation.

HOW YOUR BODY CHANGES

Uterus

Your uterus is composed of smooth muscle which stretches and grows to accommodate your growing baby. In the non-pregnant state your uterus weighs just 55 g. (2 oz.), and at the end of pregnancy it will weigh 1.2 kg. (2 lb.), which is entirely due to the increased muscle. For the first four months of pregnancy it grows within your pelvis, often pressing on your bladder so that you have to empty it more frequently. At about four and a half months the uterus grows out of the pelvis, making you begin to look pregnant and making trousers and skirts harder or impossible to do up. As the baby grows, the uterus becomes higher and higher, so that eventually you will feel kicks right under your rib-cage and may find it difficult to eat large meals. If your baby does engage at 36 weeks, you will experience what used to be called 'lightening': your uterus moves visibly downwards and you will feel much more comfortable at the top. You may, however, now experience more aches, pains, and twinges in your lower abdomen as your baby squirms and presses on nerve-endings. At this stage you may again need to empty your bladder more frequently, as

(Opposite)
By 36 weeks you may be anticipating the birth of your baby with pleasure, excitement, and a degree of apprehension

the baby presses down on it. During the last month of pregnancy the uterus becomes thinner at the bottom and thicker at the top, preparing itself for labour.

BRAXTON HICKS CONTRACTIONS You may notice 'Braxton Hicks' contractions as your pregnancy progresses, so-called after the doctor who first described them. These are practice contractions, toning your uterus up for labour, and, though they may sometimes be uncomfortable, they are rarely painful, which distinguishes them from true labour contractions. You might feel them as a sudden tightening and hardening of the uterus, or it may feel as though the baby has moved into an awkward position and stuck there for a while. If you feel your abdomen during a Braxton Hicks contraction, it will feel rock-hard.

You may well not notice your Braxton Hicks contractions, but this does not mean that you are not getting them.

Hormones

Oestrogen and progesterone soften the smooth muscles of the uterus, bladder, intestines, and veins, enabling your uterus to grow with your baby. Unfortunately, sometimes their effects give rise to varicose veins or constipation. The production of progesterone is taken over by the placenta once it has developed, at about 14 weeks, which may be why many women find their pregnancy nausea improves about this time.

The hormone relaxin is also produced by the placenta and causes the soft connective tissues of your body to become softer and more elastic. This enables the bony joints of the spine and pelvis to become flexible for birth, and the ligaments supporting the uterus to expand during labour. The increased mobility of the joints may lead to discomfort in the pelvic area, but backache is more often due to poor posture. Progesterone also contributes to the softening of the pelvic connecting tissue by increasing the amount of extracellular fluid present. This increase in extracellular fluid also enables expansion of the uterus, but can be associated with general fluid retention in pregnancy.

Lungs

Your lungs achieve a more efficient exchange of gases during pregnancy, ensuring that your baby gets enough oxygen with no extra effort from you. You may find you get breathless very easily when the growing baby fills your abdomen and presses under your diaphragm. If this happens, it is a good idea to relax and breathe as slowly and deeply as you can, concentrating on emptying your lungs thoroughly, so they automatically take in fresh air without your having to gulp it down.

All your organs have to work harder in pregnancy to support two of you. This is why your blood pressure is checked regularly and why some women develop pregnancy diabetes. During pregnancy the volume of blood circulating round your body increases by 40–50 per cent to service the baby, the uterus, the placenta, and the enlarged breasts. Since the red blood cells, which carry oxygen round your body, increase by only 18 per cent, and the baby needs to establish its own blood supply, it is important that you have sufficient iron in your diet, supplemented by iron tablets if your doctor or midwife thinks it really necessary, to prevent anaemia. This increased circulation of blood accounts for many women feeling warmer than usual during pregnancy and uncomfortable in very hot weather. The fluid from the increased circulation will be excreted as urine and perspiration in the first few days after birth.

Blood supply

Often the increase in your breast size will be one of the earliest signs of pregnancy, and there is a further increase at around 32 weeks. You may need to buy new bras to feel comfortable when your breasts grow. From 36 weeks an NCT-trained bra-fitter can fit you for a bra which will also be suitable for breastfeeding after the birth. Whether or not you wear a bra at all is entirely up to you; some women never wear one; others only feel properly comfortable in a supportive well-fitting bra; others wear one only during the last few weeks of pregnancy and the early weeks of breastfeeding, when their breasts feel particularly heavy. You may find your breasts leak towards the end of pregnancy: this is colostrum, which will provide your baby with food and more essential immunities in the first few days after birth until your milk comes in. Leaking colostrum is quite normal, and does not mean your baby will miss out once she is born.

Breasts

The two large muscles down the centre of your abdomen (the recti abdominis) will separate to make enough room for your expanding uterus. For a few weeks after your baby is born you will be able to feel this 'gap' in your abdominal muscles by feeling around your navel with the fingers of one hand to see how wide your gap is. Eventually your gap should narrow to about 1 cm. — more would suggest your abdominal muscles are still rather weak and need gentle treatment. It is because these muscles need to be well knitted together again after birth that you will have to be very careful indeed about doing any vigorous abdominal muscle-strengthening exercises postnatally (see Chapter 27, Looking After Yourself Postnatally, for further information).

Rectus abdominis muscle

Weight gain   Weight gain varies from one woman to another, but the following table will give you some idea of how much weight you might expect to put on.

Average weight gain during pregnancy

Where the weight is gained	lb.	kg.
The baby	7	3.4
Placenta	1½	0.8
Amniotic fluid	1½–2	1.0
Uterus	2	1.2
Breasts	1	0.4
Extra blood	3–4	1.5
Extra body fluid	3–3½	1.4
Fat deposits	10–12	3.5

The fat gained is used for making breast milk after the birth. Weight gain over the amounts mentioned here will mean you are putting on excess fat, or storing a lot of fluid.

Pregnancy alters the way you metabolize your food, but the effects will vary. You may find you have to eat a great deal more to achieve a good weight gain, but it may be that you find your body is able to use your food more efficiently so you do not have to eat any more than usual.

You should be able to take all these changes in your stride, particularly if you eat a good varied diet, rest when you feel tired, and respect the fact that you are living for two!

❛ *I love waking up every morning to feel the baby kicking and wriggling inside me.* ❜

❛ *Once I got over that stage of looking fat but not yet pregnant, I really enjoyed my growing abdomen. I feel proud of it, and I love to feel how round and strong it is.* ❜

❛ *I do find the physical restrictions frustrating now: not being able to cut my own toe-nails, run upstairs, or bend over properly.* ❜

LOOKING AFTER YOURSELF

6

Until now, you may not have thought terribly seriously about how you treat yourself and your body, content to let things jog along from day to day, assuming all will be well. You may, however, have found that pregnancy brings a sudden realization that it is not really quite fair to take your body for granted, when it will be changing so dramatically over the next few months. You may also be aware that how you look after yourself will affect your developing baby, and you will want to give both of you the best opportunities for growth. This chapter looks at all the positive things you can do to help yourself feel good, to provide a healthy environment for your fetus, and to prepare your body for the events ahead of you: the labour and birth, followed by your recovery during the postnatal period, and the strenuous task of caring for a new baby.

POSTURE

The word posture may have a rather old-fashioned ring to it, but in fact it is extremely important that you check your posture during pregnancy, because of the extra strain being put on your body. Pregnancy itself adds strain to your joints, ligaments, and muscles, partly because of the weight they are supporting, and partly because the hormones produced during pregnancy are softening your ligaments ready for the birth. The idea is to be supple without overstretching yourself: many of the irritating aches and pains associated with some pregnancies can be avoided or improved by paying attention to your posture.

As well as considering your own comfort, it is also a good idea to think about whether your posture is enabling your baby to adopt a good position in your pelvis. The position in which your baby lies at the end of pregnancy can have a strong influence on the kind of labour you have, and a baby who is lying in the anterior position (see Chapter 3, Antenatal Medical Care, p.45) is likely to enjoy a smoother entry into the world. It may be that some of the postures you take up mean that your pelvis is often tilted backwards making it more difficult for your baby to get into an anterior position. Choosing some of the more upright postures suggested on the following pages, so that your pelvis tilts forwards, may have a beneficial effect on your labour as well as on your well-being during pregnancy.

Lying down   You may find that you sometimes feel breathless or dizzy when you are lying flat, or you may suffer from heartburn. If this happens, you might be more comfortable propped up, with plenty of pillows supporting the upper half of your body, your neck, and head. Adding a pillow under your head alone is liable to give you nothing more helpful than a stiff neck!

In the later stages of pregnancy, it is better to avoid lying flat on your back altogether, as this position affects circulation and can make you feel faint. You may be able to prevent this by raising your head, or by lying with your knees raised. If possible, find a different position.

When getting out of bed, or off the doctor's couch — tricky manoeuvres in late pregnancy — try swinging your legs over the side of the bed first, then sit for a moment in case you feel dizzy, and stand up only when you feel ready.

Sleeping positions If you find it difficult to get off to sleep because of the discomfort caused by your large abdomen, try lying in the 'recovery' position, with extra pillows under your upper arm and knee. Turning over in bed may take on aspects of a full military-style manoeuvre, but you may feel slightly more comfortable.

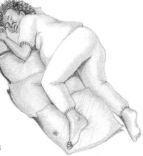

Women who normally sleep on their stomachs have a tough time in late pregnancy. You could try balancing your abdomen by adding extra pillows under your chest, hips, and thighs. It may not feel quite right, but still be the best compromise. Returning to your normal sleeping position may be the thing you most look forward to once your baby is born!

Sleeping in the recovery position may help you to feel more comfortable

Sitting down   When you sit down, check that your spine is well supported, either by your own muscles or by your chair. Many pregnant women prefer to sit upright on a hard chair with a straight back, so that the uterus is not squashing everything else uncomfortably, causing heartburn or pressure under the ribs. If you sit in car seats, an armchair, or a sofa where your knees are higher than your hips, it may help to tilt your pelvis forwards again if you try putting one firm cushion under your bottom and another against your lower back. This will not only make you more upright, but may well be much more comfortable. It is also significantly easier for most women to get up again from an upright chair. If you experience discomfort under your ribs or below your shoulder blades, try sitting 'cowboy-style' astride the chair, arms resting on its back, and keep your shoulders slightly raised when walking about.

AT WORK If you are still working and your job involves long periods of sitting, you may find it hard to get comfortable. If you are having problems, it may be worth asking your employer for a better chair. Many employers are now aware of the need to provide good, supportive equipment for their employees, as it is not only in pregnancy that good posture is essential for general good health. As well as checking that your chair allows your spine to be well supported, it is just as important to make sure you get up and move around at least once every hour — just a quick stretch or a few exercises to loosen up can make all the difference to your comfort and concentration.

TRAVELLING The same holds for any situation when you may be sitting for long periods — travelling, especially by car, can become extremely uncomfortable, and a good long stretch or loosen up is vital. If you are making a long car journey, it is best to stop at least once every two hours. Apart from anything else, your bladder will probably not hold out for much longer than that!

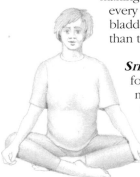

SITTING 'TAILOR-FASHION' A comfortable position for many women, and one which allows your muscles to stretch in preparation for labour, is to sit tailor-fashion, cross-legged on the floor or on cushions. Sitting like this for at least half an hour every day for a few months before your baby is due could make all the difference to your suppleness.

Sitting 'tailor-fashion'

THE 'COBBLER'S POSE' You can achieve further stretching by practising the cobbler's pose. This position not only stretches your joints and widens the front of the pelvis, it also increases the circulation to your pelvic region, benefiting all the pelvic organs. It will also help to correct the pelvic tilt (see below).

- ○ **SIT WITH A STRAIGHT BACK WITH KNEES BENT AND YOUR FEET TOGETHER, SOLES TOUCHING.**
- ○ **GENTLY BRING YOUR FEET TOWARDS YOUR GROIN UNTIL YOU FEEL THE PULL.**
- ○ **LET YOUR THIGHS OPEN UP, PUT YOUR HANDS UNDER YOUR KNEES, AND PRESS DOWN AGAINST YOUR HANDS UNTIL YOU CAN FEEL A GENTLE BUT DEFINITE STRETCH IN YOUR INNER THIGHS, HIP JOINTS, AND GROIN.**

The 'cobbler's pose'

Kneeling

Because kneeling on all fours takes the pressure of the uterus off the back, many women find kneeling positions very comfortable during pregnancy and labour. You could kneel supported either by your arms or by leaning on to a low chair or bean-bag.

If you want to kneel right down, it is better to have a cushion between your buttocks and heels, or a small stool or toddler step supporting your buttocks, to avoid pressure. Getting down on hands and knees to wash the kitchen floor can become a surprisingly pleasant activity for many women in the later stages of pregnancy. Kneeling is also a comfortable position in which to practise pelvic rocking (see opposite).

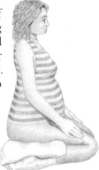

Kneeling with a cushion between buttocks and heels to avoid pressure

Lifting

Although it is safer to avoid lifting anything heavy during pregnancy because of the possibility of damage to softened ligaments and already stressed muscles and joints, it is sometimes unavoidable, particularly if you have a toddler to care for. As long as you make sure you always bend your knees before picking anything up, and use your centre of gravity to take the strain, by holding any heavy object close to your body, you should be able to minimize the risk of serious problems. Many problems associated with incorrect posture or added stress to your body during pregnancy, unfortunately, do not give you enough of a warning during the pregnancy — in fact, it may not be until your baby is a few months old that problems with your body, especially your back, manifest themselves. Being aware of your body and respecting its needs can make all the difference.

Standing

Good posture at all times will help to avoid back strain

The weight of the uterus can easily pull your abdomen forward and down in pregnancy, placing excessive strain on your spine. Try to imagine your pelvis as an egg-cup in which you have to balance the egg, your uterus. Standing or sitting, you will need to keep the egg in the cup! This exercise helps to correct the tilt of your pelvis, inevitably altered during your pregnancy.

Bending

Your waist is unfortunately not hinged, and, if you treat it as though it were, your back will eventually complain. If you need to bend down to pick up your child, collect her toys, hang out the washing, or make the beds, make sure you *always* bend at the knee.

Check that any work surfaces, changing-mats,

etc., are at an appropriate height for you too, so that you are not adding to any strain on your back by bending over, even slightly.

SOME BASIC EXERCISES

If you decide never to do any other exercise whilst pregnant, it is important to do the following exercises as part of your daily routine. They will help your body adapt to its changing shape and size, will help relieve some of the aches and pains, will improve circulation, and will strengthen your abdominal and pelvic-floor muscles ready for labour and afterwards.

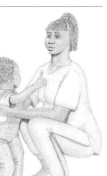

Bend at the knees rather than at the waist

PELVIC TILT You can do exercises to correct the pelvic tilt in almost any position, but, to start with, try sitting on the front of a chair with your knees apart.

○ **GENTLY HOLLOW YOUR BACK — YOUR PELVIS WILL TILT DOWN IN FRONT.**

○ **NOW ROUND YOUR LOWER BACK, PULLING IN YOUR ABDOMINAL MUSCLES.**

○ **ONCE YOU HAVE THE FEEL OF IT, YOU CAN ALSO TRY PELVIC TILTING STANDING UP, TILTING YOUR PELVIS GENTLY BACKWARDS AND FORWARDS, THEN ROUND AND ROUND AS WELL, AS IF YOU WERE BELLY-DANCING.**

Tilts on all-fours are wonderful if you are suffering from a tired aching back.

○ **KNEEL WITH YOUR KNEES SLIGHTLY APART, THEN HUMP YOUR BACK LIKE AN ANGRY CAT, DRAWING YOUR ABDOMEN IN.**

○ **NOW RELAX AND LET YOUR BACK FLATTEN — JUST ENOUGH TO BE COMFORTABLE — AND REPEAT THE EXERCISE.**

Practising the pelvic tilt on all-fours: the 'angry cat'

PELVIC ROCKING Many women find pelvic rocking very comforting and soothing during pregnancy, labour, and in the postnatal period, particularly if they have backache, so it is worth practising.

○ LIE WITH YOUR KNEES BENT AND TOUCHING EACH OTHER.

○ BREATHE IN, AND, AS YOU BREATHE OUT, PULL IN YOUR ABDOMINAL MUSCLES, PRESSING THE SMALL OF YOUR BACK FIRMLY INTO THE BED.

○ HOLD THIS FOR A COUNT OF FOUR, THEN RELEASE.

○ REPEAT FREQUENTLY, HOLDING FOR LONGER (UP TO A COUNT OF TEN) AS YOUR MUSCLES GROW STRONGER.

○ YOU CAN DO THIS EXERCISE SITTING OR STANDING ONCE YOU ARE USED TO IT.

PERINEAL MASSAGE The perineum is the area between the back of the vagina and the anus. It is the area which fans out most as your baby's head is being born. If you squat down and look in a mirror, you will be able to see the perineum, and can feel the thickness of the skin by putting your thumb inside your vagina, against the back wall, and placing a finger outside (rather like feeling a piece of material between your thumb and finger). As your baby's head is born, this skin will thin out and open an amazing amount, returning to its normal size afterwards.

Massaging your perineum during pregnancy may help it become more supple and stretchy, and also help you be more aware of sensations around your vagina.

○ PLACE YOUR THUMB INSIDE THE VAGINA AGAINST THE BACK WALL, WITH YOUR FOREFINGER ON THE PERINEUM, AND MASSAGE GENTLY, TRYING GRADUALLY TO STRETCH THE VAGINAL OPENING.

○ SOME PEOPLE LIKE TO USE WHEATGERM OR VITAMIN E OIL TO LUBRICATE THE PERINEUM WHILE MASSAGING.

○ YOU CAN DO PERINEAL MASSAGE YOURSELF, OR SUGGEST YOUR PARTNER DOES IT FOR YOU. YOUR PARTNER CAN TRY GRADUALLY INCREASING THE NUMBER OF FINGERS INSIDE THE VAGINA, STRETCHING THE SKIN.

Whether it is you or your partner doing it, you might like to make sure that all fingernails are nice and short, as well as clean, before you begin!

FOOT EXERCISES Foot exercise is essential for anyone with even a hint of varicose veins, leg cramps, or swollen ankles, and for anyone who has a sedentary occupation. It helps to improve circulation in the foot and leg, and to protect the arches from being flattened by the extra weight they are supporting.

○ BEND AND STRETCH YOUR FEET BRISKLY UP AND DOWN THIRTY TIMES (USE YOUR WHOLE FOOT, NOT JUST THE TOES).

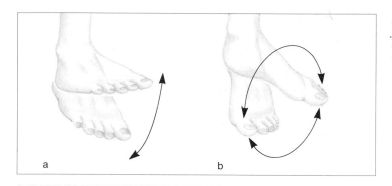

Exercises for the feet:
a. up and down
b. foot circling

○ NOW MOVE EACH FOOT ROUND IN A CIRCLE TEN TIMES IN
EACH DIRECTION, ALWAYS COMING UP IN THE MIDDLE AND
THEN OUT AND ROUND TO STRENGTHEN THE LONG ARCH.

○ WITH YOUR FEET RESTING ON THE FLOOR, DRAW UP YOUR
TOES AS THOUGH TRYING TO SCUFF UP THE CARPET; THIS
EXERCISE IS ESSENTIAL FOR STRENGTHENING THE MUSCLES
SUPPORTING THE ANTERIOR ARCH OF YOUR FOOT.

PELVIC-FLOOR EXERCISES

Your pelvic floor forms a firm but supple base to your pelvis. It is
made up of three layers of interwoven muscles which form a 'sling'
supporting the bladder, uterus, and bowel. A woman's pelvic floor
has three openings: at the urethra, the vagina, and the anus.

***Reasons for
exercising
the pelvic
floor***

SUPPORT Exercising your pelvic-floor muscles will tone them up,
so that they give good support to your growing baby and uterus,
and can help you feel more comfortable during pregnancy.

STRESS INCONTINENCE Women often find, towards the end of
pregnancy, that they have slight leaking from the bladder
when coughing, sneezing, or laughing. This is called stress
incontinence.

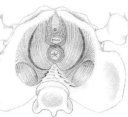

PROLAPSE Some women suffer from a prolapsed uterus. Here, the
uterus has slipped downwards in the vagina, possibly due to
weaknesses in the pelvic floor following a delivery.

*The pelvic-floor
muscles*

Some factors which can contribute to both of these distressing
conditions are:

○ BEING OVERWEIGHT
○ PERSISTENT COUGHING, SUCH AS A SMOKER MAY SUFFER

○ **WEAKNESS IN THE PELVIC-FLOOR MUSCLES**
○ **CHRONIC CONSTIPATION, CAUSING STRAINING OF THE PELVIC FLOOR WHEN OPENING THE BOWELS**

If you learn how to draw up and tighten the muscles before any pressure is put on them, you can help reduce the problem of stress incontinence. Exercise will also help you know how to relax your pelvic floor when you are giving birth to your baby.

Once your baby is born, exercise will help you regain good muscle control, which can reduce stress incontinence, reduce the likelihood of a prolapse occurring, and will increase both partners' enjoyment of love-making.

Learning pelvic-floor exercises

You may already be aware of your pelvic-floor muscles — you pull them up or tighten them to control your bladder or bowel when they are full. If you experience orgasm, you may feel the spontaneous contraction and relaxation of your vaginal walls as well as some of the pelvic-floor muscles. You may already be using them if you squeeze your partner's penis, giving 'internal kisses', when you are making love. You may have used them to stop a tampon sliding out at an inconvenient moment! These are the muscles which need to be strong and supple for pregnancy, for giving birth, and for the rest of your lives!

A BASIC EXERCISE

○ **SIT IN A COMFORTABLE POSITION WITH YOUR LEGS UNCROSSED AND SLIGHTLY SEPARATED.**
○ **NOW PULL UP AROUND THE VAGINA AS IF TO HOLD IN A TAMPON, OR AROUND THE URETHRA AS IF TO STOP YOURSELF EMPTYING YOUR BLADDER.**
○ **ONCE YOU HAVE GOT THE FEEL OF THIS AREA, TRY PULLING UP FROM THE FRONT, AROUND YOUR URETHRA, RIGHT ROUND TOWARDS YOUR ANUS.**
○ **HOLD IT FOR A COUNT OF FOUR, THEN RELEASE.**
○ **YOU SHOULD TRY NOT TO HOLD YOUR BREATH WHILE DOING THESE EXERCISES, BUT IT MAY TAKE TIME TO MANAGE THIS.**
○ **TRY TO TIGHTEN ONLY YOUR PELVIC-FLOOR MUSCLES, MAKING SURE THE MUSCLES OF YOUR BUTTOCKS, INNER THIGHS, AND ABDOMEN REMAIN RELAXED.**

Some people will find it relatively easy to hold their muscles tight to a count of four. Remember that you will be starting at a different point from everyone else, so assess how long you can hold your muscles for before you feel them starting to relax again. Your aim is to increase your own count as the weeks pass.

A useful test You may well be feeling unsure about whether or not you are doing the exercise correctly, so you can test it for yourself in this way:

- ○ WHEN YOU GO TO THE LAVATORY, START TO EMPTY YOUR BLADDER, THEN DRAW UP YOUR PELVIC-FLOOR MUSCLES TO STOP THE FLOW.
- ○ COUNT TO FOUR, THEN RELAX AND FINISH EMPTYING YOUR BLADDER. (YOU MAY HAVE HAD TO DO THIS FOR A MID-STREAM URINE SAMPLE.)

To be really effective, you need to practise your pelvic-floor exercises frequently — preferably four or more times *an hour* during the day. Once your baby is born, this needs to be increased to six times an hour until you feel happy that you have regained good muscle tone.

Further pelvic-floor exercises

The basic pelvic-floor exercise is essential, but does not necessarily tone up all the different layers of muscle, so, once you feel confident about doing the basic pelvic-floor exercise, try the following exercises as well:

VARYING THE EXERCISE

- ○ DO FOUR TIGHTENINGS, HOLDING TO A COUNT OF AT LEAST FOUR AS BEFORE.
- ○ NOW DO FOUR QUICK PULL-UPS, AS IF YOU WERE 'FLICKING' THE MUSCLES IN YOUR VAGINA.
- ○ NOW DO FOUR TIGHTENINGS AGAIN.

THE LIFT

- ○ BEGIN BY IMAGINING THAT THE MUSCLES AROUND YOUR VAGINA ARE A LIFT WHICH IS IN A RELAXED POSITION AT THE GROUND FLOOR.
- ○ TIGHTEN THE MUSCLES A LITTLE AND PULL THEM UP INSIDE THE VAGINA TO THE FIRST FLOOR.
- ○ TIGHTEN A LITTLE FURTHER, UP TO THE SECOND FLOOR.
- ○ AS YOU GROW MORE EXPERIENCED, TRY MOVING ON UP TO THE THIRD FLOOR.
- ○ NOW, HOLD YOUR MUSCLES TIGHT TO A COUNT OF FOUR-PLUS, BEFORE MOVING SLOWLY TO THE GROUND FLOOR AGAIN.

Your pelvic-floor muscle should not start to tremble; if it does, rest and then try again. Remember to keep your buttock, thigh, and abdominal muscles relaxed while you are doing the exercise. Remember to breathe as well!

RELAXING THE PELVIC FLOOR Now, without tensing your pelvic floor, cough, or blow into your fist. Could you feel the pelvic floor moving outwards? This is very similar to the movement it makes when the baby's head reaches it during the second stage of labour. Knowing how to relax these muscles completely will help you give birth to your baby. It is easier to relax your pelvic floor if you relax your mouth, jaw, and tongue, drop your shoulders, then breathe out slowly.

O   **RELAX YOUR PELVIC-FLOOR MUSCLES SO THAT THEY FEEL QUITE SOFT, AND ALLOW THEM TO BULGE SLIGHTLY DOWNWARDS. (IF IT HELPS, YOU COULD TRY THINKING OF THIS AS YOUR LIFT GOING DOWN TO THE BASEMENT.)**

O   **MAKE SURE YOU ALWAYS BRING YOUR MUSCLES BACK TO THE GROUND FLOOR BY GENTLY SQUEEZING THE MUSCLES TOGETHER AND LIFTING THEM SLIGHTLY.**

It is best to do these exercises at intervals during the day, and you will find they do become easier the more you practise. You could try involving your partner while you are making love, by getting him to test how strong your muscles are becoming. Many women find it helpful to do pelvic-floor exercises at specific times or occasions during the day so that they remember to do them as often as possible. You could try:

O   **WHILE WASHING UP**

O   **WHILE CLEANING YOUR TEETH**

O   **WHILE WASHING YOUR HANDS AFTER GOING TO THE LAVATORY**

O   **WHILE DRIVING THE CAR**

O   **WHILE WAITING AT TRAFFIC LIGHTS**

O   **DURING YOUR JOURNEY TO AND FROM WORK BY PUBLIC TRANSPORT**

O   **EVERY TIME YOU THINK ABOUT YOUR PREGNANCY, YOUR BABY, OR ITS BIRTH**

O   **WHENEVER YOU THINK ABOUT SEX**

You will find further information on exercising the pelvic floor, and specific exercises for stress incontinence, in Chapter 27, Looking After Yourself Postnatally.

EXERCISE

Pregnancy is not the time to take up an energetic new sport which will use muscles you never knew you had, but exercise is enjoyable and good for you, especially if you can combine it with some fresh air. Exercising helps you feel good, can lift depression, and helps to keep your body strong and supple. Most forms of exercise are also good for toning your pelvic floor.

If you are used to exercising regularly, carry on for as long as you feel comfortable or safe. You might feel happier avoiding activities which could involve a fall, such as horse-riding, skiing, or parachuting!

WALKING Regular brisk walks are good — though sometimes you might have to weigh up the benefit of the exercise against the possibility of inhaling lungsful of traffic fumes. However, during the later weeks you may find walking longer distances becomes increasingly uncomfortable.

SWIMMING Swimming is a particularly useful exercise in pregnancy, as it is an exercise which involves many muscle groups whilst relieving the body of any strain. Swimming on your front also helps to keep your pelvis tilted forwards. Many pools and leisure centres now hold regular exercise or swimming classes for pregnant women, so it is worth finding out what is on offer locally. Some classes are water classes, not requiring you to be able to swim, which many women find an excellent source of gentle exercise.

YOGA Some yoga teachers also hold classes specifically for pregnant women, though do check that *any* exercise teacher is qualified to deal with pregnant women before signing on.

ACTIVE BIRTH CLASSES Many areas now run active birth classes, which aim to prepare women's bodies for an active labour as well as providing exercise during pregnancy. You can find out more about these classes, either by ringing a local teacher direct (try the phone book), or by contacting the Active Birth Centre (you will find the address listed at the back of this book).

REST

For those of you with busy jobs or a child or two to care for, there may not seem to be much opportunity for rest during the day. (You may feel you are not getting much at night either, if you are going to the lavatory two or three times, or have a child who wakes regularly.) If you can, it is worth resting whenever the opportunity arises, making your own opportunities if you are feeling really tired. Some restful periods every day can save you becoming overtired and possibly ill or overstressed later.

WORKING MOTHERS If you are at work, you could try putting your feet up during your lunch break; take sandwiches so you do not have to spend time waiting for a meal. If the weather is nice, combine lunch with a walk to find somewhere pleasant to sit and eat. If you are usually rushing round doing the shopping in your lunch-hour, try organizing your weekly chores differently, or arrange for your partner to shop.

MOTHERS WORKING AT HOME If you are at home with other children, rest may be equally elusive. If your toddler is still sleeping during the day, use that time to rest yourself rather than trying to squeeze in hundreds of jobs. If she is not too keen on sleeping any more, could you suggest both of you having a quiet lie down together, perhaps with a story first to help you both relax? If a sleep during the day means she is up for hours in the evening, this may cause more problems than it solves. Some children do not want to rest in the daytime; perhaps you could arrange a child-swap with a friend for an afternoon or two a week to give you some time to yourself.

SOCIAL LIFE If you do not feel up to evening activities, say so; do not force yourself to carry on, but accept that pregnancy can be tiring and let your body decide when it has had enough. Should you need to go to bed at 8.30 each evening, then you can do so, knowing that this is your body's way of coping with the natural stresses of pregnancy.

RELAXATION

Relaxation is not necessarily the same as resting — your body can be rested but tense. If you are normally busy without much time for a proper rest, a few minutes' relaxation can make all the difference to how you cope with the rest of the day.

Pregnancy is an ideal time to learn the skill of relaxation: you are aware of your body, you have an increased need for rest and relaxation, and you may be willing to try all sorts of new ideas.

RECOGNIZING STRESS It is a good idea to start by being aware of your own body's reactions to stress.

- O **DO YOU TENSE YOUR SHOULDERS?**
- O **DO YOU CLENCH YOUR TEETH OR FISTS?**
- O **DO YOU GET A TIGHT FEELING IN YOUR THROAT?**
- O **DO YOU BECOME VERY IRRITABLE?**
- O **DO YOU CURL UP YOUR TOES?**
- O **DO YOU SIGH FREQUENTLY?**
- O **DO YOU OFTEN HAVE A TIGHT HEADACHE AT THE END OF THE DAY?**

○ **DO YOU NOTICE THAT YOUR JAWS ACHE?**
○ **DO YOU FEEL THE NEED OF A DRINK OR CIGARETTE TO CALM YOU DOWN?**

WHY RELAX? Relaxation can help you get off to sleep, or back to sleep if you have woken up and cannot drop off again. It can help you keep your blood pressure down while waiting for an antenatal appointment or any stressful situation, and relaxing can help you prepare for an examination by your doctor or midwife. Using relaxation in labour will help you work with your uterus rather than fighting it, and will help you conserve energy. Once your baby is born, relaxation will help you cope with the demands of early parenthood — a tiring and stressful time for all parents, as well as a happy one.

Fathers as well as mothers find that relaxation helps them cope, not only with the immediate effects of pregnancy, labour, and life with a new baby, but also their lives beyond:

○ **COPING WITH STRESS AT WORK**
○ **COPING WITH FRACTIOUS CHILDREN**
○ **HANDLING AWKWARD SITUATIONS OR PEOPLE**
○ **DEALING WITH ALL SORTS OF MINOR IRRITATIONS IN LIFE**

Relaxation is not something you can only do sitting or lying down for ten minutes every day. It is a technique you can practise actively:

○ **DRIVING**
○ **PREPARING MEALS**
○ **SHOPPING**
○ **AT WORK**
○ **ANYWHERE**

Relaxation does not mean losing concentration or just letting go; it can mean being active without being tense. If you take exercise, like going for a walk or gardening, you are active but relaxed and will feel good afterwards. If you learn to relax effectively, you will always have a skill to be summoned up in any situation, or as an excellent means of giving your mind and body a regular treat. Teaching your children to relax as well can help them cope when they come up against pressures in life.

PREPARING FOR RELAXATION

○ **SIT IN A COMFORTABLE CHAIR WITH YOUR BACK, NECK, AND HEAD WELL SUPPORTED AND COMFORTABLE. YOU WILL NEED TO BE QUITE FIRM RATHER THAN SAGGING.**

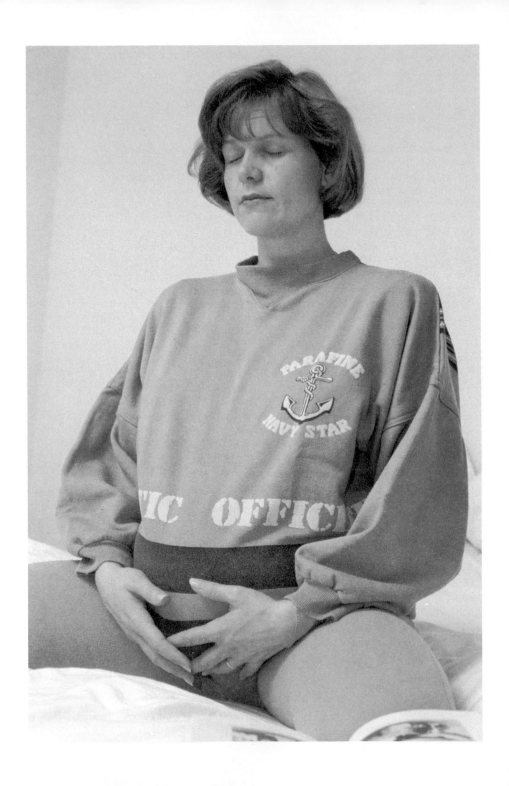

○ CHECK THAT YOU ARE REALLY COMFORTABLE. WRIGGLE
    AROUND UNTIL YOU ARE.
○ REST YOUR FEET ON THE FLOOR AND YOUR HANDS LOOSELY
    IN YOUR LAP OR ON YOUR THIGHS.
○ CHECK THAT YOU HAVE NOT GOT YOUR ANKLES CROSSED.
○ CLOSE YOUR EYES, OR LEAVE THEM OPEN BUT NOT FOCUSED
    ON JUST ONE SPOT; A BLANK STARE IS BETTER.
○ BREATHE OUT SLOWLY, NOTICING HOW YOU CAN FEEL YOUR
    BODY BEGINNING TO LET GO AS YOU BREATHE OUT. THE
    OUT-BREATH IS THE RELAXING BREATH, AND THIS IS WHAT
    YOU WILL CONCENTRATE ON TO HELP YOU RELEASE
    TENSION.

RELAXING YOUR BODY It is useful to be able to tell the difference between your muscles in their relaxed state and your muscles when they are tense; this simple exercise will help you think about how your muscles work.

You can start this exercise at your head and work downwards, as here, or reverse the order so that you start at your feet and work upwards if that feels better for you.

○ BEGIN BY CONCENTRATING ON BREATHING SLOWLY AND
    EVENLY, AS DEEPLY AS IS COMFORTABLE FOR YOU, UNTIL
    YOU FEEL YOUR BREATHING HAS SETTLED INTO A NICE,
    REGULAR, EASY RHYTHM.
○ CONCENTRATE ON YOUR FOREHEAD. FROWN SLIGHTLY
    UNTIL YOU FEEL IT WRINKLE, THEN LET IT GO, RELAXING
    IT. NOW FEEL YOUR FOREHEAD SMOOTHING OUT, BECOM-
    ING SOFTER, EASING DOWN TOWARDS YOUR TEMPLES.
○ THINK ABOUT YOUR FACE. LET YOUR LOWER JAW DROP
    SLIGHTLY, ALLOWING YOUR LIPS TO REST SLIGHTLY
    PARTED, NOT PRESSED AGAINST EACH OTHER. CHECK
    THAT YOUR TONGUE IS NOT CLAMPED ON THE ROOF OF
    YOUR MOUTH AND THAT YOUR TEETH ARE NOT
    CLENCHED. FEEL YOUR WHOLE FACE BECOMING SOFTER
    AND SMOOTHER.
○ NOW MOVE YOUR SHOULDERS AROUND A LITTLE. SHRUG
    THEM UP AND DOWN, MOVE THEM ROUND AND ROUND,
    RELEASING TENSION. MOVE YOUR HEAD UNTIL IT FEELS
    REALLY COMFORTABLY POSITIONED. MAKE YOUR NECK AS
    LONG AS YOU CAN, THEN LET IT SINK BACK GENTLY SO IT
    IS SUPPORTING YOUR HEAD WITHOUT STRAIN.
○ ARCH THE SMALL OF YOUR BACK TO STRETCH IT, THEN LET
    GO. PULL YOUR SHOULDER BLADES TOGETHER, STRETCH-
    ING AND TIGHTENING THE UPPER BACK, THEN LET GO,
    FEELING THE TENSION FLOWING FROM YOUR BODY.

○ TIGHTEN YOUR ABDOMINAL MUSCLES, NOTICING WHAT HAPPENS TO YOUR BREATHING AS YOU DO SO. NOW LET YOUR BREATH OUT AND RELAX YOUR ABDOMINAL MUSCLES AS YOU BREATHE OUT.

○ NOW TIGHTEN THE MUSCLES OF YOUR BUTTOCKS AND PELVIC FLOOR. AS YOU BREATHE OUT, LET THESE MUSCLES RELAX AND FEEL YOURSELF SINKING BACK DOWN INTO THE CUSHIONS.

○ TIGHTEN YOUR THIGH MUSCLES, THEN FEEL THE TENSION FLOW OUT AS YOU BREATHE OUT.

○ DO THE SAME WITH YOUR CALF MUSCLES.

○ PULL YOUR FEET UPWARDS, BENDING AT THE ANKLE SO THAT YOUR TOES ARE POINTING UPWARDS. ALLOW THIS TENSION TO FLOW OUT OF THEM AS YOU BREATHE OUT.

○ CURL YOUR TOES UP TIGHT, THEN RELAX THEM AS YOU BREATHE OUT.

○ CONCENTRATE ON LISTENING TO YOUR BREATHING, USING EVERY OUT-BREATH TO RELEASE TENSION. AS YOU BREATHE OUT, FEEL THE TENSION FLOWING AWAY FROM EACH PART OF YOUR BODY, ALLOWING YOU TO SINK FURTHER AND DEEPER INTO YOUR RELAXED STATE.

RELAXING YOUR MIND You may find that, once your body is relaxed, your brain goes into overdrive, thinking of all the things you ought to be doing. It can be helpful to try and still your mind by focusing on a place you find enjoyable — your own bedroom, a garden, somewhere in the country or by the sea, a warm bath. Try to recreate your special place in every detail, as if painting a mental picture of it. This technique of visualization also takes time to acquire, so keep practising it. You may also find it helpful to imagine yourself placing all your worries, concerns, and irritations into a box or basket, with the lid firmly shut. This container can then be put away somewhere safe to be brought out, opened up, and the problems dealt with only when the relaxation is over!

Once you are feeling well relaxed, sit or lie back and enjoy the feelings of calm and peace that you have created within yourself, and stay like this for a while, in complete quiet. Just enjoy the way your body feels when it is relaxed, and get to know it so that you will know immediately any part of you becomes tense again.

When you are ready to get up, slowly wriggle your fingers and toes, stretch or yawn if you need to, then, when you are fully ready, slowly get up.

You should never try to get up quickly from a relaxed position — your blood pressure will have been lowered and you will risk feeling very dizzy or faint. For this reason, some people prefer to unplug their phones while they are relaxing.

Many women find that it is through careful relaxation of their bodies like this that they become more fully aware of their body's responses and how they can affect these responses. Relaxation comes more easily to some than to others, but it is a skill which needs to be worked at and to be practised regularly until you feel thoroughly in tune with your body in all its moods.

If you find it difficult to attempt to relax whilst reading the instructions, you could either tape yourself reading them through beforehand, or ask your partner or a friend to read them or tape them for you.

There are relaxation tapes available to buy, though you may need to search before finding one that suits you.

DIET

What your body needs

Contrary to what some people you meet might say, there is no need to eat for two when you are pregnant — bodies metabolize very effectively in pregnancy. It is better to make sure you are eating a moderate, well-balanced diet to ensure optimum growth for both of you. Simply following your appetite is fine, provided your appetite does not lead you to believe that several chocolate bars a day are the best form of nutrition for the two of you. You may feel concerned that your diet is not supplying all the essential nutrients during pregnancy. Choosing a wide variety of foods from the five groups listed below will ensure that you are providing a good nutritional balance for yourself and your growing baby.

Vegetarians and vegans should also be able to choose a healthy diet from the main food groups. Vegans may, however, need a Vitamin B12 supplement, as this is mainly found in animal foods. You can ask a dietician for advice if you are at all worried that your diet may not be adequate in any way.

MILK AND MILK PRODUCTS

The main food groups

Fresh milk, yoghurt, and cheese

One pint of milk a day provides both calcium and protein. Skimmed and semi-skimmed milk contain just as much calcium and protein but less fat. If you dislike the idea of drinking this much, or any, milk, you can get calcium from other dairy sources. A third of a pint of milk is equivalent to one small carton of yoghurt or 1 oz. of hard cheese such as Cheddar or Edam.

If you are a vegan, or you cannot eat dairy products at all, it may be a good idea to ask to see a dietician to check that your diet contains enough calcium. There are plenty of other, non-dairy sources of this mineral (sesame seeds or sardines, for example).

MEAT AND ALTERNATIVES

Lean meat (e.g. lamb, beef, or pork)
Poultry (e.g. chicken or turkey)
White fish (e.g. cod, haddock), or oily fish (e.g. mackerel,
    herring, tuna, trout, salmon)
Eggs
Beans, peas, lentils, nuts

Choosing two or three foods from this group each day will provide you with protein and iron.

FRUIT AND VEGETABLES

Fresh fruit
Potatoes, green, leafy, and root vegetables, including all ,
    salad vegetables

Making sure you have at least five portions of fruit or vegetables each day will help to ensure you have a good intake of vitamins, minerals, and fibre in your diet. To make sure you have sufficient vitamin C, it is a good idea to choose one citrus fruit every day, or drink a glass of citrus fruit juice instead.

BREAD AND CEREALS

Bread, breakfast cereals, rice, pasta, crispbreads, biscuits

One or more of these foods at every meal (about 4–6 portions per day) will provide you with all the necessary carbohydrates.

FATS AND OILS

Butter, margarine, vegetable oils, animal fats

Only a small amount of fat is needed daily. There is no need to have any more fat than is already present in the rest of your daily diet, as fats are naturally found in many other foods, such as meat or dairy products. Many snack foods, such as crisps, chocolates, pastries, cakes, and biscuits, have a very high fat content, which you may prefer to avoid. Generally speaking, cutting down on fats as much as possible, and using low-fat alternatives, as well as choosing fats or oils which are rich in polyunsaturates, are useful guidelines for good health.

Food for thought

○ IF YOU ARE WELL NOURISHED, YOU ARE LESS LIKELY TO HAVE A PREMATURE BIRTH OR LOW-BIRTH-WEIGHT BABY, BECAUSE YOU ARE LESS VULNERABLE TO THE EFFECTS OF INFECTION AND ENVIRONMENTAL POLLUTION. THE WELL-NOURISHED BABY WILL WITHSTAND LABOUR BETTER, ENTER THE WORLD STRONGER, AND BE LESS PRONE TO SUFFER FROM INFECTIOUS ILLNESSES AND ALLERGIES.

○ PREGNANCY IS NOT A GOOD TIME TO DIET.

○ IF YOU DO, OR DID, SMOKE OR DRINK ALCOHOL, YOU MAY BE DEFICIENT IN VITAMINS B AND C AND MAY NEED TO MAKE SURE YOU HAVE PLENTY IN YOUR DIET NOW.

○ IF YOU FIND YOU ARE HUNGRY BETWEEN MEALS, OR IF YOU CANNOT MANAGE THREE LARGER MEALS A DAY AS YOUR UTERUS GROWS, ALTERING YOUR DIET TO HAVING SEVERAL (SIX OR MORE) SMALLER, SNACKIER MEALS A DAY MIGHT SUIT YOU BETTER. AS LONG AS THE SNACKS ARE STILL NUTRITIONALLY BALANCED, YOU WILL NOT BE DOING YOURSELF ANY HARM AND MAY FEEL A LOT MORE COMFORTABLE.

○ USING WHOLE FOODS (I.E. NON-REFINED — BROWN RICE RATHER THAN WHITE; WHOLEMEAL BREAD RATHER THAN WHITE) IN YOUR COOKING WILL NOT ONLY FILL YOU UP BETTER, BUT WILL ALSO BE BETTER FOR YOU GENERALLY. WHOLE FOODS CONTAIN MORE FIBRE, VITAMINS, AND MINERALS.

○ THE FRESHER FOOD IS EATEN THE BETTER — RAW WHENEVER POSSIBLE, WHERE FRUIT AND VEGETABLES ARE CONCERNED. IF YOU DO COOK VEGETABLES, YOU CAN CONSERVE THE VITAMIN AND MINERAL VALUE BY USING AS LITTLE WATER AS POSSIBLE AND COOKING FOR THE SHORTEST TIME POSSIBLE, SO THEY REMAIN SLIGHTLY CRISP RATHER THAN SOFT AND SOGGY. WHEN YOU CAN AVOID COOKING, DO SO; EAT PLENTY OF SALADS AND BE ADVENTUROUS IN YOUR CHOICE OF SALAD VEGETABLES, INVENTING ALL SORTS OF NEW AND EXCITING COMBINATIONS WITH DIFFERENT DRESSINGS.

○ DRINKING PLENTY OF FLUIDS (WATER, FRUIT JUICES) IS IMPORTANT TO AVOID BECOMING DEHYDRATED.

○ MANY PROCESSED FOODS CONTAIN HIGH QUANTITIES OF 'HIDDEN' FATS. CUTTING DOWN ON, OR AVOIDING THESE MAY REDUCE YOUR FAT INTAKE CONSIDERABLY. READING FOOD LABELS WILL HELP YOU DISCOVER WHICH FOODS YOU MIGHT BE BETTER OFF WITHOUT.

If you have not thought very much about the food you eat up to now, this can be an opportunity to move towards a healthier eating style, ready for your baby to enjoy also.

You will also find information on specific foods that are best avoided or treated with caution during pregnancy in Chapter 1, Beginning a Pregnancy.

TIME FOR YOURSELF

Finding time for yourself is essential if you are to enjoy life to the full. It is difficult to keep giving yourself to your work, your children, your partner, your home, or your other relatives without spending some time recharging your batteries. Perhaps you could reassess how much you are doing and how much is truly essential. How much can you bear to put off for a bit longer?

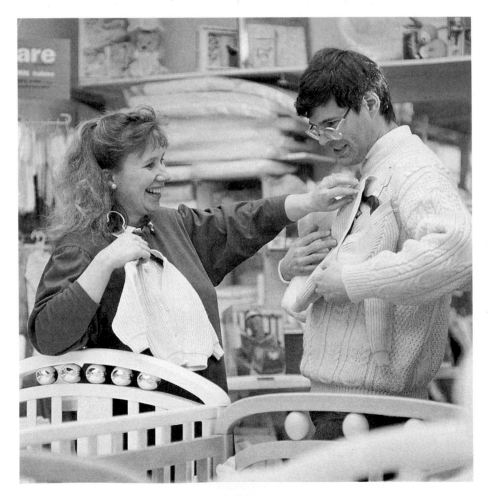

Enlist the help of your partner (and your children if they are old enough). Explaining that the more they help with the mundane chores, the more time and energy you will have for the interesting things, the more receptive they are likely to be.

You may find that you feel guilty when, having coped all day at work or with the children, you are finally too tired for your partner once you are together for the evening. If you find this happening, try reorganizing your day or your week so that you have something left both for yourself and your relationship. Above all, discuss how you are feeling. There may be ways he could help: by coming home a little earlier; by caring for the children or doing the shopping while you go and have your hair cut. He may not realize how tired you are feeling, especially if you usually manage to put a good face on things.

Tiredness is also sometimes a matter of routine or habit. Though you may not feel like it beforehand, it is amazing how often some exercise or an evening out can buck you up when you actually embark on it.

Most of all, you need not feel guilty about taking time for recharging your batteries, for doing the things you enjoy that make you feel better. If you are feeling good in yourself and you are looking after yourself well, you are likely to get very much more out of every facet of your life, and you will enjoy your pregnancy that much more as well.

I got thoroughly fed up with being made a fuss of and being told I must look after myself. Of course I was looking after myself. It made me feel like a little girl, the way they all treated me as though I wasn't responsible now I was pregnant.

I had a somewhat ambivalent attitude towards my food. On the one hand I was eating very well, lots of fresh fruit, salads, whole grains and so on. On the other hand, I was also enjoying a doughnut or bar of chocolate every day. I thought, it's only while I'm pregnant that I can justify eating these "naughty" things, so I'm going to enjoy them.

I've never been very good at relaxing and sitting quietly, and it took a lot of effort before I could force myself to take things easy, but I did and felt a lot better for it.

7   PREGNANCY DISCOMFORTS

Taking care of yourself will not actually eliminate or alleviate all of the common discomforts of pregnancy, but you may be able to do something towards helping yourself cope with them, or, in some cases, improve the way you feel.

To hear some people talking, you could imagine that pregnancy is entirely composed of problems and ailments almost too awful to mention. If you are actually feeling well, there is a suggestion that you will feel the effects sooner or later. Conversely, if you are failing to bloom during your pregnancy, there may be little sympathy around. You may, however, find yourself suffering aches and pains you have never experienced before and which may mar your enjoyment of the pregnancy. Such problems are often described as 'minor', which technically they may be, yet they may seem very far from minor to you. All is not doom and gloom, however. The majority of these problems can indeed be relieved in some way, if not entirely avoided, and, as a general rule, the symptoms have a limited life-expectancy, disappearing once your baby is born.

It is wisest not to take any drug or medication for a problem unless it has been prescribed for you by a doctor who knows you are pregnant.

COMMON PROBLEMS

SICKNESS The cause of pregnancy sickness is probably hormonal; it mostly seems to settle down once the placenta has taken over hormone production at around 12–14 weeks.

Symptoms may begin even before the first missed period, and are often at their worst around the ninth and tenth weeks. Some women are unfortunate enough to suffer from sickness throughout the pregnancy.

The common term — morning sickness — is not a terribly apt name for something which can as easily occur at any time of day or evening as in the morning. It can vary from mild nausea to frequent vomiting.

You may feel concerned that the endless 'little-and-often' nibbling to attempt to counteract nausea or sickness is leading to a faster weight-gain than you were hoping for. Most women find that this evens out, and weight-gain slows right down, once the problem with sickness subsides.

If you are very sick, you may be worried about losing weight, or failing to gain any. Your body reserves should normally be able to cope with weight loss of up to half a stone (2.5 kg.), but if you are particularly worried, do consult your midwife or doctor.

There are many suggestions for alleviation of sickness and nausea, but these are the most common remedies:

○ IF YOUR PROBLEM OCCURS IN THE MORNING, TRY TO START YOUR DAY WITH A DRINK AND A PLAIN BISCUIT *BEFORE* YOU EVEN CONSIDER GETTING OUT OF BED. IF A MORNING CUP OF TEA IS WHAT YOU FANCY, YOU WILL NEED TO ENLIST YOUR PARTNER'S HELP.

○ EAT FREQUENT SMALL SNACKS CONTAINING CARBOHYD-RATES DURING THE DAY, SO THAT YOUR BLOOD-SUGAR LEVEL DOES NOT FALL TOO LOW — MANY WOMEN FEEL WORSE WHEN THEY HAVE NOT EATEN FOR A WHILE. FRUIT, ESPECIALLY BANANAS, TOAST, CRACKERS, OR SEMI-SWEET BISCUITS CAN ALL HELP. IF YOU SUSPECT LOW BLOOD SUGAR COULD BE THE REASON FOR YOUR MORNING SICKNESS, TRY EATING SOMETHING BEFORE GOING TO BED AT NIGHT AS WELL.

○ HAVE PLENTY TO DRINK BETWEEN MEALS; FIZZY DRINKS OF ALL SORTS SEEM TO HELP — TRY LOW-CALORIE CANNED DRINKS, OR COMBINE FRUIT JUICES WITH CARBONATED WATER.

○ TRY TO AVOID HAVING TO PREPARE CERTAIN FOODS FOR OTHER PEOPLE, ESPECIALLY FOODS WITH STRONG SMELLS.

○ GINGER CAN BE A VERY EFFECTIVE REMEDY IN COMBATING SICKNESS. AS WELL AS IN ITS NATURAL FORM OR IN COMBINATION WITH OTHER FOODS, YOU CAN BUY GINGER CAPSULES FROM HEALTH FOOD SHOPS. CRYSTALLIZED GINGER, POWDERED ROOT GINGER, GINGER BISCUITS, AND GINGER ALE HAVE ALL BEEN USED EFFECTIVELY AS SICKNESS REMEDIES FOR MANY WOMEN.

○ THERE IS ALSO A RANGE OF HOMOEOPATHIC REMEDIES SUITING DIFFERENT TYPES AND TIMES OF SICKNESS.

○ TRY TO AVOID DRINKING LIQUIDS WITH YOUR MEALS — KEEP 'WET' AND 'DRY' SEPARATE.

○ TRY TO AVOID BECOMING OVERTIRED.

HEARTBURN Heartburn can occur when the muscle between the oesophagus (food pipe) and stomach relaxes due to high levels of progesterone and other hormones. It can also be the result of the enlarged uterus pressing on to the stomach in late pregnancy. In either case, acid from the stomach rises into the oesophagus and produces a burning sensation.

It may help this distressing problem if you try the following suggestions:

○ **EAT LITTLE AND OFTEN.**
○ **AVOID HIGHLY SPICED, ACIDIC, OR FATTY FOODS.**
○ **RAISE THE UPPER PART OF YOUR BED IF THE PROBLEM IS WORSE AT NIGHT.**
○ **DRINK PEPPERMINT, FENNEL, OR CHAMOMILE HERB TEAS AFTER MEALS AND INSTEAD OF YOUR USUAL HOT DRINKS.**
○ **AVOID ANTACIDS GENERALLY, AS THE STOMACH WILL EVENTUALLY PRODUCE EVEN MORE ACID TO COUNTERBALANCE THE ANTACID YOU ARE TAKING, THOUGH THESE MAY WORK ON A VERY SHORT-TERM BASIS.**
○ **MILK OR YOGHURT MAY RELIEVE SYMPTOMS.**

CRAMP No one really knows the reason for cramp, though all sorts of possibilities have been suggested. Cramp in the legs seems to happen more frequently when you point your toes, usually in bed at night, and often during sleep.

Rather than treat the problem once it has occurred, you can avoid it by trying the following exercises:

An exercise which stretches the calf to avoid cramp

○ **STRETCH WITH YOUR TOES PULLING TOWARDS YOUR HEAD.**
○ **EXERCISE YOUR CALF MUSCLES DURING THE EVENING BY DOING YOUR FOOT EXERCISES OR BY ROLLING YOUR FOOT OVER A TENNIS BALL OR MILK BOTTLE SEVERAL TIMES.**
○ **STRETCH YOUR CALF MUSCLES BY LEANING YOUR HEAD AND ARMS AGAINST A WALL WITH ONE LEG FORWARDS, THE OTHER STRETCHED STRAIGHT BEHIND YOU. YOUR STRETCHED LEG SHOULD HAVE THE TOE ON THE FLOOR, THE HEEL PULLING AWAY SO YOU CAN FEEL THE STRETCH. GENTLY BOUNCE YOUR BACK LEG SO YOU CAN FEEL THE CALF MUSCLE PULLING AND STRETCHING SLIGHTLY. REPEAT FOR YOUR OTHER LEG.**

If you do get cramp:

○ **SIT WITH YOUR LEGS STRAIGHT AND PULL YOUR TOES TOWARDS YOUR FACE, WITH YOUR HEELS ON THE GROUND OR THE BED.**

> ○ NOW BEND YOUR KNEE AND STROKE YOUR CALF MUSCLES FIRMLY
>   UPWARDS; RUBBING THEM CAN DAMAGE THE TISSUES.
> ○ CIRCLE YOUR FOOT TEN TIMES IN EACH DIRECTION — THIS WILL
>   HELP PREVENT YOUR LEG FEELING SORE IN THE MORNING.

ABDOMINAL OR ROUND LIGAMENT PAIN Pain in the groin, below your abdomen, is due to stretching, or possibly straining, of the round ligaments which help to support the uterus. You may notice it if you turn over awkwardly in bed (though by the end of pregnancy it is hard to be anything but awkward when turning over!), or if you stand up suddenly. You may also find it hard to walk for very long if your lower abdomen aches or pulls constantly.

The following precautions should help you avoid round ligament pain:

> ○ TAKE CARE NOT TO MAKE SUDDEN JERKY MOVEMENTS
>   WHICH MAY STRAIN THE LIGAMENT.
> ○ PROTECT THE LIGAMENTS BY DRAWING YOUR KNEES UP
>   BEFORE TURNING OVER IN BED.
> ○ BEND FORWARD FROM THE HIP BEFORE COUGHING,
>   SNEEZING, OR LAUGHING.
> ○ TAKE ESPECIAL CARE WHEN WALKING DOWNSTAIRS OR
>   DOWNHILL, PARTICULARLY IF YOU ARE CARRYING A HEAVY
>   LOAD OF SHOPPING, WASHING, OR A TODDLER.
> ○ WEAR A MATERNITY PANTY-GIRDLE WHEN YOU ARE BUSY. IF
>   THAT DOES NOT HELP, ASK THE HOSPITAL TO PRESCRIBE A
>   SPECIAL LIGHT-WEIGHT ELASTIC SUPPORT-BELT
>   (FEMBRACE).

BACKACHE Few women manage to get through a whole pregnancy without some sort of backache. Most problems are fortunately easily avoided or remedied.

There are suggestions for improving or maintaining good posture in Chapter 6, Looking After Yourself. If you do suffer from an aching back, you could try the following suggestions:

> ○ GENTLE PELVIC-TILTING EXERCISES ARE HELPFUL. IF YOU
>   HAVE PRACTISED THEM STANDING AS WELL AS SITTING OR
>   KNEELING, YOU WILL BE ABLE TO DO THEM SURREPTI-
>   TIOUSLY ON OCCASIONS WHEN YOU HAVE TO STAND FOR
>   A LONG TIME.
> ○ IF THE PAIN COMES IN THE HIP JOINT RATHER THAN IN THE
>   LOWER BACK, LIE ON THE FLOOR OR BED, WITH YOUR
>   HANDS ON YOUR SHOULDERS, ONE LEG STRAIGHT, THE

OTHER BENT AT THE KNEE. TUCK THE BENT LEG UNDER
THE THIGH OF THE STRAIGHTENED LEG, THEN TWIST
YOUR BODY ROUND TOWARDS THE SIDE WITH THE BENT
LEG, KEEPING YOUR SHOULDERS ON THE FLOOR.

O   CONSIDER BUYING A MATERNITY GIRDLE IF YOUR BACK-
    ACHE IS VERY SEVERE. (DO MAKE SURE IT FITS PROPERLY
    BEFORE YOU BUY IT!)

O   SUPPORT YOUR BACK WITH A SMALL CUSHION OR ROLLED
    UP TOWEL IN THE SMALL OF YOUR BACK IF YOU HAVE TO
    SIT FOR ANY LENGTH OF TIME — THIS IS ESPECIALLY
    USEFUL ON CAR JOURNEYS. CHECK THAT THIS DOES NOT
    MAKE YOUR ANKLES SWELL; IF IT DOES, TRY SITTING ON
    YOUR CUSHION INSTEAD, TO MAKE MORE ROOM BETWEEN
    YOUR THIGHS AND YOUR ABDOMEN.

O   PUT A BOARD UNDER YOUR MATTRESS, IF YOU SUSPECT
    YOUR MATTRESS MAY BE TOO SOFT AND SAGGY.

Soothing an aching back by practising pelvic-tilt exercises

CONSTIPATION Constipation in pregnancy is caused by the hormone relaxin, which slows down the digestive and excretory systems as well as loosening joints. Constipation is best avoided whenever possible, as it is not only uncomfortable but it can also exacerbate or cause problems with piles, and any straining puts undue pressure on the pelvic floor.

You could try the following remedies to prevent constipation:

O   MAKE SURE YOU DRINK PLENTY OF WATER. .

O   EAT SMALLER, MORE FREQUENT MEALS.

O   EAT PLENTY OF ROUGHAGE: EAT RAW FRUITS AND VEGETA-
    BLES, AND USE FIBRE-RICH INGREDIENTS IN YOUR DIET,
    ESPECIALLY WHOLEGRAINS.

O   CHANGE TO HERBAL TEAS OR OTHER DRINKS IF YOU DRINK
    A LOT OF TEA, AS TEA CAN BE A CAUSE OF CONSTIPATION.

If you have persistent constipation, try eating plenty of dried fruits or taking senna powder. If you are being prescribed iron tablets and suspect that these may be partly to blame, you could ask your doctor if he thinks they are really necessary for you, or if it would be worth changing to a different kind.

VARICOSE VEINS Varicose veins can occur in either the legs or the vulva. They are caused by pregnancy hormones together with the weight of the abdomen making the vein walls bulge and causing the blood flow from the legs to become sluggish.

You can reduce the discomfort in the following ways:

> ☒ DO NOT STAND IN ONE POSITION FOR ANY LENGTH OF TIME.
>
> ☒ DO NOT WEAR 'POP-SOCKS', STOCKINGS, OR OTHER TIGHT RESTRICTING CLOTHES.
>
> ☒ DO NOT SIT WITH YOUR LEGS CROSSED OR PRESSING ON TO THE EDGE OF YOUR CHAIR.
>
> ☑ ALWAYS SIT WITH YOUR FEET UP.
>
> ☑ DO YOUR FOOT EXERCISES REGULARLY AND VIGOROUSLY TO IMPROVE CIRCULATION.
>
> ☑ TAKE PLENTY OF EXERCISE EVERY DAY — WALKING IS PARTICU-LARLY USEFUL.
>
> ☑ WEAR SUPPORT TIGHTS — THESE ARE SUPPOSED TO BE PUT ON BEFORE YOU EVEN GET OUT OF BED IN THE MORNINGS.
>
> ☑ RAISE THE FOOT OF YOUR BED A LITTLE IF YOUR VARICOSE VEINS ARE IN YOUR VULVA. (YOU MAY NEED TO FIND A VERY FINE BALANCE, IF YOU HAVE ALREADY RAISED THE HEAD OF THE BED TO AVOID HEARTBURN OR DIZZINESS!)

HAEMORRHOIDS (PILES) The object of many jokes, but most unpleasant for the sufferer, piles are really varicose veins of the rectum. They can cause itching or soreness and may bleed. They are aggravated by constipation because of the extra strain put on the rectum.

Your doctor or midwife may be able to help by prescribing a cream, ointment, or suppositories to ease discomfort, or Vitamin E capsules or homoeopathic remedies to reduce the piles. To help yourself, you can try the following:

> ○ TAKE MEASURES TO AVOID CONSTIPATION.
>
> ○ RUB THE AFFECTED AREA WITH AN ICE-CUBE OR SPECIAL ICE-PACK AS A TEMPORARY MEASURE TO EASE THE ITCHING AND SORENESS.

SKIN-CHANGES Pregnancy hormones can cause your skin to change in many ways. It may be particularly healthy during pregnancy, but it may become unusually dry or greasy. You may find patches of red or brown colour appearing, or stretch marks may appear on thighs, buttocks, abdomen, or breasts. Occasionally, a brown line may form from the navel down to the pubic hair, or the skin, particularly on the abdomen or legs, may itch intolerably. Apart from the stretch marks, all of these will disappear once the baby has been born.

The following hints may help you care for your skin during your pregnancy:

○ IF YOU HAVE BROWN PATCHES, IT IS BETTER TO AVOID SUNBATHING.

○ RUBBING CREAM INTO STRETCH MARKS CANNOT PREVENT THEM OCCURRING, BUT MAY HELP KEEP YOUR SKIN MORE SUPPLE. IT WILL FEEL NICE BUT WILL NOT STOP THE MARKS APPEARING; EVENTUALLY THEY WILL FADE TO FINE SILVERY STREAKS, WHICH MAY NOT TAN QUITE AS WELL AS THE REST OF YOU! VITAMIN E OIL ENCOURAGES THE GROWTH OF NORMAL SKIN CELLS, AND MAY GET RID OF ANY SCARRING.

○ NOTHING CAN BE DONE ABOUT THE BROWN ABDOMINAL LINE — IT SHOWS THAT YOUR RECTUS MUSCLE IS PARTING TO CREATE MORE SPACE FOR YOUR BABY, AND IT WILL DISAPPEAR AFTER PREGNANCY.

○ YOU CAN SOMETIMES RELIEVE ITCHING BY RUBBING IN OIL OR MOISTURIZING CREAMS AND BY WEARING LOOSE CLOTHING THAT IS MADE OF NATURAL FIBRES. ADDING SOME GENTLE, AROMATIC OIL TO YOUR BATHWATER CAN BE VERY SOOTHING, OR TRY SPLASHING YOUR SKIN WITH COLD NETTLE LOTION (STEEP NETTLES IN BOILING WATER, THEN COOL).

INSOMNIA Sleep difficulties for pregnant women have a variety of causes, and are distressingly common. Any of the following may lead to disturbed or sleepless nights:

○ THE INABILITY TO FIND A COMFORTABLE POSITION

○ YOUR BABY CHOOSING ITS MOMENT FOR PRACTISING GYMNASTICS AGAINST YOUR ABDOMEN

○ VIVID DREAMS OR NIGHTMARES

○ WORRY

○ ENDLESS TRIPS TO THE LAVATORY

You might either find it difficult to get off to sleep in the first place or, having woken at 3.00 a.m., find it impossible to drift off again.

You could help yourself deal with insomnia in the following ways:

○ MAKE SURE YOU HAVE TAKEN SOME FORM OF EXERCISE DURING THE DAY.

○ HAVE A WARM DRINK BEFORE BED. SOME WOMEN FIND A MILKY DRINK HELPS, OTHERS FIND HERB TEAS, ESPECIALLY CHAMOMILE OR VERVAIN, ARE USEFUL.

> ○ LISTEN TO CALMING MUSIC — YOUR BABY MAY ENJOY THIS TOO. READ A DULL BOOK.
>
> ○ CONSCIOUSLY PRACTISE YOUR RELAXATION — YOU WILL BE RELAXED EVEN IF NOT ACTUALLY ASLEEP.
>
> ○ USE EXTRA PILLOWS TO SUPPORT YOURSELF (SEE THE ADVICE ON POSTURE, IN CHAPTER 6, LOOKING AFTER YOURSELF).
>
> ○ TALK OVER ANY WORRIES YOU MAY HAVE WITH YOUR PARTNER, FRIEND, MIDWIFE, DOCTOR, OR ANTENATAL TEACHER.

FEELING FAINT It is not at all unusual to feel faint during pregnancy, particularly in the earlier months. This may be due to lowered blood pressure, or low blood sugar, as many women find they feel faint just before a meal.

You should avoid the following:

> ☒ STANDING FOR PROLONGED PERIODS
> ☒ SMOKY ATMOSPHERES OR HOT, ENCLOSED PLACES
> ☒ LYING FLAT ON YOUR BACK
> ☒ WEARING TIGHT CLOTHES
> ☒ WAITING TOO LONG BETWEEN MEALS
> ☒ SITTING OR STANDING UP VERY SUDDENLY

If you do feel faint, you should try the following:

> ☑ SIT DOWN.
> ☑ GET FRESH AIR AS SOON AS POSSIBLE.
> ☑ BREATHE SLOWLY AND DEEPLY.
> ☑ LOOSEN ANY TIGHT CLOTHING.
> ☑ PUT YOUR HEAD DOWN AS LOW AS POSSIBLE, IF NECESSARY.

VAGINAL DISCHARGE Normal vaginal discharge is always increased during pregnancy, however minimally, and any white, slightly thickened fluid is not a cause for concern. If, however, the discharge is thicker, curdy, or yellowish, if it has an offensive smell, or if it is combined with itching or irritation, you could have a vaginal infection. If you suspect an infection, consult your doctor or midwife.

You can help yourself cope with any discharge in the following ways:

> ☑ WASH YOUR GENITAL AREA AT LEAST TWICE A DAY WITH PLENTY OF WARM WATER; IF YOU USE FLANNELS, REMEMBER TO KEEP THEM SCRUPULOUSLY CLEAN.
> ☑ DRY YOURSELF WELL.

☑ WEAR COTTON PANTS AND CHANGE THEM REGULARLY.
☑ WIPE YOURSELF FROM FRONT TO BACK WHEN GOING TO THE
    LAVATORY.
☑ DRY ALL TOWELS AND FLANNELS THOROUGHLY EACH TIME
    YOU USE THEM—BACTERIA MULTIPLY RAPIDLY IN MOIST
    CONDITIONS.
☒ AVOID SCENTED OILS OR POWDER IN YOUR BATH WATER.
☒ AVOID SO-CALLED 'FEMININE' TALCS OR SPRAYS.

If you do have a thrush infection — very common during pregnancy — natural live yoghurt, both applied directly to the vagina and also eaten, helps your body regain the bacteria normally found in the vagina. Natural yoghurt is not easy to insert into the vagina; try asking your chemist for a syringe and inserting it that way. Thrush infections like warm, damp conditions, so it is advisable to avoid wearing clothing which does not allow the skin to breathe freely, such as tights and leggings, or tight trousers. Check that any towels, sponges, or flannels you use can be dried completely between each use, or even try to manage without sponges or flannels at all. It may help to keep the infection under control if you use paper towels or tissues to dry yourself rather than towels. Cutting out all sugar in your diet will also help to get rid of the infection by starving the bacteria of its favourite food.

CARPAL-TUNNEL SYNDROME Carpal-tunnel syndrome is an acutely painful condition, causing numbness and pain in the hand and possibly the arm. It may be caused by fluid retention pressing on nerve endings round your wrist, but can also be caused by wearing a bra with narrow stretchy straps which dig into your shoulders, resulting in nerve pressure.

Putting a folded tissue or special pad under the strap on your shoulder to relieve pressure, and sleeping with a pillow hugged between your top arm and your ribs, should alleviate this condition. You may need to seek medical advice as well.

FATIGUE For many women, fatigue is the most difficult aspect of pregnancy to cope with, as it is often surprisingly overwhelming.

Considering any possibilities for rest and relaxation may help you find extra time to recover from activities which you find tiring. Let your body decide how much you can cope with, and do not let yourself in for any commitment you cannot get out of should you feel too tired at the last moment. Accept all offers of help to relieve some of the pressures on you.

As with any of the common pregnancy problems, it is important to listen to what your body is telling you and deal with it in a way that is appropriate for you.

* *I think the worst thing for me was feeling rotten, but not being able to take anything to help me feel better.* '

* *I spent a fortune buying bunches of seedless grapes, which I kept in the fridge to keep me going.* '

* *I was sick at a different Underground station every day for six weeks.* '

* *One night my back seized up entirely so when I had to get up to go to the lavatory, I ended up crawling there on hands and knees.* '

* *Paul's never quite got over all the times I woke up shrieking in the night, hopping round the bedroom, and shouting at him to come and massage my leg.* '

* *I'm on to four pillows propping me up at night to ease the heartburn. If it gets any worse, I might as well stay downstairs in the armchair all night.* '

* *They kept telling me I'd be blooming during the middle months. Well, I'm still waiting!* '

* *I was sick every night for the first 8 months of my first pregnancy. Then I gave up work, and the sickness stopped—just like that.* '

* *It was a tremendous relief to talk to the other women I met at my antenatal classes and find that I wasn't the only one to be having these horribly vivid dreams that were so strange.* '

8 SEX IN PREGNANCY

Having a baby is an exciting event, but it is also a major change which brings challenges and may cause stress. When relationships are changing because of life events, sex is likely to be affected in some way. Some couples do manage to go through pregnancy and the time after birth making very few sexual adjustments, but many women and their partners find that pregnancy brings to the surface a need and opportunity to reassess their sexual relationship, in the context of their wider relationship.

ALTERED ATTITUDES

Positive reactions

Many of the changes which a pregnancy brings have a very positive and beneficial effect on a couple's sex life. The new image which you have of yourselves and the different image which society has of you may open up new aspects of your sexual relationship. As a woman you may find you feel able to be more womanly and sexual with this new life inside you. You may both be feeling exhilarated at the prospect of becoming parents, and the baby growing inside may bring you closer together than ever before. Many men feel especially tender towards their partners during pregnancy, which may add yet another new dimension to your relationship. You may simply enjoy the bond of having created a new human being from your loving relationship.

Many women do also find that the hormones produced during pregnancy have the effect of stimulating their sexual appetite throughout pregnancy, which is usually regarded by the couple as an advantage, if potentially a little exhausting by the time the nine months are up! A woman's heightened awareness of her own body and her creative powers can also help her to enjoy every aspect of her body while she is pregnant.

Many couples find the freedom from the need to think or do anything about contraception is a delightful bonus to be made the most of. If you have been trying to become pregnant for some while, you may also discover that the sense of freedom from trying as well as the excitement of achievement give your love-making a welcome boost now that you are pregnant.

Partly because pregnancy brings physical changes for a woman, and emotional adjustments for both partners, this may also be an opportunity for you to explore different ways of making love. There may well be times when either one or both of you does not feel like having full sexual intercourse with penetration. There may be times when you feel it would be more judicious to avoid intercourse for a while. If you decide this, it need not mean your sexual relationship has to shut down completely for the time being. It is a chance to enjoy making love in other ways.

○ **BY CUDDLING**
○ **BY STROKING**
○ **THROUGH ORAL SEX**
○ **THROUGH MASTURBATION**
○ **BY FINDING ALL SORTS OF DIFFERENT MEANS OF GIVING AND RECEIVING PLEASURE WITH EACH OTHER'S BODIES.**

These months of pregnancy can be some of the most exciting in a relationship because of the new stimulation the life changes have to offer.

Not-so-welcome reactions

Whilst many couples find much that is positively refreshing in their sex lives during a pregnancy, they may also, at times, find other aspects less stimulating. Because emotions and physical experiences change so often during pregnancy, nothing is ever cut and dried. Few couples experience only positive or only negative feelings — for the majority, feelings alter and vary throughout the pregnancy: whereas some couples' relationships are enhanced by being pregnant, others may feel a loss of purpose once pregnancy has occurred. You may feel that pregnancy means the beginning of having to put behind you some of the freedom and spontaneity you have enjoyed up until now. Either or both of you may feel angry and resentful that this pregnancy is forcing you into a maturity and responsibility you are not sure you are ready for, particularly if there are financial or other domestic worries overshadowing your whole relationship. You may be finding your pregnancy tiring, and then feel guilty that the effects of your tiredness are being taken out on your partner.

Your partner may understand and accept all this and support you, or he may feel resentful at being taken for granted.

As a woman, you too, of course, may feel you are taken for granted and expected to cope, with no allowance being made for your pregnancy and the adjustments you are having to make. You may feel equally irritated at being treated as though you were fragile or ill, when you are basically feeling well.

A man may find it difficult to adjust to his partner's new image as a mother rather than a lover, especially if he has never thought of 'mothers' as sexually desirable. These feelings may put some men off sex, and need to be talked through, rather than left to simmer away, causing a build up of resentment and anxiety.

PHYSICAL FACTORS

Physical factors also play a large part in determining how one feels about sex during pregnancy. During the early weeks and months you may be feeling too utterly exhausted or too sick even to contemplate making love. Then, later in pregnancy, you may feel heavy, tired, and uncomfortable, so that love-making begins to seem like a chore to be got through rather than a pleasurable activity. You may have tender breasts for many months, or find any pressure on your abdomen quite unbearable at times. Whilst you may find that your increased awareness of your physical self positively reinforces your sexuality, you may nevertheless find it hard to feel sexy if you are conscious only of feeling lumpy and ungainly. You may, in common with many women and men, like the softness, the rounded contours of pregnancy, but on the other hand you may fail to be turned on by the woman's changing shape.

There is quite a tricky balance to be manoeuvred during pregnancy, and it is only by both of you talking about all your feelings at different stages that you will manage to understand how the other is feeling and how you can adjust to improve your relationship. Sex is not something that can be taken separately from all the other aspects of your lives together; it is an integral part of your relationship as a whole.

MAKING ADJUSTMENTS

CARING FOR YOURSELF If you find you are feeling low, and you have the resources, it can help to treat yourself to something which will boost your own self-esteem: something new to wear; something luxurious for the bath; even a visit to the hairdresser can all help at low moments. Maybe just a quiet day spent doing things entirely for yourself can give tremendous encouragement if you are fed up with yourself and your pregnancy. If you are going through a period when you have a low opinion of your own worth and desirability, it may be difficult to respond positively in your love-making, so anything which helps to boost your own self-image will do you good all round.

FINDING TIME As pregnancy progresses, your usual positions, and possibly occasions, for love-making may no longer feel comfortable, and you may have to start rethinking your whole approach. This is where your joint creative ingenuity comes in! If you are feeling tired by the end of the day, sleep or a quiet read may seem infinitely preferable to any activity involving physical and emotional effort. Is there any other time of the day or night when you feel more alert and responsive, when you could make love? If you have children already, opportunities may be rather more seriously limited, especially if they are early risers.

Many women find it hard to sleep if they wake during the night in pregnancy — perhaps you could use this time for love-making? Your partner might not actually mind too much being woken for a pleasurable purpose.

Finding a comfortable position It is better to choose a position which leaves the woman's abdomen and breasts free of pressure — it is hard to enjoy sex either if you are aware that a part of you is uncomfortably squashed, or if you are worried you might be doing the squashing. It is also a good idea to leave the woman's pelvis free to move. Some women experience strong Braxton Hicks contractions during love-making as the oxytocin released during arousal causes the uterus to contract. If you do have a frequently contracting uterus during intercourse, you will prefer it to be very gentle. It may help you to practise relaxation techniques (see Chapter 6, Looking After Yourself), to help ease any discomfort.

Suitable positions

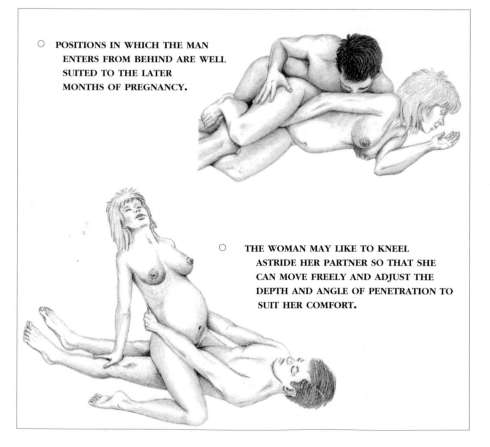

○ POSITIONS IN WHICH THE MAN ENTERS FROM BEHIND ARE WELL SUITED TO THE LATER MONTHS OF PREGNANCY.

○ THE WOMAN MAY LIKE TO KNEEL ASTRIDE HER PARTNER SO THAT SHE CAN MOVE FREELY AND ADJUST THE DEPTH AND ANGLE OF PENETRATION TO SUIT HER COMFORT.

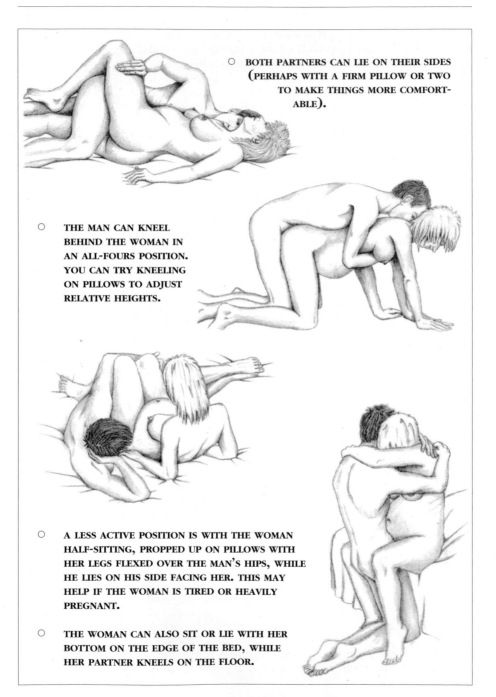

○ BOTH PARTNERS CAN LIE ON THEIR SIDES (PERHAPS WITH A FIRM PILLOW OR TWO TO MAKE THINGS MORE COMFORTABLE).

○ THE MAN CAN KNEEL BEHIND THE WOMAN IN AN ALL-FOURS POSITION. YOU CAN TRY KNEELING ON PILLOWS TO ADJUST RELATIVE HEIGHTS.

○ A LESS ACTIVE POSITION IS WITH THE WOMAN HALF-SITTING, PROPPED UP ON PILLOWS WITH HER LEGS FLEXED OVER THE MAN'S HIPS, WHILE HE LIES ON HIS SIDE FACING HER. THIS MAY HELP IF THE WOMAN IS TIRED OR HEAVILY PREGNANT.

○ THE WOMAN CAN ALSO SIT OR LIE WITH HER BOTTOM ON THE EDGE OF THE BED, WHILE HER PARTNER KNEELS ON THE FLOOR.

COMMON WORRIES

Many men and women have some anxieties about sex during pregnancy. Making sure you have accurate information, sensitively offered, and talking over any worries with your partner will help to reduce your anxiety levels and allow you to relax.

WILL IT HARM THE BABY? Many women and men fear that sex may somehow harm either the baby or the woman. In fact, the baby is very well protected by the muscular walls of the uterus, by the cushioning effect of the amniotic sac, and by the mucus plug which seals the cervix, so that no harm can occur during gentle, loving sex.

WILL IT TRIGGER LABOUR? As previously mentioned, many women experience contractions during arousal, and also during orgasm. These contractions will not be powerful enough to start a labour unless it is imminent. A woman who has had previous miscarriages might prefer to avoid sex during the first few months, however, especially around the times when her period would have been due. A woman with a history of premature labour may decide with her partner to avoid sex in the later stages of her pregnancy, until her baby would no longer be pre-term.

THE BABY IS THERE! Some men and women find the thought of the baby's presence disturbing, so that they are always conscious of another person being there and feel somewhat inhibited as a result. Others are aware of this but are unconcerned by it, even relishing the baby's presence.

If you do have any worries or fears, talk to each other and share your feelings. You may not be able to take away the source of your concern, but sharing it will make it seem less threatening.

Pregnancy can provide a real opportunity to explore various aspects of your sexual relationship, to find what is satisfying and pleasurable for both of you. It offers a chance to discover other ways of making love than simply having full, penetrative intercourse. Talking together, looking at different approaches, explaining clearly what you do and do not enjoy, and allowing each other time to adjust are all important ways of helping you enjoy your relationship to the full.

If you feel worried about the changes in your sex life since becoming pregnant, there are positive ways of dealing with any potential problems:

- ○ **TALK IT OVER WITH YOUR PARTNER.**
- ○ **FIND PLENTY OF TIME FOR CUDDLES, NOT NECESSARILY LEADING TO INTERCOURSE.**
- ○ **SPEND TIME DOING SOMETHING YOU REALLY ENJOY.**
- ○ **EXPLORE ALTERNATIVE WAYS OF ENJOYING LOVE-MAKING**

> WITHOUT NECESSARILY HAVING FULL INTERCOURSE.
> ○ FIND A DIFFERENT TIME DURING THE DAY FOR MAKING
>   LOVE.
> ○ DISCOVER SOME VARIATIONS IN POSITION FOR INTERCOURSE
>   WHICH MIGHT HELP YOU FEEL MORE COMFORTABLE.
> ○ DO NOT LOSE HEART — ACCEPT CHANGES AS A NORMAL
>   PART OF ADJUSTMENT TO YOUR PREGNANCY.

' *We collapse in giggles at the contortions we have to get into to make it possible.* '

' *My midwife suggested we try to induce the labour by making love frequently. We tried and had a very tiring weekend, but the baby stayed put.* '

' *George was extremely relieved when I went into premature labour. I'd been so turned on during the pregnancy, he was exhausted.* '

' *I went right off sex almost the minute I became pregnant, and that's the way I stayed until the baby was three or four months old.* '

TWINS AND SUPERTWINS 9

Having already gone through the process of finding out that you are pregnant, with the mixture of feelings that this discovery brings, you discover that you are expecting, not one, but two, or maybe three or more babies. Not many parents are prepared for this news. Some may be aware that twins run in the family, and some may have been on a course of fertility drugs which raise the likelihood of it occurring, but for most parents it comes as a bolt from the blue.

A multiple pregnancy will most often be detected at a first scan, but it is possible for ultrasound to miss one of a set of twins if one baby is lying behind the other, and for there to be some confusion over the number if there are more than two babies. You may, of course, have been sent for a scan specifically because your doctor or midwife has suspected there is more than one baby, in which case the news will not have come as quite so much of a surprise.

Many mothers say that it was a good job they were lying down when they heard the news, because it came as such a shock. The next reaction is often laughter and delight, after which the excitement calms down, and they are seized with panic, and questions such as, 'How ever will I cope?' as the reality sinks in. Luckily you usually have a few months to adjust to the idea and make arrangements for a very different life-style. This may even go as far as planning to build an extension or getting a larger car to accommodate your dramatically growing family, but perhaps the most important thing to try and arrange is the extra help you will almost certainly need in the early days after the birth. Once you have started adjusting to the idea of having more than one baby, it is sensible to try to rest as much as possible and enjoy the remainder of your pregnancy, before the hard work begins.

HOW TWINS AND SUPERTWINS ARE CONCEIVED

FRATERNAL TWINS Fraternal, or non-identical twins are formed when two sperm fertilize two eggs released simultaneously (or three eggs or more for larger fraternal multiple births), so the babies conceived this way have different genetic compositions and are no more alike

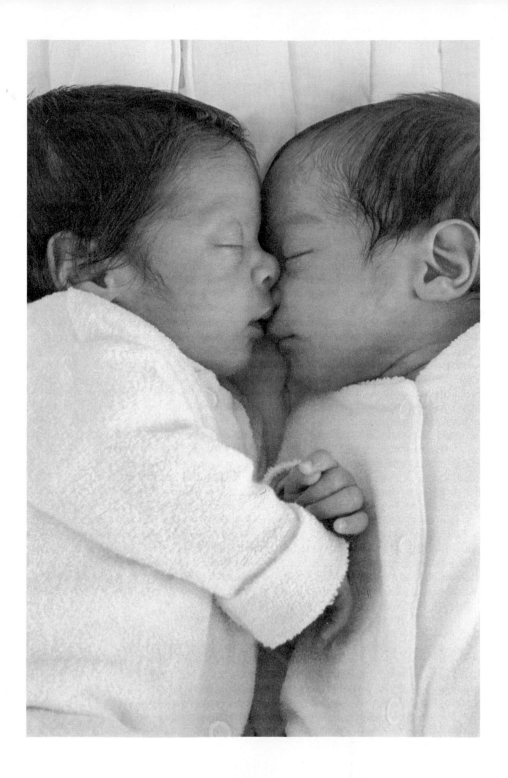

than any other siblings. Obviously if a boy and girl arrive at birth, they are fraternal rather than identical, but it is not always so easy to tell. In the uterus, fraternal twins have separate placentae, but sometimes these lie so close together that they fuse and look like one, so the appearance of the placenta at the birth is not necessarily a sure sign. Sometimes, too, the babies look very similar indeed, and only a complex blood test would determine whether they developed from one fertilized egg (identical) or from two (fraternal).

There are several factors which can influence the chances of conceiving fraternal twins:

○ **THE INCIDENCE VARIES FROM RACE TO RACE. A PARTICULAR TRIBE IN AFRICA, THE YORUBA, HAS THE HIGHEST TWINNING RATE IN THE WORLD AT 42.3 TWIN BIRTHS PER 1,000 AND THE RATE OVER ALL AFRICAN BIRTHS IS 25 PER 1,000. IN WESTERN EUROPE IT IS 11 OR 12 PER 1,000, WHILE IN JAPAN IT IS VERY LOW AT ONLY 3 PER 1,000.**

○ **A MOTHER'S PROPENSITY TO PRODUCE TWO EGGS AT EACH OVULATION INCREASES OVER THE CHILD-BEARING YEARS UP TO THE AGE OF 35, THEN GRADUALLY DECREASES.**

○ **TWINS RUN IN FAMILIES AND THE TENDENCY TO RELEASE MORE THAN ONE EGG AT A TIME IS PASSED ON GENETI-CALLY FROM MOTHER TO DAUGHTER.**

○ **A WOMAN IS MORE LIKELY TO PRODUCE TWO EGGS IF SHE HAS HAD SEVERAL CHILDREN ALREADY.**

IDENTICAL TWINS Identical twins begin as a single egg; a single ovum is fertilized by a single sperm in the usual manner, but in the very early stages of cell division this egg splits completely in half, and each of these halves develops into a whole human being. These babies have identical genetic formation, but, again, it is not always easy to tell at birth, as one may be very much bigger than the other. They are more likely to share a single placenta, though if the division happened while they were still in the Fallopian tube, they may have embedded separately. The great similarity between them tends to become more marked as they grow and develop.

The incidence of identical twins is the same throughout all races, and over different ages and parities of women, and no hereditary factor is involved. It is also a far more rare event, occurring at a rate of only 3.7 births per 1,000 throughout the world.

LARGER MULTIPLE BIRTHS Larger multiples can be either fraternal or identical, or even, possibly, a mixture of both, although those resulting from fertility drugs will usually be fraternal, since the point of the drugs is to stimulate ovulation.

Twin pregnancies which do not develop

With the development of ultrasound it has become apparent that many more pregnancies start out as twins than actually develop to term.

REABSORPTION OF ONE EMBRYO An early scan may show two embryos, but later on in pregnancy one has disappeared and labour produces only one baby. The second twin seems to have been reabsorbed into the uterus. This is known as the 'vanishing twin syndrome'.

MISCARRIAGE In other cases, one baby may be lost through a miscarriage, while the other goes on to full development and a healthy birth. A mother who had been unaware that she was carrying twins may suspect that her pregnancy is at an end, but a scan will detect an intact baby still growing inside her. It may feel very strange to her to be mourning the loss of one baby through miscarriage, whilst still carrying the other. It may make it harder than after a straightforward miscarriage for the parents to grieve for the one lost baby. There may also be a period of several days or weeks between the miscarriage and the confirmation of a continuing pregnancy. If a woman is still feeling sick and 'pregnant', this will be a particularly confusing and distressing time for her. You will find further information about miscarriage in Chapter 10.

COPING WITH PREGNANCY

A pregnancy with twins may be as straightforward as a singleton pregnancy, and you may sail through it feeling better than you have ever done before. The human reproductive system is, however, basically geared towards one offspring at a time, and carrying two or three babies is far harder work for your body. You may feel this

The most common positions for twins:
a. Both twins cephalic, or head down
b. The first twin cephalic, the second in the breech position

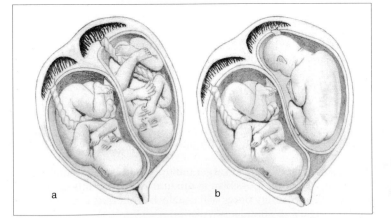

a   b

quite early on, as there is often rapid weight gain and the uterus enlarges more quickly (this may well also happen to a woman expecting a fourth or subsequent baby). The usual discomforts of pregnancy may be more pronounced; the sickness and tiredness in the early days are often worse, and as time goes on there is more likelihood of indigestion, heartburn, and swelling of feet and ankles. You may suffer from breathlessness, and in the last trimester of pregnancy the sheer size of a very full uterus may seriously limit your movements and make you feel tired and cumbersome.

The discomforts of increased size come earlier with a multiple birth. It is not only the weight of the babies, but the two, three or more placentae and correspondingly more amniotic fluid and extra maternal body fluids that you are having to cope with. The size and shape that you would be at 20 weeks for a singleton baby, you might reach at 16 weeks with twins. The uterus reaches the rib-cage by 32 weeks instead of the customary 36, and your overall weight gain can be half as much again as your pre-pregnancy weight!

A pregnancy with twins or more does not usually last as long as one for one baby; 36–37 weeks is an average gestation, and 5 lb. 6 oz. (2,500 g.) an average weight for each twin.

CARING FOR YOURSELF

Uncomfortable though many of these factors may be in a multiple pregnancy, they are normal, and are not worrying in medical terms. Some of the discomforts — the sickness and the extreme tiredness — may pass after 12–16 weeks and then you may have two or three months of feeling really well and not too uncomfortable because of sheer size and weight.

It is particularly important to look after yourself properly when you are expecting more than one baby, and to do everything you can to help your body cope with the additional strain.

REST Perhaps the most important change you have to make to your life-style is finding time to rest. Most mothers of twins say that they felt particularly conscious of the care they must take of their babies while *in utero*, so that they listened to their bodies and gave in graciously when they felt physically weary, even if mentally they were keen to carry on with their activities. Rest can help to prevent many serious problems that sometimes occur in multiple pregnancies, such as:

- ○ **SLOW GROWTH OF THE BABIES**
- ○ **INADEQUACY OF THE PLACENTAL SYSTEM**
- ○ **HIGH BLOOD PRESSURE IN THE MOTHER**
- ○ **PREMATURE BIRTH**

It used to be the case that all mothers of twins were prescribed bed rest in hospital for several weeks towards the end of pregnancy, but not everyone needs this, and, since some women find it more difficult to rest and relax in hospital than at home, a compromise is often reached, so that a mother needing more rest can stay at home but either make more frequent visits to the antenatal clinic (not very restful) or, preferably, have frequent home visits from her community midwife. If extra rest is recommended by the doctor, this often does mean spending most of the day in bed, which can be exceedingly difficult to manage at home if there are other children to care for.

Even if rest is not actually prescribed, it is helpful for you and the babies to have a good hour or two with your feet up in the middle of the day. You may need longer if you are not sleeping well at night.

EXERCISE The same principles apply to multiple pregnancies as to any pregnancy (see the sections on exercise in Chapter 6, Looking After Yourself), though you may be particularly thankful to take up exercises in the water and thus relieve your body of some of the strain.

DIET Two or more babies need a lot of nourishment to grow well, and for you too, at a time when you are making incredible physical demands on your body, good nutrition is a priority. The same guidelines for good eating will hold as for a singleton pregnancy (see Chapter 6, Looking After Yourself), but, since a woman expecting more than one baby is prone to anaemia, iron-rich foods are especially important in your diet.

In the early months, when you may be suffering from nausea, and during the last few weeks, when there may be a lot of pressure under your stomach, food may lose its appeal, so it is especially important to eat well while you are enjoying your food. Eating small snacks of whatever you can stomach during any very uncomfortable times may help keep your strength up.

ANTENATAL CHECKS Besides looking after yourself properly, you will probably be expected to attend more often for check-ups than if you were expecting only one baby. Many of the problems associated with multiple births can be detected early on before they become serious, and for some of them the prime treatment is simply more rest.

YOUR EMOTIONS As well as the overwhelming physical experience of being pregnant with twins or more, there are a multitude of emotional factors, and, in working through these, expectant parents often find the most help in talking to other parents-to-be, in making contact with other parents of twins or triplets, and in talking through their feelings with sympathetic medical staff and antenatal teachers.

FINDING SUPPORT

There may be a Twins Club in your area; your health visitor or local NCT branch will be able to give you details.

The Twins and Multiple Births Association (TAMBA) produces some helpful leaflets, and may be able to put you in touch with other parents in the same situation as you. You will find the address at the back of this book.

Most people are fascinated by twins, triplets, and even more babies arriving all at once, and will give the new parents a lot of friendship and practical help too, especially if there are other children who need to be looked after. You will find further information on twin births and on caring for more than one baby, in Chapter 17, Complications in Labour, and Chapter 30, Twins and Supertwins: Life after Birth.

' *I found it a time of mixed emotions. I was ecstatic to be preg-nant after trying for six years, at the same time as being extremely tired and very sick. I couldn't believe that after all this time of waiting we were actually going to be parents to two babies!* '

' *I couldn't say that it was comfortable being pregnant with three babies. At 26 weeks I was the size of a normal 40-week preg-nant mum. I was getting terrible heartburn and being very sick. In fact I could hardly eat, but drank a lot of milk to compensate. Other problems arose as I got even bigger. I couldn't sit with my feet raised — there was too much tummy in the way. So I had to sit upright in a chair. But then the weight of my tummy on my legs badly affected circulation so my feet swelled up, and that had to be righted by a spell of lying flat on the bed.* '

' *I was incredibly relieved when I found out I was carrying twins. I knew the tiredness and heaviness weren't normal for an ordinary pregnancy — I never felt like this with my other daughter. So the shock of discovering it was twins was offset by knowing there was a good reason for why I'd been feeling so totally exhausted and fed up with myself. I felt a lot better once I knew.* '

' *My pregnancy wasn't very good; I was sick a lot and felt extremely tired. As a result I started resenting these babies who were growing inside me, who made me feel so ill. But then I discovered the NCT classes, which helped me feel more positive about being pregnant. We used to laugh a lot at the classes, because, as we learned more about the birth, it was always different for twins. Our group also helped me through the early months, as we still kept in touch, meeting once a week until just recently (over two years later). It was always nice to have somebody else who was going through the same problems and stages with her baby, to confide in.* **'**

MISCARRIAGE

10

Miscarriàge is a very common occurrence — recent studies have suggested that as many as 43 per cent of all pregnancies end in miscarriage before 20 weeks. Many of these miscarriages will, of course, have taken place very early in pregnancy, often before a woman is even sure she is pregnant, and a late, rather heavy period could mark the end of as many as one in three pregnancies. The most usual time for a miscarriage to occur is during the first trimester of pregnancy, frequently taking place when a woman would normally have expected her period if she were not pregnant. Only 3 per cent of all miscarriages take place during the next fourteen weeks, the second trimester, and once the fetus has reached 28 weeks, when it would be possible for the baby to survive outside the uterus, it is called a stillbirth rather than a miscarriage.

The possibility of a pregnancy ending in miscarriage is a very real worry for many women, who find that every twinge and ache fills them with some anxiety. Even women who have begun feeling rather ambivalent towards the whole pregnancy often feel unexpectedly sad, with a strong sense of loss, should they miscarry. There is now, fortunately, much more information available on miscarriages and the subject is discussed more openly than even a few years ago. There are also support groups around if you feel the need to talk to someone, whether you have had a miscarriage or one is threatened.

THREATENED MISCARRIAGE

VAGINAL BLEEDING For most women who miscarry, the first sign is usually bleeding from the vagina, often a dark red-brown colour. Although any vaginal bleeding should be taken seriously in pregnancy and medical advice sought, it does not necessarily mean a miscarriage will follow. In fact, fewer than 50 per cent of women who experience bleeding in early pregnancy go on to miscarry.

There are a number of possible reasons for vaginal bleeding:

o   **THERE MAY HAVE BEEN A PARTIALLY SUPPRESSED PERIOD, WHICH HAPPENS WHEN THE BODY HAS MADE INSUFFICIENT**

PREGNANCY HORMONE TO STOP THE PERIOD COMPLETELY.
○ **SMALL PIECES OF THE PLACENTA MAY HAVE SEPARATED FROM THE WALL OF THE UTERUS.**
○ **POLYPS MAY BE PRESENT; THESE ARE NON-CANCEROUS GROWTHS IN THE VAGINA OR ON THE CERVIX.**
○ **THERE MAY BE CERVICAL EROSION; THIS IS A SMALL MUCUS-PRODUCING AREA OF THE CERVIX WHICH CAN BLEED EASILY.**
○ **THE BLEEDING MAY NOT BE FROM THE VAGINA AT ALL, BUT FROM THE URETHRA, AND YOU MAY HAVE AN INFECTION SUCH AS CYSTITIS.**

As it is not always easy to find the specific cause of bleeding, the term 'threatened miscarriage' tends to be used to cover virtually any bleeding in early pregnancy. If the bleeding stops and you continue the pregnancy, delivering the baby as normal, there is absolutely no increased likelihood of abnormality or problems as a result of any bleeding.

INEVITABLE MISCARRIAGE

BLEEDING If the bleeding is a sign of an inevitable miscarriage, it is usually accompanied by other symptoms. Many women experience shivering and sickness, while others report feeling 'less pregnant'. Some women pass pieces of tissue resembling lumps of liver. The bleeding will increase, becoming brighter in colour, and there will usually be some degree of discomfort or pain. The blood will be mixed with the amniotic fluid which surrounded the fetus, and this may make the amount of blood lost appear frighteningly large.

PAIN Most women feel any pain directly above the pubic bone, rather like strong menstrual cramps, but pain may also be felt in the stomach, the lower back, or the thighs.

The pain is caused by the uterus contracting to open the cervix in order to expel the fetus. It may vary from mild, period-type cramps to severe pain. As a miscarriage is now quite certain, you need not put up with any pain if you do not want to, and should ask for effective pain relief. For some women, miscarriage is over in about an hour, but for others it may take many hours, even days, with pain and bleeding that can be either continuous or intermittent. The pain and bleeding will cease once the miscarriage is complete.

THE FETUS It is unusual to see the fetus — often it will not have developed properly and will have been reabsorbed by your body, or it may still be too small to be seen easily. Sometimes, however, and more frequently in miscarriages which happen during the latter part of the second trimester — after about 20 weeks — the fetus can be seen quite clearly. Women who have seen their babies after a miscarriage describe them as being beautiful and perfectly formed. It is far easier to grieve for a baby you have seen than for one who exists only in your imagination and memory. So, although at the time it may be a great shock to see your baby, in the long run it may help you to come to terms with your loss. If you miscarry when you are in hospital, any tissue expelled from the uterus will be routinely incinerated. For women who feel that a body is unimportant once they know the fetus is dead, this is the ideal solution. It is, however, important to be aware that parents have the right both to see the fetus, and to bury it, if that is their wish.

Medical help

If you think you may be miscarrying, you can phone or visit your GP, when you will need to describe all your symptoms fully. If you are feeling unwell, your GP should visit you at home. As with all other situations, you can keep asking until all the questions you have are answered to your satisfaction. If you feel you are not receiving satisfactory help or advice, you can ask to be transferred to the hospital obstetrician.

Some women who contact their GPs because they have begun to bleed in early pregnancy are upset because their problem seems to have been treated so lightly. What may seem like an unexceptional matter to a GP can be a very frightening and distressing experience for a woman who has just begun to enjoy the idea of a pregnancy and a baby. Many women find they are given insufficient information about what they should do and what they might expect to happen, and feel they have been treated unsympathetically. There may in fact be nothing that a woman or her doctor can do, either to save the pregnancy or make a threatened miscarriage any less distressing. It may simply be a matter of waiting, and slowly coming to terms with the possibility that this pregnancy may be lost. Many women feel something ought to be done immediately, and GPs sometimes fail to reassure women that it is normal procedure to let nature take its course.

If you feel your GP is unable to give you the time to listen to your fears, and you think it would be helpful for you to talk to someone, you could try contacting the NCT, a local NCT teacher, or The Miscarriage Association (you will find details listed at the back of this book). This can be a difficult, stressful time, and it can be very reassuring to have a non-medical but knowledgeable person to speak to who will not simply dismiss your worries, but will offer support and a friendly ear.

It does not appear to make any difference to the outcome of a threatened miscarriage whether or not the mother or doctor takes specific action. Some doctors will take tests to try to discover what is happening; others will observe, but let nature take its course. Some mothers feel they would rather be in bed resting, while others are happy to carry on as normal while they wait. What you decide to do will usually depend on how you are feeling in yourself; if you feel ill enough to go to bed, you will be better off there, even though resting will not affect the outcome. Similarly, if you feel well and active, you will not be damaging your chances by being up and about.

DIAGNOSIS Your doctor may use an obstetric stethoscope or Sonicaid to listen for the fetus's heartbeat, or he may perform a pregnancy test to establish whether the fetus is still alive (this test is not 100 per cent reliable at all stages of early pregnancy). He may suggest doing an internal examination to find out whether or not the cervix has begun to dilate. An ultrasound scan can be used to give a more accurate picture of what is happening, though most obstetricians prefer to avoid ultrasound scans on any fetus in the first trimester. If you are sent to hospital for a scan, you may prefer not to look at the screen, as seeing the fetus at this stage can be very distressing indeed. If it is alive and well, the sight of it moving about is most reassuring, but you may want to be told the probable outcome before having a look. In many areas, cost-cutting measures mean that hospitals now no longer offer a scan to determine whether or not a miscarriage is inevitable.

AFTER A MISCARRIAGE

Incomplete miscarriage

Sometimes a miscarriage is incomplete, when some, or part, of the placenta or fetus is left in the uterus.

D AND C If an incomplete miscarriage is suspected, you will probably have to have a Dilation and Curettage (D and C) or 'scrape' to make certain that nothing is left in the uterus to cause infection or further bleeding. Under general anaesthetic, the cervix is stretched (dilated) and the inner lining of the uterus scraped (curettage). The operation only takes a few minutes and you will be able to go home later that day or early the next if all else is well.

Missed abortion

Occasionally, when a fetus dies, there may be a little bleeding, but miscarriage does not actually occur. This is termed a missed abortion. After discussion with the mother, the doctor may decide to wait and see if the body reabsorbs the pregnancy, or if miscarriage occurs later. But they may both decide that the uterus should be emptied, by means of a D and C if the pregnancy is less than 16 weeks, or by induced labour if it is over 16 weeks.

Labour is induced by administering the hormone prostaglandin by passing a catheter (a fine tube) into the uterus through the cervix, or via an intravenous drip into the back of the hand. Oxytocin will sometimes be used with the prostaglandin to make the uterus contract. This can cause strong, painful contractions and you should be offered pain relief such as Entonox or Pethidine to help you cope.

TAKING IRON If, during the course of your miscarriage, you have lost a lot of blood, it may be necessary for you to be prescribed iron in the form of capsules or injections to restore your haemoglobin levels.

After care

RHESUS-NEGATIVE BLOOD Your blood group may be rhesus-negative, in which case you will need to make sure you are given the Anti-D injection. This will destroy any antibodies you may have produced if the fetus's rhesus-positive blood mixed with yours during the miscarriage. The injection, which should be given within seventy-two hours of the miscarriage, will safeguard any future babies you have against any antibodies you might have produced.

TIREDNESS You may feel surprisingly tired after a miscarriage, and it is important to allow yourself plenty of time to recover, both emotionally and physically, before resuming your normal activities.

BREAST MILK The later in pregnancy your miscarriage occurs, the more likely you are to produce milk. At 12 weeks only 10 per cent of women do so, but this figure rises rapidly with the length of the pregnancy until 19 weeks, when the majority of women produce milk. If your breasts are going to produce milk, they will do so between two and five days after the miscarriage. Your breasts may swell and there may be a tingling or even painful sensation. It is better not to squeeze your breasts to express milk as this will only increase milk production. Instead, you could try wearing a fairly tight, firm bra, and splashing your breasts with cold water to relieve discomfort. You may also find that taking a pain-killer such as paracetamol or a homoeopathic remedy is helpful. You may find that the arrival of milk in your breasts comes as a painful physical and emotional reminder of your baby's death — a powerful and poignant recognition of what should have been.

YOUR EMOTIONS After a miscarriage, the emotions women experience may often be confusing and astonishingly intense. Initially, the dominant emotions may be shock and grief, but to their surprise many women also feel a sense of relief — the stress and pain of the actual miscarriage is over and they have come through it. Whatever you do feel, it is important to acknowledge all your feelings, to discuss them with your partner, who will also have his share of distress and grieving to cope with. Many women will not have told relatives or work colleagues about the pregnancy yet, so it will be difficult to share any feelings about the miscarriage with them.

All too often the response, even from doctors and nurses, is, 'Well, that's that. Pull yourself together. Plenty of time to have another baby.'

In these circumstances, it is easy to feel isolated and unsupported, even angry. Your partner may also find it hard to understand why you are feeling so upset if, for him, the baby had not yet taken on any reality. Nothing can replace the baby you have lost, or make up for all those plans that have to be abandoned for the time being. It is useful to acknowledge these feelings too and to find ways of moving forward once you have managed to deal with all that the miscarriage has brought.

Coming to terms with a miscarriage

Some couples find their grieving process has been helped by creating their own small ritual, such as planting a shrub or tree in the garden. Others have found that writing down their feelings and experiences has helped enormously. Talking to another woman who has also had a miscarriage but has now come to terms with her own situation, yet can understand yours, can be both helpful and supportive. Both the NCT and the Miscarriage Association have networks of women across the country who are willing to talk to anyone, usually by phone, offering woman-to-woman support to anyone who would like their help in finding ways of accepting the feelings of sadness, loss, anger, and guilt that can follow a miscarriage. (The address of the Miscarriage Association is listed at the back of this book.)

ANOTHER PREGNANCY

TRYING AGAIN When you make the decision to try to become pregnant again is entirely a matter for you and your partner. Only you will know when your body has recovered sufficiently to embark on another pregnancy. Only you as a couple will know when your own grieving processes are completed so that you can happily start again. Discuss it between yourselves and ignore well-meaning outside advice — when to conceive again is something for you to choose. You may find that, if you are in a hurry to become pregnant again, it will be difficult to enjoy this next pregnancy fully, while you are still mourning the loss of the previous pregnancy and your baby. Anniversaries, both of the expected date of delivery and of the miscarriage itself, may be especially hard to deal with, even when you feel you are basically over the miscarriage. It is most unlikely that you will ever quite forget the baby who should have been. So, allow yourself time to mourn, and set aside some time for this baby, before beginning the next. Try also not to conceive on a date such that the expected birth of the next baby coincides with the date of the loss of your previous one.

Fear of another miscarriage

One of the great sadnesses surrounding miscarriage, and one aspect which can be difficult to accept, is that, except for a small minority of cases, the reason for the miscarriage is unknown. When you become pregnant again, you may well be fearful that you will again miscarry. This response is perfectly understandable; talk about it to your partner, your GP, your midwife, an NCT teacher. Their emotional support and understanding will help you, especially around the time you previously miscarried. The likelihood is that this next pregnancy will be successful, but if you have had several miscarriages you may feel that it would be helpful to have specific or genetic counselling. You can ask your doctor or gynaecologist to refer you for this, though you may have to press rather hard to get this service, as some doctors are reluctant; if you want it, then it may well be worth persisting to help set your mind at rest.

REPEATED MISCARRIAGES Repeated miscarriages may be due to a variety of reasons. One possible cause is 'cervical incompetence', when the cervix is too weak to support the weight of the uterus and its contents. This can be corrected by a running suture ('purse string' or Shirodker Stitch), which will hold the cervix closed. This needs to be removed before labour is due. Another cause is incorrect hormone balance, and injections of progesterone may be needed to maintain the pregnancy.

TAKING MISCARRIAGE SERIOUSLY

Miscarriage is still something which many people, including the medical profession, find hard to discuss or take seriously. For the women who have gone through it, this lack of concern may make it much harder to grieve. It may also make it harder to get all the information and support you need. If you find yourself feeling unsupported, your experience trivialized in some way, do continue to talk about it, to express your feelings and your anger. Letting those around you know how strongly you feel may not only help you to recover fully from the miscarriage, but may also make the way a little easier for those women who will be following you.

• *When I lost the baby at 12 weeks, nobody knew — I didn't even miss work because it was half-term. Consequently, there was nobody outside my family to understand my sense of loss, nobody to share my sorrow. My urgent need to become pregnant again as quickly as possible is difficult to describe. When you've had a miscarriage and it's your first baby — you've not yet had a chance to join the ranks of motherhood — it can be a very lonely, frightening experience.* •

• *Friends' attitudes were mostly, "Well, you were only 7 weeks pregnant." I felt that was irrelevant — I had lost my baby, but I also felt I shouldn't make a fuss for the very reason that I was early on in my pregnancy. My other feeling was of failure; me, a woman, unable to accomplish the most natural function in the world.* •

11 COMMUNICATING WITH HEALTH PROFESSIONALS

Although it may seem surprising to devote an entire chapter to communicating with health professionals, this is an extremely important area, and one which does worry many expectant parents. When women in antenatal classes are asked about their fears and worries during pregnancy, one of the commonest is fear of the hospital itself and of the attitudes of the staff who will be attending them. Many pregnant women and their partners are concerned that they will not get on with the staff caring for them in labour and want to know how they can express their own views and preferences whilst building up a good relationship.

Some people have little difficulty in dealing with medical personnel, while others find the fact that someone wears a uniform

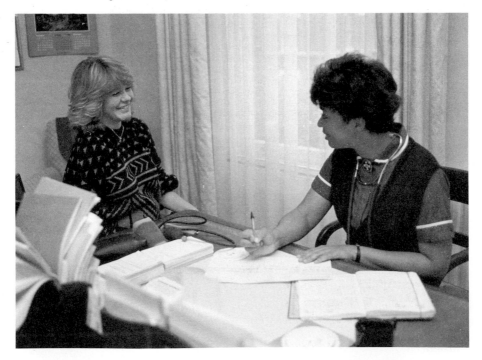

or is in a position of medical authority utterly daunting, which can lead to a loss of confidence. This confidence may be further eroded by the atmosphere in some hospitals and GPs' surgeries, particularly the antenatal clinics. If doctors and midwives appear intent on rushing you through with little regard for you as a person; if you are not offered any real opportunities for asking questions; if the clinic is apparently run for the convenience of the staff rather than for the comfort and reassurance of the women attending it, you may understandably feel undermined and unsure of how to approach your medical carers.

CHANGING ATTITUDES

During the latter half of the twentieth century there has been a progression from a position where no one would dream of questioning the word of a doctor or midwife, to a situation where many women would like to be treated as part of the team caring for them. Women and their partners have begun to take back much of the responsibility for their babies' births, expecting to be consulted about any decision-making. They are no longer dependent on medical staff to take charge and to know what is best. Alongside this desire to play a full part in determining the course of pregnancy and birth comes a fear that, because medical staff are in positions of power, they should not be upset. The wish to be involved may be tempered with anxiety that someone who has control over you might be antagonized.

Much of this anxiety is groundless. Midwives and doctors are now being trained and encouraged to care for the whole woman, not to regard her simply as a patient. (After all, pregnancy is not a disease; pregnant women are fulfilling a natural function.) You may well be greeted by your midwife asking you what kind of birth you would like and how she can help you achieve it. While this attitude is encouraged by many midwives and doctors, some have found it more difficult to adapt, and there is still a good deal of mistrust and contention amongst medical professionals themselves, which can be both confusing and frustrating for the expectant parents.

If you are already finding it difficult to communicate with those who are caring for you during your pregnancy, or if you are concerned to find the most effective ways of expressing your needs and feelings without causing antagonism, this chapter may offer you some ideas for opening up channels of communication.

IMPROVING YOUR OWN SITUATION

CONTINUITY OF CARE Much of the distrust and unease between expectant parents and their carers would disappear if they could get to know each other. It is rarely possible to have any sort of open, friendly relationship with someone you met only half an hour ago.

Getting to know the professionals

Many women are lucky enough to be cared for by a small team of community or hospital midwives. Some attend a hospital where they are always seen by the same doctor or midwife, or they regularly see their GP. Others will be delivered by their GP or community midwife in a small maternity unit where everyone has time to get to know each other properly. These women can form relationships with that person or team of people, which means they can negotiate the sort of care they want during birth and can openly share any fears or worries.

Unfortunately, many women do not enjoy continuity of care, but see different faces at each antenatal appointment, some of which are friendlier than others. They may wait in some trepidation to see who will be delivering them, knowing that, even though they may meet a friendly face at first, a change of shift could bring someone very different.

You may be one of the lucky ones who meets very few people during pregnancy and birth, in which case you should have ample opportunities to ask questions, listen to explanations, and put forward your own ideas. If you do find you are meeting an endless stream of new individuals or cannot easily communicate with your carers, you may have to take some more positive steps towards achieving your preferences. It is important that you believe you can influence what happens to you during pregnancy and birth, so that you are working on positive assumptions from the beginning.

Some practical hints

○ MAKE AN EFFORT TO GET TO KNOW WHOEVER YOU MEET DURING PREGNANCY. ASK PEOPLE'S NAMES AND TRY TO IMPRESS YOURSELF UPON THEM AS A PERSON, NOT AS 'THE WOMAN IN ROOM 2'.

○ ESTABLISH EYE CONTACT AND USE NAMES ONCE YOU HAVE LEARNED THEM; THIS IS A USEFUL MEANS OF GETTING THROUGH TO THE PERSON, RATHER THAN SIMPLY RESPONDING TO HIS OR HER POSITION.

○ PUT ANY QUESTIONS YOU HAVE TO THE DIFFERENT PEOPLE YOU MEET AND COMPARE ANSWERS. REALIZING THERE ARE DIFFERENT APPROACHES WILL HELP YOU FEEL LESS PART OF A TREADMILL.

○ IF SOMEONE DOES NOT HAVE THE TIME TO TALK TO YOU, THEN MAKE ANOTHER APPOINTMENT OR ASK WHO WOULD BE THE MOST APPROPRIATE PERSON TO SPEAK TO.

○ WAIT UNTIL YOU ARE SURE YOU HAVE SOMEONE'S FULL ATTENTION BEFORE SPEAKING. WAIT UNTIL THE DOCTOR HAS FINISHED WRITING AND LOOKS UP. SAY, 'GOOD MORNING, DR X', IF HE DOES NOT ACKNOWLEDGE YOUR PRESENCE IN THE ROOM.

○ IF YOU ARE NERVOUS (AND MOST OF US ARE), TAKE YOUR

PARTNER OR A FRIEND ALONG WITH YOU.

O WRITE DOWN ANY QUESTIONS YOU MIGHT HAVE, SO THAT
YOU WILL NOT FORGET THEM IN YOUR NERVOUSNESS AT
THE TIME. IT MAY ALSO BE USEFUL TO TAKE NOTES OF
WHAT HAS BEEN SAID, AS DETAILS MAY BECOME A BLUR
ONCE YOU GET BACK HOME.

O IF YOU WILL NOT HAVE A CHANCE TO MEET THE MIDWIFE
WHO WILL BE DELIVERING YOU BEFOREHAND, WRITING A
BIRTH OR CARE PLAN TO PUT IN YOUR NOTES, WHICH CAN
THEN BE DISCUSSED WITH WHOEVER CARES FOR YOU IN
LABOUR, IS A USEFUL STARTING-POINT. YOUR MIDWIFE
WILL GET A GOOD IDEA OF WHAT YOU WOULD LIKE AND
YOU WILL NOT HAVE TO REMEMBER ALL THE DETAILS AT A
TIME WHEN YOU ARE CONCENTRATING ON YOUR LABOUR.
YOU WILL FIND SOME SUGGESTIONS FOR WRITING A BIRTH
PLAN AT THE END OF THIS CHAPTER.

Talking to professionals

Some people's circumstances — their personalities or previous experiences — make it easier for them to communicate with health professionals. Whilst attitudes amongst medical personnel do differ, pregnant women also have to take some of the responsibility for how good or bad communications are.

You will find it easier to communicate if you are:

O WELL INFORMED FROM READING AND ASKING QUESTIONS
ABOUT THE SORT OF ISSUES THAT ARE IMPORTANT TO YOU

O FRIENDLY AND ACCESSIBLE YOURSELF, NOT AGGRESSIVE AND
DOGMATIC

O ABLE TO THINK OF THE PERSON YOU ARE DEALING WITH AS
A PERSON, NOT SIMPLY A BODY IN UNIFORM

O WILLING TO LISTEN AS WELL AS EXPLAIN YOURSELF AND, IF
NECESSARY, NEGOTIATE

RETAINING YOUR DIGNITY The most articulate, well-informed, confident person is liable to feel daunted when undressed and exposed, lying supine in front of sundry clothed experts. If you find yourself in this position, you can make some basic changes. It may be more difficult when you are actually in labour, but recovering some of your dignity and asking your partner to liaise for you will help.

O FIRSTLY, SIT UP AND COVER YOURSELF.

O ESTABLISH EYE CONTACT.

O ESTABLISH THAT THE PERSON DOES HAVE TIME TO TALK TO
YOU AND CAN GIVE YOU FULL ATTENTION.

O BE CLEAR ABOUT WHAT YOU WANT TO SAY; IF NECESSARY

OR APPROPRIATE, HAVE A LIST OF QUESTIONS.
- ○ DO NOT BE FOBBED OFF, BUT PERSIST UNTIL YOU HAVE HAD YOUR QUESTIONS ANSWERED OR REQUESTS CONSIDERED. NO MEDICAL EXPERT WILL LOSE HIS OR HER EXPERTISE BY EXPLAINING THINGS IN A WAY WHICH YOU CAN UNDERSTAND.
- ○ DO NOT BE HURRIED INTO MAKING DECISIONS YOU ARE UNSURE OF; ASK FOR TIME TO CONSIDER OR DISCUSS THEM WITH YOUR PARTNER OR OTHERS, AND, IF NECESSARY, ASK FOR FURTHER INFORMATION OR CLARIFICATION.
- ○ MAKE IT CLEAR FROM THE OUTSET THAT YOU CONSIDER YOURSELF A FULL PART OF THE TEAM CARING FOR YOUR PREGNANCY AND BIRTH, AND THEREFORE EXPECT TO BE CONSULTED THROUGHOUT. THIS WAY, YOU ARE LESS LIKELY TO HAVE SURPRISE DECISIONS THRUST UPON YOU.

BEING ASSERTIVE

In order to be assertive, you need to make a clear calm statement of what you think or wish to know. Do express your feelings about an issue; feelings matter; they are not irrelevant to any discussion, and they cannot be denied. The person you are speaking to may disagree with you or may try to ignore emotional considerations, but they are nevertheless real and important for you.

Do not make the mistake of attacking the person, or allowing yourself to be sidetracked by other issues, but reiterate what it is you need to know until you are satisfied you have an answer. Nor need you feel embarrassed into giving up before you are satisfied. This is *your* pregnancy, *your* birth, *your* body, and *your* baby, and these are *your* feelings and concerns; you have a right to find out whatever you need to know so that you can make a properly informed decision when the time comes. Being assertive does not mean you have to be dogmatic or aggressive. Your ideas may change as your situation changes or as more information becomes available to you. Whatever decisions you, your partner, and your medical carers come to should feel right at that moment.

The following exchange illustrates how you might handle a situation assertively, stating your case whilst remaining polite and non-threatening to the midwife:

Midwife: In a minute I am going to put a clip on the baby's head.
Woman: Why are you going to do that?
Midwife: We need to check that the baby is all right.
Woman: Is there any reason to believe that it is not?
Midwife: We think it is safer for the baby.

Woman: Could you explain to me exactly what it is that you are concerned about?

Midwife: Well, you would not want to put your baby at risk, would you?

Woman: Is there any reason to believe that there is any problem with the baby right now?

Midwife: Not at the moment, but just in case . . .

Woman: Thank you, but I would rather not have a clip put on just yet. I should like to get up and walk around for a while now. I shall be happy to talk it over with you again if you feel concerned later on.

This woman has been able to take responsibility for her own decisions whilst still considering the midwife's feelings and position. She was not deflected by the implied but unsubstantiated threat to her baby, but was clear in her line of questioning and was able to make a decision which was right for her at the time, but without closing her options for later.

CHANGING YOUR CARER

Occasionally, a woman finds she is unhappy with someone caring for her during her pregnancy.

If you do not like one of the people who is responsible for part of your care, then the chances are that he or she will not be happy with the relationship either. If possible, in such a situation, if discussing the problem does not resolve matters, the best thing you can do is to change your carer.

GP If you wish to change your GP for good, you will need to approach your new doctor first to see if he will be able to take you on his list, then ask your former GP to sign your medical card, releasing you from his list. If you have any problems with the change-over, you should contact your Family Health Services Authority, which is there to deal with just this sort of problem. If it is unable to help, it may be worth trying your Community Health Council.

How to go about changing your carer

You could ask your GP if there is someone else in the practice or nearby whom he could recommend, who would be likely to meet your needs. Make sure you have talked to a new GP before signing on, or your situation may not be improved at all. You might find it useful to contact other local women to check on their experience of local GPs. Local pharmacists are also often a good source of information about GPs in the area.

MIDWIFE If you wish to change your community midwife, you can ring or write to your local Director of Midwifery Services — the hospital will give you her name. You can then explain your problem and ask for her help in changing the situation.

If it is your hospital midwife with whom you are unhappy, you may feel very diffident about asking to change, but most midwives will understand and will try to accommodate your wishes. Asking if there is another midwife available to continue with your delivery will make your point clearly but not aggressively. Many hospitals make it clear to women when they are on their tour of the labour ward that they are at liberty to ask to change their midwife if they are at all unhappy.

CONSULTANT Changing your consultant and/or your hospital may prove much more difficult, and will certainly vary from area to area. If you are having problems, however, it may be worth persisting by, firstly, finding another consultant who will accept you, and, secondly, writing letters to the consultant or hospital of your choice stating clearly why you wish to change. Your local Association for Improvement in Maternity Services (AIMS) group should be very helpful in supporting you through this. (You will find the address at the back of this book.)

PARTNERS

These days, few women are alone in their labours. The role of the known and trusted local midwife has been taken, in non-medical areas, by a partner, relative, or friend. The value of having a familiar, caring face, and, moreover, one who has discussed at length your wishes for the birth, preferably also having attended antenatal classes with you, should not be underestimated. This person may also attend some or all of your antenatal appointments where he (or she) can ask some of the questions, raise issues, and discuss them later. Partners are an invaluable liaison between you and your medical attendants, able to negotiate on your behalf. Women who feel that they will not be in a position to ask questions or explain what they would like when concentrating on labour, can feel reassured by knowing that they have with them someone who will be their partner and friend throughout.

If your partner is someone who finds communications with medical staff difficult or who tends not to want to discuss or negotiate matters, you will need to explain your wishes very clearly and make it plain that he is there to support you, and to be involved in the decision-making with you. If you have written a birth plan between you, this will also be a good reference point for you all.

However your birth proceeds, you will want to be able to look back on it afterwards knowing that you felt in control of your environment throughout, that you were included in decisions, and that your wishes were always taken into consideration. If you have been able to communicate with those caring for you throughout the antenatal and birth periods, the experience will be a positive one, reinforcing your self-confidence.

WRITING A BIRTH PLAN

Some women are happy to accept whatever routine procedures the hospital has laid down for labour and, where a labour is not straightforward, to leave all decision-making to the medical staff concerned. Others prefer to accept some routine procedures and reject others; if their labour is not straightforward, they would prefer to share in the decision-making, keeping themselves fully informed, and regarding the recommendations of the medical staff as advice which they may either accept or reject, or, if a second opinion has been sought, choose between. The sort of course you decide to follow is, naturally, up to you. However, if you would prefer to take an active part in any decision-making, you may find it helpful to prepare a 'birth plan' in which you state your preferences.

KNOWING YOUR HOSPITAL A birth plan is generally unnecessary if you have booked a home birth, domino, or GP delivery, since you will have plenty of opportunities for discussing your preferences during your antenatal care. Some hospitals have prepared their own standard birth plan consisting of a form with boxes to tick; this may be sufficient for your needs, but do feel free to add a letter or plan of your own if it is not. Other hospitals provide women with a suggestions leaflet, or sheet, which is given out towards the end of pregnancy, and on which women can write their preferences for the coming labour and stay in hospital.

A birth plan can be of any length, and in it you may write which routine procedures you would rather avoid, and anything about the way in which you intend to give birth which may be different from the way in which labours at the hospital are usually conducted. It is important in writing it that you familiarize yourself with standard procedures at your hospital. You can do this by asking questions at antenatal classes, both NCT and hospital; by asking questions at antenatal appointments, both at hospital and with your GP; and by contacting the supervisor of midwives at your hospital if you need further information. By finding out all you can about how labour is conducted, you can make your birth plan as brief as possible, concentrating only on those areas where your preferences differ from what is normally offered. By reading this book — particularly the chapters entitled Preparing for Labour, Medical Procedures, Pain Relief in Labour, Complications of Labour, Caesarean Section, The First Few Hours, and Early Days, and by talking to other women who have had their babies at your hospital, you will become clear about the range of possibilities and begin to evolve preferences of your own. You may well wish to involve your labour partner in this.

It helps if the plan is written in as non-aggressive a tone as possible, and makes it clear that you are familiar with hospital policies. A birth plan cannot, of course, guarantee a normal labour, so should contain a statement to the effect that you realize that you may have to rely on immediate action by medical staff in the event of an emergency. You should also reserve the right to change your mind, showing that you are aware that the course of any labour and a woman's reactions to it may be unpredictable.

Once you have written the plan, you might wish to show it to your NCT teacher or community midwife for comments. The plan can then be taken along to an antenatal appointment at some time during the last two months of your pregnancy, and discussed with either your consultant, an obstetrician on his team, or a midwifery sister from the labour ward. It might be advisable to arrange with the antenatal clinic in advance to ensure that there will be the time available to do this. You might like to have your partner or a friend or relative with you for support.

Once your plan has been agreed, it will be attached to your notes, and the doctor will usually make a note of the discussion there. The notes will be used by the medical staff during your labour, and you will need to keep a copy to bring in with you as well. If you are unable to agree the plan, you have a number of options:

○ **YOU MAY DECIDE TO GO ALONG WITH HOSPITAL POLICY.**
○ **YOU MAY DECIDE TO CHANGE YOUR CONSULTANT.**
○ **IF THE DISAGREEMENT IS FUNDAMENTAL, YOU MAY DECIDE TO CHANGE YOUR HOSPITAL.**

This last option should theoretically be feasible even in the last month of pregnancy, but is becoming more difficult as hospitals increasingly refuse to take women from outside their boundaries.

Birth plan check-list

Areas you might think about are listed here, but the list is by no means exhaustive:

○ **BEING ACCOMPANIED BY MORE THAN ONE LABOUR PARTNER**
○ **ROUTINE INDUCTIONS**
○ **ADMISSION PROCEDURES**
○ **EATING AND DRINKING DURING LABOUR**
○ **WEARING OWN CLOTHES FOR LABOUR**
○ **POSITIONS FOR LABOUR**
○ **VAGINAL EXAMINATIONS**
○ **ROUTINE ACCELERATION (I.E. ARTIFICIAL RUPTURE OF MEMBRANES AND SYNTOCINON DRIP)**
○ **MANAGEMENT OF BREECH LABOUR**

○ ROUTINE OFFERING OF PAIN RELIEF (I.E. PETHIDINE, EPIDURAL, GAS AND AIR)

○ AVAILABILITY OF EPIDURAL ANAESTHESIA FOR PAIN RELIEF AND CAESAREAN SECTION

○ AVAILABILITY OF TENS MACHINES AND/OR MIDWIVES TRAINED IN THEIR USE

○ POLICY TOWARDS USE OF ALTERNATIVE METHODS OF PAIN RELIEF (E.G. HOMOEOPATHIC REMEDIES, HYPNOSIS, ACUPUNCTURE)

○ TIME-LIMITS FOR FIRST, SECOND, AND THIRD STAGES OF LABOUR

○ MANAGEMENT OF SECOND STAGE: WHETHER PUSHING DIRECTED BY MIDWIFE OR BY MOTHER'S URGE TO PUSH; WHETHER EPIDURALS ALLOWED TO WEAR OFF FOR SECOND STAGE

○ ROUTINE EPISIOTOMY AND POLICY ON TEARING

○ AVAILABILITY OF LOCAL ANAESTHETIC FOR EPISIOTOMY AND/OR STITCHES

○ POSITIONS FOR DELIVERY

○ MANAGEMENT OF THIRD STAGE: WHETHER MIDWIVES ARE TRAINED IN PHYSIOLOGICAL MANAGEMENT IF THIS IS PREFERRED

○ MANAGEMENT OF BABY IMMEDIATELY AFTER BIRTH: SUCKING OUT OF MUCUS, WHETHER HANDED TO MOTHER IMMEDIATELY, BREASTFEEDING IN DELIVERY ROOM, VITAMIN K INJECTION/DROPS

○ THE STAY IN HOSPITAL: HOW LONG, SUPPORT FOR BREASTFEEDING, ROOMING-IN, VISITING, PRIVACY

• *My GP just sits there. He hardly bothers to examine me, let alone talk to me, so I can't bring myself to ask him any questions. I have wondered why he does antenatal clinics at all.* •

• *I feel I've really got to know my midwife during this pregnancy. She understands me too, and I trust her to look after me in labour and afterwards as I want.* •

• *We were glad we'd written our birth plan, because, when it came to the crunch in labour, I wasn't in any frame of mind to bother with explaining how I'd like it to go.* •

• *We both knew we should keep asking questions, but it is difficult when they're the experts. We're articulate, intelligent people, but we both felt overawed by being in the hospital and off familiar territory.* •

12 GETTING READY FOR THE BIRTH

Most women feel an urge to get themselves organized ready for the baby's birth. As the expected date of delivery draws closer, many couples find a certain mild panic creeping in when they begin to wonder whether they will ever actually be ready. The panic usually disappears as the birth approaches, being replaced by a more relaxed feeling that, even if the decorating is not quite finished, the larder still rather empty, it no longer matters; the birth becomes the important event to look forward to. In order to enjoy this relaxation fully, however, it does help to have prepared yourselves in some fairly specific ways. This might take the form of a consideration and discussion of issues related to birth and parenthood which are important for you — a physical and mental preparation for labour — or it might involve basic, practical domestic arrangements. Anything which helps to ease your mind in these last weeks, so that you can go into labour feeling reasonably confident, well informed, and ready for the events ahead, can be immensely reassuring. This chapter will deal with some of the preparations you might wish to make to help yourself feel as ready as possible for your baby's birth.

ANTENATAL CLASSES

Attending antenatal classes is the best possible way of preparing for your baby's birth. They will provide you with an opportunity to give some thought to the birth and your baby — a chance to concentrate fully on the coming events. Most classes will provide information about all aspects of pregnancy, labour, delivery, and the postnatal period, in particular covering the range of options available to you locally. They will cover the basic physiology of labour, normal and abnormal, as well as some physical preparation for your labour, including relaxation and breathing techniques, massage, and a chance to try out a variety of different positions for use in labour. They will also provide information, and possibly discussion, on many aspects of pregnancy, birth, and parenthood. The best classes will offer you an opportunity to share your feelings and experiences with other parents in the same group. If you are finding it difficult to think what you ought to be doing in preparation for the birth and the arrival of a baby in your home, antenatal classes will help you focus on what it is that you want and how you are going to achieve it.

Classes vary in approach, in quality, and in precise objectives, and you may decide to go to more than one set. You may be offered a choice between courses for mothers and those for couples. Some men are reluctant to attend antenatal classes, viewing them as potentially embarrassing, too likely to make them feel squeamish, or simply not for them. If you would like the baby's father to go with you, discuss with the teacher or midwife what is liable to be included in the course, and discuss how you both feel once you have a better idea of what will be involved. Classes normally start about three months before your baby is due, but this will vary with local circumstances. It is well worth finding out about the options early in your pregnancy to be sure you do not miss anything.

You can find local information on classes from:

- ○ **YOUR GP'S SURGERY**
- ○ **YOUR MIDWIFE**
- ○ **THE COMMUNITY HEALTH COUNCIL**
- ○ **YOUR LOCAL NCT BRANCH (TRY YOUR LOCAL PHONE BOOK OR NCT HEADQUARTERS; YOU WILL FIND THE ADDRESS LISTED AT THE BACK OF THIS BOOK)**

Hospital classes

Hospital antenatal classes are offered to all women intending to have their babies at that hospital. They are normally for mothers only, with one or two sessions to include fathers. Most last for six or eight weeks, with weekly classes covering a variety of topics. They are usually run by a midwife, who may invite colleagues from the hospital to give talks. You might hear a midwife from the Special Care Baby Unit one week, a physiotherapist another time, or an anaesthetist talking about pain relief in labour on another occasion. Often, though, the midwives themselves take all the classes.

The classes should give you a good idea of hospital procedures, so you will know roughly what to expect and what is expected of you. The main drawback of hospital classes is usually their sheer size, and the formality of the occasion. Sometimes as many as thirty or even fifty people attend a class. This makes asking questions almost impossible, particularly if there is a strong 'lecturing' atmosphere. There may not even be time allocated for questions. The size and formality of some groups also makes it hard to get to know other women very well.

Hospital classes are free.

Clinic classes

These are NHS classes held at a local clinic, GP's surgery, or community health centre, usually run by the local health visitor or community midwife. Although there will be classes on pregnancy, labour, birth, and preparations for birth, there is sometimes a greater emphasis on caring for a new baby, as this is where a health visitor's expertise lies. They may be somewhat less formal than hospital classes, as well as being more accessible for most women. You will probably be offered opportunities for relaxation, plus a chance to get to know other mothers from your locality.

The direct knowledge of current hospital practice may not always be quite so up to date, but clinic classes may be able to present a more objective view of policies and procedures. It is also useful to get to know the community midwife and health visitor who may well be attending you once your baby is born.

These classes are also free.

There is a wide variation in both content and standard of both hospital and clinic classes: some are excellent, others disappointingly poor. It is a good idea to ask other local mothers who have recently had babies for their impressions of what is on offer in your area.

NCT classes

Although they cover similar ground in preparing parents for birth and parenthood, the approach of NCT classes is rather different from hospital and clinic classes. The emphasis here is on learning through informal, discussion-based classes in a small group. All NCT teachers are parents themselves and their approach is from the lay or consumer perspective. Classes are very often held in the teacher's own home, creating a different atmosphere altogether. NCT classes will provide extremely detailed information on all issues surrounding pregnancy, birth, and parenthood, so that you are able to make your own informed decisions when the time comes.

As well as information, relaxation, and discussion, most courses will involve a local breastfeeding counsellor, who will discuss breastfeeding your baby and will be available for help and support afterwards. You will also be allocated a postnatal supporter, usually a mother with a young child herself, who can offer you support and friendship on a mother-to-mother basis.

Because groups are small and informal, there is a good chance to get to know each other reasonably well over the eight or nine weeks that the course lasts, and many groups continue to meet for years afterwards, providing welcome peer-group support.

Although all teachers have trained with the NCT, all work in slightly different ways according to personality and circumstance. Some teach courses mainly for mothers, with two or three fathers' evenings; others teach courses for couples. Some teachers also run refreshers' classes for those who have previously attended NCT classes.

You do not have to be a member of the NCT to attend its antenatal classes; NCT facilities are there for everyone.

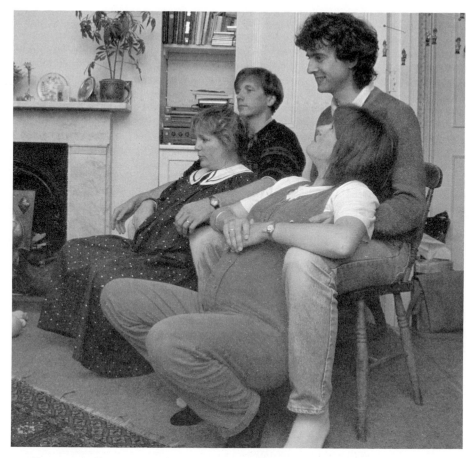

There is a charge for NCT classes, but the fee will always be waived or reduced if finding the full amount is difficult. You will, however, need to book early to make sure of a place — classes are often full five or more months in advance, so it is unwise to leave booking until you give up work or suddenly realize that it is time you ought to be starting the course. Booking a place as soon as you know you are pregnant is a wise move. You could also ask if there is a local support network through which you could meet mothers with small babies.

An NCT antenatal class offers many opportunities for you to prepare fully for the birth of your baby

As mentioned in Chapter 6, Looking After Yourself, active birth classes are exercise-based classes aiming to keep you fit and supple during pregnancy, in preparation for labour and birth. The emphasis will normally be on exercising, but most teachers also cover essential information about labour and early parenthood.

Active birth classes

VISITING THE HOSPITAL

If your baby will be born in hospital, you will be invited to go on a tour of the hospital at some point during your pregnancy, often as part of the NHS antenatal classes. Not all hospitals invite fathers as well, so, if you are expecting your partner to take you into hospital when you are in labour, it is useful for you both to visit the hospital at some time, so that he at least knows where the Maternity Unit is, and if there is a separate, different door to be used at night.

Even if you are not attending the hospital classes, a tour of the Maternity Unit will give you a good feel of the place, provide an opportunity to ask questions and see the rooms and equipment, and help you feel familiar with the place where your baby will be born. Most parents find the tour reasonably reassuring, though the appearance of the delivery rooms, delivery bed, and sometimes the wards can come as a surprise. It is probably preferable to experience that moment of surprise before you enter the hospital in labour.

ARRANGEMENTS FOR WHEN YOU GO INTO LABOUR

Contacting your partner

You may feel anxious that you might be unable to contact your partner when you eventually go into labour, particularly if your partner commutes, travels frequently, or is often away from his main place of work. In fact, most men actually spend more time at home than away over the whole week, if you include weekends and night-times. If you are worried, it is possible to hire radio-pagers for a month or so around your expected date of delivery. Some men also prefer to limit their travelling when the baby is due, if they are often several hours' journey away. For most, it should be enough to make sure you know where he expects to be, or where he can be contacted day by day.

If you are concerned that your partner may not be available immediately, you might like to consider if there is anyone else you might ask to take you into hospital and perhaps act as your labour companion if you would like that.

Transport

If you are expecting to travel to hospital in your own car, you will need to make sure your petrol tank is going to manage the journey too.

Care of your other children

This can be a source of worry, especially if you have no nearby relatives who can readily look after your children. You could ask a friend or neighbour to look after the children or, if you go into labour during the night, to come and sleep at your house. Few people refuse such a request.

Some parents arrange to drop their child off *en route* for the hospital, but not all young children are happy to be left in someone else's house for a long while without mummy or daddy. There may also be occasions when there is little time for anything but heading straight for the hospital!

The arrangements which work best are those of which you feel confident, so that you can relax and concentrate on your labour without worrying about your other children.

If you are intending to give birth at home, you may also like to consider having a friend or relative in to look after your children, even during the night, in case they wake up and need attention. You may be needing your partner at that particular moment, and not wish him to have to leave you for the child.

It is useful to keep a list of 'emergency' telephone numbers next to the phone for a week or two beforehand — hospital, GP, midwife, your parents, neighbours — so that, when anything does happen, you will not have to go rummaging around the house searching for the right telephone number while coping with contractions. Your partner may find the list useful too, should he have to make the calls when you are busy concentrating on your contractions.

Phone numbers

It is also useful to have phone numbers in your diary by any appointments you or your partner makes over these weeks; that way you can contact him quickly should he not be at his usual number; and he can cancel any appointments you are unable to keep because you are in hospital.

PACKING YOUR BAGS

It is wisest to have your bags packed by 37 weeks, to avoid last-minute panics. You will need a suitcase or holdall of things for your stay in hospital, a separate carrier of any items you want for the labour, and a bag of going-home clothes for yourself and your baby. If you are going in on a six-hour discharge, you will obviously need going-home clothes in your suitcase.

For the hospital stay

Most hospitals issue a reasonably comprehensive list of necessities for the stay, and obviously different hospitals have different arrangements for the provision of nappies, sanitary towels, baby clothes, and the like.

Suggestions for your suitcase:

- ☑ **MONEY**
- ☑ **WASHING-KIT**
- ☑ **NIGHTDRESSES**
- ☑ **DRESSING-GOWN**
- ☑ **SLIPPERS**
- ☑ **BRAS**

☑ **SANITARY TOWELS**
☑ **PANTS**
☑ **DAY CLOTHES FOR YOURSELF**
☑ **BOX OF TISSUES**
☑ **BOOK, MAGAZINES, ETC.**
☑ **LETTER-WRITING EQUIPMENT**
☑ **ADDRESS BOOK AND LIST OF PEOPLE TO RING WITH YOUR NEWS!**
☑ **CLEANING MATERIALS FOR BATHS, BIDETS, ETC. (SEE CHAPTER 22, EARLY DAYS)**
☑ **ANTISEPTIC OR ALCOHOL WIPES FOR LAVATORY SEATS, AND/ OR PAPER LAVATORY-SEAT COVERS**
☑ **A CLEAN WASHING-UP LIQUID CONTAINER TO USE AS A WATER SPRAY (SEE CHAPTER 22, EARLY DAYS)**
☑ **CARTONS OF FRUIT DRINK**
☑ **NAPPIES**
☑ **BABY CLOTHES**

MONEY You will need plenty of change for the phone, but otherwise money is best kept to a minimum.

NIGHTDRESSES Choose light cotton nightdresses, as hospitals are notoriously hot, sticky places. If you will be breastfeeding, choose ones which will be easy to feed in. You may prefer not to wear your very best nightdress in the first twenty-four hours or so after delivery, as it may become rather blood-stained. You will probably need more nightdresses than you imagine, unless you have very good arrangements for getting your clothes washed.

DRESSING-GOWN A dressing-gown is not an essential, but is useful as a cover-up. Again, choose a light one.

BRAS Most women prefer to wear a well-fitting bra when they first start breastfeeding. You will need at least two and preferably more to avoid hurried washing and drying. Do make sure you try a bra on before buying it, as the fit will be important. The NCT sells feeding bras in various styles and sizes which can be fitted any time after 36 weeks, ready for when you begin feeding. You may also like to wear a 'sleep' bra at night for comfort.

SANITARY TOWELS Most hospitals only provide a few sanitary towels, if any, nowadays; maybe the first ten, or the first day's worth. Choose heavy-duty ones for the first few days.

PANTS Your pants are liable to become rather stained in the early days after giving birth, so you might take old ones you do not mind throwing out afterwards, or use disposable ones (difficult to find a comfortable fit for most people, but men's sizes tend to be marginally better). Those supplied by the NCT Maternity Sales Ltd. are excellent. They are not glamorous by any stretch of the imagination, but will comfortably and securely hold a sanitary towel in place without putting pressure on your abdomen. They can also be washed out and dried quickly and easily.

DAY CLOTHES Many hospitals now encourage mothers to wear their own clothes rather than nightdresses during their stay. This helps women feel less like patients recovering from an illness and more like human beings. Loose-fitting, light, comfortable clothes with easy access for breastfeeding are best. Tracksuits, baggy T-shirts, leggings, light dresses are all useful.

Some women prefer to wear nightdresses anyway, as they will be either in or on the bed much of the time and feel clothes may be too warm. Women who choose to go home early often stay in their nightclothes for a few days in case other members of the family should think they might be ready to carry on as normal!

Labour bag

If you keep this separate, it will not matter if there is no room for your suitcase in the delivery room. You will find suggestions for what you might like to take in your labour bag in Chapter 14, Preparing for Labour.

Coming home

Unless your partner is very clued up as to the whereabouts of all your clothes and the baby's, it is reasonable to get these ready yourself before you go in. Clothes for the baby are fairly obvious: nappy, vest, and stretch suit, plus a cardigan if it is cold, and an outdoor suit or warm wrap, remembering that she will be going outside for the journey home.

For yourself, if you have been wearing your own clothes in hospital anyway, there is no problem. If you have not, this is not the best time to try on your really tight, close-fitting clothes, slim though you may feel, and delighted though you may be at the loss of your 'bump'. It takes the majority of women many weeks and months to regain their previous figures, and it is safer to allow for the worst rather than risk severe disappointment or an extremely uncomfortable journey home in tight trousers.

PREPARING FOR LIFE WITH A NEW BABY

It is virtually impossible to imagine the precise impact your baby will have on your domestic arrangements until she arrives. However you currently organize your household chores — the cooking, shopping, cleaning, washing, etc. — you will inevitably have less time once there is a baby to care for. Most mothers find they can manage little more than simply looking after themselves and the baby in the early weeks and have neither time, energy, nor inclination for housework.

With this in mind, it may be useful to discuss in advance how you and your partner each feels about the state of the house. In most relationships there is one who tends to mind more about the tidiness of the sitting-room or the stickiness of the kitchen floor. Perhaps sorting out priorities now, and keeping to just those one or two chores you might come to feel desperate about, would help. The main focus of concentration will be yourself and your new baby. Most other things can wait. Or be done by somebody else!

If you have a freezer, one idea is to make double quantities of pies, casseroles, or any other suitable dishes, over the last few weeks of pregnancy. Freezing half each time provides a good stock of emergency meals for those days when you cannot seem to get anything much done and you are fed up with take-aways. Meals that will not need much cutting-up are useful too, as babies invariably wake up for a bit of attention just as you are starting a meal — they seem to like the smell of food too! Few couples, if any, escape readjustments to their living arrangements when a baby arrives. The more you can discuss — and preferably agree on — some basic ground rules first, the smoother the transition can be. Once your baby is here, talking over any problems or difficulties as they crop up will prevent real resentment or annoyances building up to unmanageable proportions.

BREASTFEEDING

Alongside all these practical matters and the general preparation for your baby's birth, it is a good idea to start thinking now about how you would like to feed your baby. You will find information about both breast- and bottlefeeding in Chapter 24, Feeding your Baby, to help you make your decision.

Whatever preparations you make during pregnancy will be aimed at relieving you of any worry or anxiety to do with the birth, or how you will cope with the new baby afterwards. How much you get yourself organized, therefore, depends on how much you think your mind will be set at rest by being well organized first. Relaxing and enjoying your pregnancy, and later your baby, is ultimately far more important than having a spotless home with everything neatly in its place. Discuss your needs now, and in anticipation find out what your partner thinks, feels, and wants, and work from there. It is not all hard work — plan to enjoy it as much as you can.

* *I hadn't realized how unprepared I was till I started going to classes and found the other mothers so apparently well-organized already.*

* *It was a great relief to go to classes and find I wasn't the only one feeling like that — it put a lot of worries into perspective.* *

* *I made silly little lists all over the place: jobs to be done; phone numbers for Mike, for me, for my mother; things for my suit-case, for my labour bag . . .* *

* *Last time we talked for ages about how we'd cope after the baby arrived. In the end, Stuart took some time off immediately I came out of hospital, then my mum came to stay when he went back to work. Basically, she looked after the house and Mark [older child], while I looked after myself and the baby. It worked well enough, but this time I'd like to see if we can manage by ourselves.* *

Part 2
BIRTH

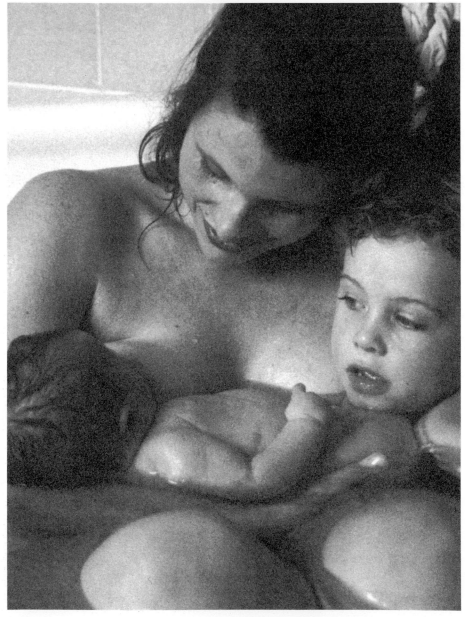

ANATOMY AND PHYSIOLOGY OF LABOUR

Labour is the process of childbirth, during which the baby is born. There are three stages to labour, each of which has a specific function. During the first stage of labour the cervix opens; during the second

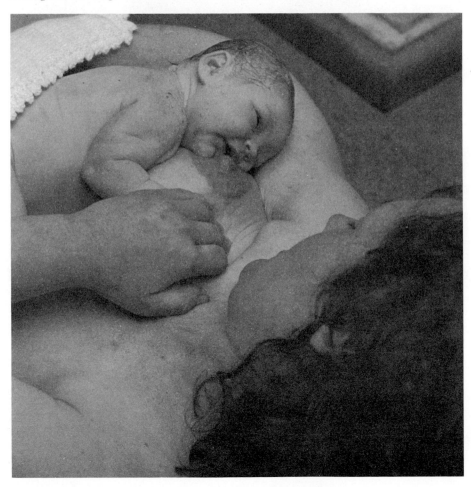

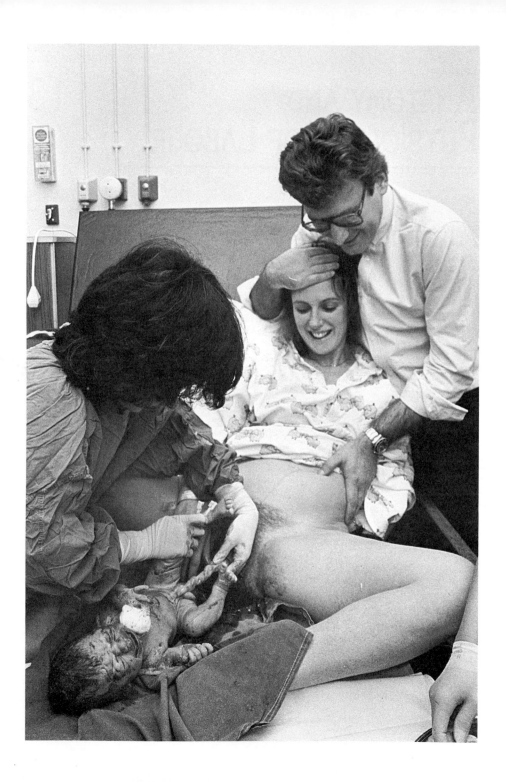

stage the uterus pushes the baby out of the pelvis and through the vaginal opening; during the third stage the placenta is delivered and the uterus begins to return to its non-pregnant state.

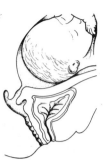

APPROACHING LABOUR

Various changes occur during the last weeks of pregnancy, not the least being the psychological changes for both partners as the baby's birth approaches.

As your hormones prepare for labour, you may experience any of the following signs:

The cervix and uterus before labour begins; the cervix is closed and hangs in the vagina

○ YOU MAY BECOME MORE AWARE OF THE BRAXTON HICKS CONTRACTIONS WHICH HAVE BEEN OCCURRING EVERY TWENTY MINUTES THROUGHOUT PREGNANCY, KEEPING THE MUSCLE OF THE UTERUS TONED. THESE MAY NOW BE MORE DEFINITELY FELT AS A TIGHTENING OF THE ABDOMEN. TOWARDS THE END OF PREGNANCY THE UTERUS WILL BECOME THICKER TOWARDS THE TOP AND THINNER AT THE BOTTOM IN PREPARATION FOR THE BIRTH.

○ YOU MAY FEEL BOTH PHYSICALLY TIRED TOWARDS THE END OF PREGNANCY AND EMOTIONALLY MORE THAN READY FOR YOUR PREGNANCY TO BE AT AN END.

○ YOU MAY EXPERIENCE A SURGE OF ENERGY A DAY OR TWO BEFORE GOING INTO LABOUR, FINDING ENERGY AND INCLINATION FOR TASKS SUCH AS CLEANING THE HOUSE, TURNING OUT CUPBOARDS, OR WEEDING THE GARDEN.

○ YOU MAY HAVE A STRONG NESTING INSTINCT, ENCOURAGING YOU TO MAKE SURE THAT EVERYTHING IS READY IN PREPA-RATION FOR LABOUR AND YOUR BABY'S BIRTH.

○ YOU MAY HAVE MILD DIARRHOEA OR, LESS COMMONLY, VOMIT-ING, FOR A DAY OR MORE BEFORE LABOUR BEGINS. THIS IS YOUR BODY'S WAY OF CLEARING OUT THE SYSTEM FOR LABOUR AND OFTEN OCCURS IN EARLY LABOUR AS WELL.

○ A SMALL WEIGHT LOSS OF 1–1½ KG. (2 OR 3 LB.) IS COMMON IN THE LAST WEEK OR TWO BEFORE THE BIRTH, AND IS CAUSED BY REDUCTION OF THE BLOOD CIRCULATION AND LESS FLUID RETENTION.

○ YOU MAY BEGIN TO FEEL EXTREMELY IMPATIENT FOR YOUR LABOUR TO START AND YOUR BABY TO BE BORN.

○ YOU MAY FEEL A SENSE OF CALM ACCEPTANCE OR RESIGNA-TION AS YOU APPROACH THE BIRTH.

○ YOU MAY ALREADY BE AWARE OF YOUR BABY'S HEAD PRESSING DOWN ON YOUR CERVIX, EVEN BEFORE LABOUR BEGINS.

THE ONSET OF LABOUR

There are three signs which signal that labour is imminent or is just beginning and these symptoms may occur in any order or combination.

THE SHOW As the cervix starts to soften (or 'ripen') and open a little, the plug of mucus which has sealed it during pregnancy comes away, and with it a little blood from between the uterus and the membranes of the amniotic sac. You may notice this as a pinkish discharge when you go to the lavatory. The show may occur up to two weeks before labour actually begins, or immediately before; it varies, but is a sign that your uterus is beginning to get ready for labour. You may not notice your show at all, as it often comes away during the actual labour, possibly when the membranes rupture.

CONTRACTIONS Contractions are the muscular tightenings of the uterus, controlled by the hormone oxytocin, which open and pull up the cervix, thus making the passage through which your baby will leave the uterus. During a contraction your uterus becomes hard and appears to bulge forward.

RECOGNIZING LABOUR CONTRACTIONS First-stage contractions might be experienced as:

○ MILD TO INTENSE PAINS IN THE ABDOMEN, RATHER LIKE PERIOD PAINS
○ BACKACHE
○ PAIN SIMILAR TO ABDOMINAL CRAMP
○ PAINS IN THE HIPS, ON THE INSIDE OR OUTSIDE OF THE LEGS, OR IN THE KNEES
○ PAINS IN THE RECTUM SIMILAR TO CONSTIPATION

THE BREAKING OF THE WATERS For 10 per cent of women, the breaking of the waters, or 'rupture of the membranes', is the first indication that labour is imminent. It occurs when the membranes of the amniotic sac, which contains the amniotic fluid, rupture, allowing the fluid to leak out. It can be either a gush or a trickle, depending on where the membranes have ruptured. If the bulge of membranes in front of your baby's head, or presenting part, ruptures, you will feel a gush of water. If, however, the hind waters further up the uterus rupture, you will notice only a gentle trickle. The breaking of the waters is painless, though you may be aware of a feeling of pressure immediately beforehand. Some women feel a distinct 'pop' or 'ping' and then a gush of surprisingly warm, clear fluid with its own distinctive smell. It may be hard to tell if your waters have really gone if you have only a trickle, as it could so easily be either urine or some vaginal discharge. If you are unsure, your doctor or midwife can test whether the fluid is amniotic fluid or not.

Once the membranes have broken, the baby's barrier against infection is no longer present, and most doctors prefer labour to have started within twenty four hours.

In the great majority of women, the waters will break spontaneously towards the end of the first stage of labour as the descending baby puts extra pressure on the membranes.

It can be difficult to be sure when you really are in labour, particularly if you have been experiencing very strong and regular Braxton Hicks contractions towards the end of pregnancy.

Recognizing labour

FALSE LABOUR Sometimes women experience 'false labour', when contractions appear to start, but then fade away without the increase in length, intensity, and frequency; this can continue at intervals for as long as two weeks, and is often due to the uterus contracting whilst manoeuvring the baby's head into a favourable position in the pelvis. These 'false-labour' contractions are usually part of the prelude to labour and an indication that the labour will get going very soon. It is, however, extremely frustrating if you keep thinking your baby is on the way, only for your contractions to die down again.

FIRST-STAGE CONTRACTIONS First-stage labour contractions differ from Braxton Hicks contractions in a number of ways:

- THE CONTRACTIONS BECOME GRADUALLY STRONGER, LONGER, AND CLOSER TOGETHER AS TIME PASSES.
- THE UPPER PART OF THE UTERUS MOVES FORWARD PERCEPTIBLY DURING CONTRACTIONS, AND BY KEEPING YOUR HAND ON YOUR ABDOMEN YOU CAN USE THIS MOVEMENT TO HELP YOU RECOGNIZE WHEN A CONTRACTION IS COMING.
- EACH CONTRACTION BUILDS UP TO A PEAK OF INTENSITY IN THE MIDDLE AND THEN DIES AWAY AGAIN.

THE FIRST STAGE OF LABOUR

In the first stage of labour contractions open or 'dilate' the cervix to 10 cm. wide, the size needed for your baby's head to be pushed out of the uterus. First stage may last eight to sixteen hours with a first baby, but may be shorter or longer than this. Labour tends to be shorter with second and subsequent babies. These timings are, of course, only a guide; each labour is entirely individual.

Contractions

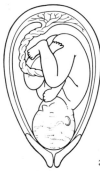

Labour contractions differ from any other muscle contractions because, as the contractions proceed, the muscle fibres of which the uterus is composed become progressively shorter and thicker, gradually reducing the size of the uterus. At the same time, the contractions thin (efface), open (dilate), and pull up the cervix. Unlike other muscular contractions, the labouring uterus will not return to its original state when a contraction is over, but will gradually continue to dilate the cervix and reduce in size, pushing the baby deeper into the pelvis.

Contractions might last ten seconds and be thirty minutes apart at the beginning of the first stage; by the end they may be lasting for sixty seconds and be only two minutes apart. You may be surprised to find your labour *begins* with contractions which are only three minutes apart, but of no great intensity. If this happens, you will need to observe the duration and strength of each contraction as your guide to your labour's progress rather than taking the gap between your contractions as your reference point. The timing of contractions varies from woman to woman, but there will usually be an increase in length, frequency, and intensity as labour progresses.

Early 1st-stage labour: the cervix is partly effaced, but dilatation has not yet begun

Most women find labour painful to some extent; contractions used to be called 'labour pains'. Pain in labour is thought to be due to referred pain from the uterus, which itself has no nerve endings so cannot feel pain, and to the ischaemia (lack of blood) in the abdominal tissues caused by the uterine contractions. The precise place where the labour contractions are experienced will depend on an individual's pain pathways, and how the baby is lying.

Early contractions may be experienced as low, intermittent backache or as resembling a period pain. As labour progresses and the contractions become more frequent and intense, they may be felt more towards the top of your uterus, demanding all your concentration and energy.

Some women, however, though they experience labour as uncomfortable, or are aware of something 'happening', would hesitate to describe their sensations as painful. Whatever the nature of the experience, most women find being in some sort of upright position reduces their pain or discomfort.

You will find further discussion of the nature of pain in labour, and how you might deal with it, in Chapter 14, Preparing for Labour, and Chapter 16, Pain Relief in Labour.

The dilatation of the cervix from 0 to 10 cm. is not an even process. Many women are 2 cm. dilated before labour even starts, but then take a long time to reach 10 cm. One woman may progress slowly from, say, 2 to 6 cm., but then swiftly to 10 cm. Another may progress quickly to 5 cm., get 'stuck' for a while, progress quickly to 8 cm. and more slowly again to 10 cm. Any pattern is possible, and every labour is unique.

A woman having her second or subsequent baby may find her cervix dilates rapidly, particularly once she has reached 5 or 6 cm. dilatation. It is possible, for instance, for the cervix to dilate from 7 to 10 cm. in only ten or twenty minutes, which may come as rather a surprise for everyone involved.

As the cervix nears 10 cm. dilatation, the baby's head will descend further into the pelvis, and at 10 cm. the cervix will usually have disappeared behind the baby's ears so that it can no longer be felt in a vaginal examination.

The baby's head pressing down on to the cervix helps the cervix dilate both mechanically (imagine it as being like pushing your head through a polo-neck sweater — both your head and the sweater play a part in the process), and also by stimulating the production of the hormone oxytocin, which strengthens contractions. Gravity can clearly assist this process, as it brings the baby's head firmly down on to your cervix.

As long as the amniotic sac is intact, it will even out the pressure on the baby's head. When the waters break, contractions often intensify as the direct pressure of the baby's head on the cervix increases the production of oxytocin, and therefore the intensity of the contractions.

Unless you have been specifically advised otherwise, you can carry on with your normal activities until your contractions are lasting for about forty-five seconds or until you feel uncomfortable and feel you would rather move to where your baby will be born. If you are unsure, phone the Labour Ward, when you will be able to talk with a midwife who can help you decide if you need to come in or will be better off staying at home for a while. You will also need to take into account the time of day, conditions, and the length of your journey when considering the best time to leave for hospital.

TRANSITION

This phase of labour, between the first and second stages, is not recognized by every midwife or doctor, or by every woman in labour. Physiologically, it is the time when the hormones are preparing the woman's uterus to change its contractions from those which dilate the cervix, to those which push the baby out — the expulsive contractions. The change in hormones can cause changes in a woman before she has reached second stage, and therefore before her cervix is fully dilated.

Cervical dilatation

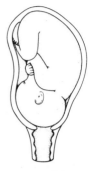

1st-stage labour: early dilatation of the cervix — the cervix is now fully effaced and dilated to approximately 4 cm.

When to go into hospital

1st-stage labour: the cervix is approximately 8 cm. dilated

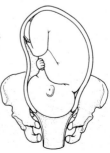

Recognizing transition

Transition may be experienced in one or more of the following ways, or not at all:

○ YOU MAY FIND YOUR CONTRACTIONS SUDDENLY HAVE NO REAL PATTERN.

○ YOU MAY SUDDENLY LOSE YOUR ABILITY TO KEEP THINGS IN PERSPECTIVE.

○ YOU MAY NO LONGER BE ABLE TO KEEP ON TOP OF YOUR CONTRACTIONS.

○ YOU MAY FEEL NAUSEOUS.

○ YOU MAY VOMIT OR HAVE DIARRHOEA.

○ YOU MAY SHAKE UNCONTROLLABLY.

○ YOU MAY EXPERIENCE EXTREME FEELINGS OF HOT OR COLD.

○ YOU MAY FIND YOURSELF VERY CONFUSED MENTALLY; YOU MAY WANT TO GO HOME, FEEL IRRITATED WITH THOSE AROUND YOU, AND FIND IT DIFFICULT TO CO-OPERATE.

○ YOU MAY EXPERIENCE A PREMATURE URGE TO PUSH THE BABY OUT BEFORE YOUR CERVIX IS FULLY DILATED. THIS MAY BE CAUSED BY THE HORMONES FOR THE SECOND STAGE TAKING OVER A LITTLE EARLY, OR A REFLEX RESPONSE TO THE BABY'S HEAD PRESSING ON TO YOUR RECTUM.

○ YOU MAY FIND CONTRACTIONS MAY STOP COMPLETELY FOR AS LONG AS 30–40 MINUTES; TAKE THIS OPPORTUNITY TO REST.

Although many of the symptoms of transition sound rather unpleasant, you are most unlikely to experience all of them, and if your midwife or companion can remind you that they indicate that your baby will soon be born, this can ease some of the negative feelings you may experience.

Your labour companions may observe such strong emotional reactions and wish to help in a positive and supportive way. It is, however, very common for a woman not to want to be touched at this time, which can be particularly difficult for a labour partner who would like to comfort her.

A 'LIP' Sometimes, with or without the premature urge to push, the cervix may have dilated unevenly around the baby's head, leaving a 'lip' which can still be felt: the lip is 'anterior' if it is at the front of your pelvis, and 'posterior' if it is at the back. If you do push vigorously on to an incompletely dilated cervix, it might become swollen and thus take a little longer to recede, but it will eventually dilate fully.

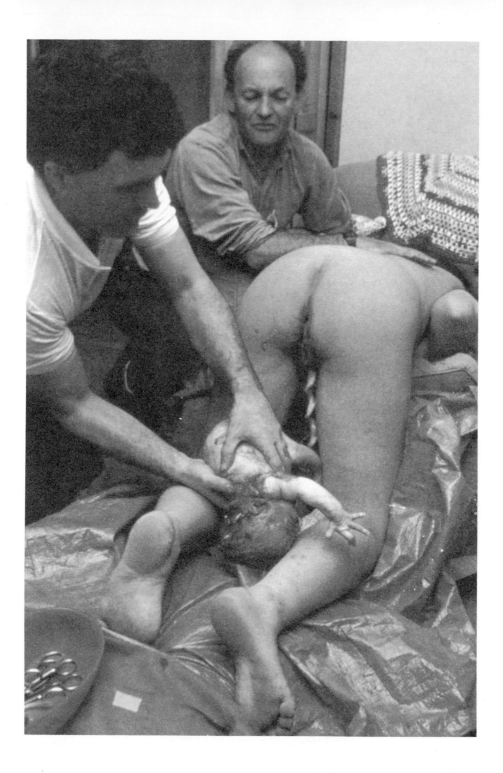

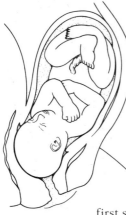

2nd-stage labour:
full dilatation of
the cervix, and
descent of the baby
down the birth
canal

THE SECOND STAGE OF LABOUR

Although some doctors will still describe the onset of second stage as being when the woman is fully dilated, many midwives consider second stage to be under way when the woman experiences a strong desire to push her baby out. Those midwives who perform very few vaginal examinations, relying instead on their knowledge and understanding of women in labour through close observation, will not know whether or not the cervix is fully dilated, but will consider second stage to have begun when the woman indicates that she wants to push.

As you move into second stage, your contractions may be further apart than at the end of the first stage; instead of having a peak of intensity, they may feel about the same all the way through.

○ **YOU MAY HAVE COMPLETELY DIFFERENT SENSATIONS OF INTENSITY OR PAIN FROM THOSE OF THE FIRST STAGE.**
○ **YOU MAY FEEL A STRONG URGE TO BEAR DOWN.**
○ **YOU MAY FEEL AS THOUGH YOU ARE ABOUT TO HAVE A BOWEL MOVEMENT.**
○ **YOU MAY FEEL VERY EXCITED, FULL OF RENEWED ENERGY, AND READY TO WORK WITH YOUR BODY IN GIVING BIRTH TO YOUR BABY.**

Recognizing second stage

There is no longer any resistance from the cervix, and each contraction will push the baby a fraction of the way along the birth canal.

From full dilatation of the cervix to the birth of the baby may take as long as four hours or may last just a few contractions. Second and subsequent babies are usually born much more quickly than first babies.

WHAT HAPPENS IN SECOND STAGE Mechanically, two things happen in second stage: first the baby comes out of the bony pelvis and round an angle into the vagina (rather like a foot going down into a Wellington boot); then it comes down the vagina, under the pubic bone, and through the opening in the pelvic floor. Midwives and doctors call this path the 'birth canal'; this sounds impressive, but it is in fact only about 10 cm. long!

The fit of the baby's head through the outlet of the pelvis is very snug and this is helped in a number of ways:

○ THE BONES OF THE BABY'S SKULL ARE SOFT AND NOT
FUSED, SO THAT, AS THE BABY'S HEAD PASSES
THROUGH THE PELVIS AND VAGINA, IT IS MADE UP
TO 1 CM. SMALLER BY CHANGING SHAPE (MOULD-
ING) WITH THE BONES OVERLAPPING.
○ THE PREGNANCY HORMONES HAVE SOFTENED THE
LIGAMENTS IN THE PELVIC JOINTS SO THAT THE
PELVIS CAN BECOME A LITTLE BIGGER.
○ THE BABY IS POSITIONED SO THAT IT CAN BEST USE
THE WIDEST MEASUREMENTS OF THE PELVIS.

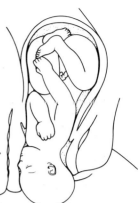

At the beginning of the second stage the baby usually has
its head down and is beginning to turn to face its
mother's back. With its head bent towards its chest (or
flexed), the narrowest part of its head will go through the
narrowest part of the pelvic outlet, and negotiate the angle
between the cervix and vagina in this sideways position. As the
head comes into contact with the pelvic-floor muscles, it rotates
to face the mother's spine, leaving the rest of the body to go
through the pelvic outlet sideways, the neck twisted 90 degrees.
The head then comes under the pubic bone and through the
vaginal opening and, as the neck unbends, the baby is born.

*2nd-stage labour:
crowning of the
baby's head*

Once the head is born, before the next contraction, the baby
turns its head to straighten its neck so it is facing to the side
again. Then, with the next contraction, the baby's shoulders are
born, one at a time, turning as the head did, and followed by the
rest of its body.

All this time, the uterus has been contracting, doing 80 per
cent of the work of pushing out the baby. Often women only
get the urge to push once the head has made contact with
the pelvic floor. The accordion-like folds of the vagina
gradually stretch as the baby's head comes down and the
outside tissues of the perineum gradually fan out. It can be
frustrating to watch the baby's head come down during
contractions and then disappear when they are over, but this
slow, gentle movement, 'two steps forward, one step back',
enables the tissues of the pelvic floor to stretch to accommodate
the baby.

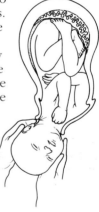

*Delivery of the
baby's head*

As the baby feels air on its skin, the change in temperature causes
it to take a breath and fill its lungs. Sometimes it takes a little time
for the baby to breathe for itself: while the umbilical cord is still
attached to the placenta, it continues to pulsate, maintaining the
baby's oxygen supply until breathing is established. When the cord
stops pulsating, the surge of oxytocin which women have at delivery
causes the now empty uterus to contract down strongly.

Delivery

THE THIRD STAGE

The final stage of labour is the delivery of the placenta. If you have been given an injection to speed up the third stage (see Chapter 15, Medical Procedures, for more information), this procedure may take as little as ten minutes. If the third stage has been a physiological, or non-managed one, it may take longer, possibly half an hour or more.

As the uterus becomes smaller, the side of the placenta attached to the uterus crumples (rather as a label stuck to an inflated balloon does as the balloon is deflated) and the placenta peels away. The 'living ligatures', the maternal blood vessels to the placenta which have been left exposed by the delivery of the placenta, are closed as the uterus continues to decrease in size. Once the placenta has dropped into the lower part of the uterus, it is expelled with the next contraction, together with the membranes. Delivery of the placenta can take anything from a few minutes to two hours; it is assisted by the mother being in an upright position and the baby being held and, if it wishes, suckled, to increase production of the mother's oxytocin and therefore the strength of the contractions. The cord can then be cut and the baby is an independent human being.

3rd-stage labour: the placenta separates as the uterus continues to contract

RETURNING TO NORMAL

For two or three weeks after delivery the uterus will continue to decrease in size, until it is slightly larger than its pre-pregnancy state. During this time the site where the placenta was attached continues to bleed, until it has healed; this blood loss is called the 'lochia' and may be found to increase during breastfeeds, when the oxytocin stimulated by the baby's suckling causes the uterus to contract down a little.

PREPARING FOR LABOUR 14

Having a baby is both hard physical work and emotionally demanding. As with any experience which involves mental and physical stamina, preparation for labour and birth can help you make the most of your experience and respond positively to the challenge. Nobody intending to run a long distance or climb a mountain would set off without having given some thought to the route, the conditions, her own physical preparedness, and her aspirations. In a similar way, preparing for labour gives you the opportunity to approach childbirth with confidence, armed with the resources that will help you cope and make whatever decisions feel right at the time.

Preparing for labour in a way which maximizes the use of your own resources involves more than attending classes and reading a few books, useful though these are. By practising the positions and breathing exercises learned in classes and from this book, and discovering from the people around you how labour was for them and what they found helpful, you can gradually build up a picture of the range of possibilities for the course of labour, and the options for dealing with them. Sometimes pregnant women are afraid of 'horror stories', and these are occasionally forced on them willy-nilly, but you will often find that every negative birth experience is balanced by a positive one, if you keep asking and listening. Being bombarded by other women's stories is not necessarily a bad thing if you are able to use them to help prepare yourself for your own baby's birth.

The important thing to remember about self-help for labour is that it can be used both at home and in hospital, and even in the car or ambulance taking you there! Different options will be helpful at different times in labour, so if something has stopped working for you, try something else; keep a wide range of tactics up your sleeve, ready to call upon at any time.

THE ROLE OF THE PARTNER
The majority of women giving birth nowadays are accompanied by the father of their child. This is a recent development and in other countries and other cultures is considered unthinkable, especially

where birth is considered to be essentially a female activity. In this country, however, most fathers and their partners have found their presence at the birth a positive, encouraging factor, and, where the father plays an active role, he is usually described afterwards by both the mother and the midwives as 'wonderful'. It is common to hear newly delivered women say they would not have managed as they did without their partner's help. Sometimes, however, the father's presence is not possible, or a woman and her partner decide it would be better for him not to be there. In such a case, the woman might choose another labour partner, such as her mother, sister, or friend, with whom she feels comfortable. Few women choose to labour alone these days, without a close and trusted companion.

Whoever the labour partner is, it is important that he (or she) is clear about his role: whether he will merely observe or will play a more positive part in supporting the woman. In the latter case, he will need to learn and work with the woman to be an effective support. Reading this book is a good start, and accompanying the woman to NCT and/or NHS classes is ideal. Many labour companions feel anxious that they may end up feeling helpless, like a 'spare part', unsure of how to help. Preparing with your partner will also help you to feel more confident of your role. Labour is certainly not the best moment to be discussing for the first time what you would like your labour companion to be doing to help and support you.

Once labour has started, it is important for the partner to be sensitive to the woman's needs whilst remaining aware of his own, in particular keeping up his energy by taking regular breaks and adequate food and drink. It is also worth remembering to dress appropriately for the heat of a hospital. It is unusual for labour companions to faint, but, if they do, it is more often the result of too little rest, too low a blood-sugar level, or simple overheating than any other cause.

Sometimes the role of the partner is to stand by and do nothing, and to remember that his presence alone makes the woman's experience a better one. Often a labour partner can talk in detail to medical staff about procedures if the woman prefers not to at that moment, or he may liaise with the medical carers on her behalf. Most women find communication with other people difficult during contractions; sometimes a partner's role is to remind other people of this. Often the partner's most important job is to remind the woman of ways in which she can help herself cope with her labour contractions: it may be easier for the partner to think of all the things they had discussed using and doing to help the progress of the labour.

Sometimes a woman goes into labour alone and then the midwife attending her plays a more actively supportive role than when a partner is present. Many midwives enjoy the chance to be a woman's sole birth attendant and use their experience to meet the woman's needs for non-medical support most effectively.

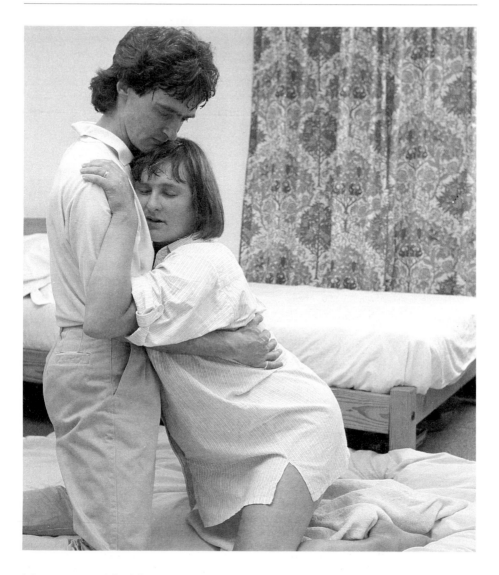

THE FIRST STAGE

There are four main ways of coping with contractions:

- ○ **MAINTAINING AN UPRIGHT POSITION**
- ○ **RELAXATION**
- ○ **BREATHING CALMLY AND REGULARLY**
- ○ **TOUCH**

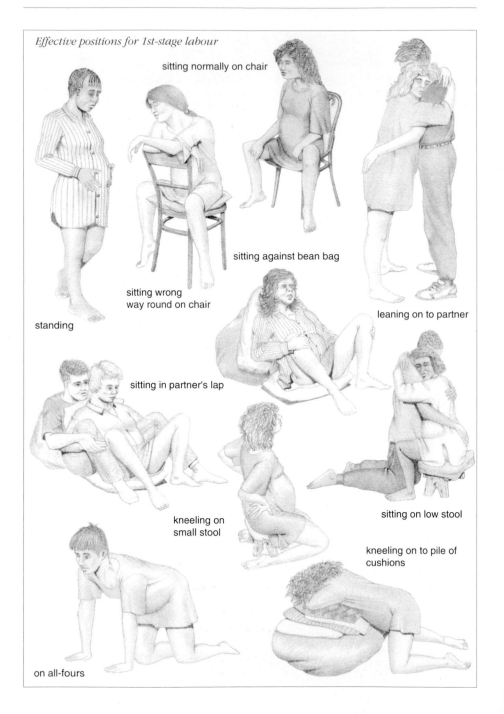

Effective positions for 1st-stage labour

sitting normally on chair

sitting against bean bag

sitting wrong way round on chair

leaning on to partner

standing

sitting in partner's lap

kneeling on small stool

sitting on low stool

kneeling on to pile of cushions

on all-fours

All of these need to be practised and thought about during pregnancy to be fully effective in labour.

In each stage of labour, being in an upright position enables a woman's body to work at its maximum efficiency, using gravity as an aid. Most women find that being in an upright position in labour is less painful than lying down. Leaning forward is also often very helpful. Lying on one's back can be positively harmful for the baby, as the weight of the uterus compresses major blood vessels, reducing the oxygen supply. If you want to lie down (perhaps if labour starts slowly and you would like to try to sleep to conserve energy for later, or if you are very tired in between contractions later in labour), remember to lie on one side rather than on your back. In early labour, walking around will help strengthen contractions, but as labour grows stronger, many women find they take up progressively lower positions and become more reluctant to move. It is important to try not to become static in any one position for too long, so that the cervix has a better chance of dilating evenly.

Hourly visits to the lavatory to keep your bladder emptied, whether you feel the need or not, can help here, as can the sensitive help of a labour partner. In fact, encouraging a woman to keep mobile during labour, to try to change her position frequently, and to remind her to empty her bladder are important roles for any labour companion. Whatever position you are in, moving your body (such as rotating your hips when standing or on all-fours), can also lessen pain and is very soothing for most women, who often find themselves moving instinctively.

Positions for labour

Positions for first stage

- ○ STANDING
- ○ LEANING FORWARD AGAINST A WALL, PIECE OF FURNITURE, OR YOUR PARTNER
- ○ SITTING UPRIGHT ON AN ORDINARY, ROCKING, OR BIRTHING CHAIR
- ○ SITTING ASTRIDE AN UPRIGHT CHAIR, LEANING ON THE BACK PADDED WITH A CUSHION OR PILLOW
- ○ SITTING ON A SOFA OR BED, LEANING ON TO A PILE OF PILLOWS ON YOUR LAP, OR ON TO A BEAN-BAG
- ○ SITTING IN YOUR PARTNER'S LAP, KNEES WELL APART
- ○ SITTING ON A LOW STOOL OR TODDLER'S STEP, OR A PILE OF CUSHIONS, AND LEANING BACK AGAINST YOUR PARTNER OR FORWARD ON TO HIS LAP
- ○ KNEELING, KNEES APART, LEANING FORWARD ON TO A PIECE OF FURNITURE, PARTNER, OR LARGE PILE OF CUSHIONS
- ○ KNEELING ON ALL-FOURS
- ○ KNEELING DOWN WITH A SMALL STOOL OR TODDLER'S STEP SUPPORTING YOU UNDERNEATH YOUR BUTTOCKS

PRACTISING POSITIONS Practise positions in pregnancy (with your partner if possible); use the furniture at home and, on your tour of the labour ward, look at how you would use the furniture of the delivery room. This way your body will learn all sorts of ways of getting comfortable in labour. Remember to practise moving your body as well. You may find you and/or your partner invent positions of your own; many people do.

* *The contractions were coming every four or five minutes, and I found brisk walking up and down the best way to combat the pain.* *

* *At 10.00 they started again. Contractions every five minutes, some short, some up to fifty seconds. I was breathing deeply through them but found it easier to use a bending-over-the-bed or all-fours position to take them in.* *

* *The only position I was comfortable in was sitting on the edge of the bed, and I wouldn't move from there.* *

* *Ann [midwife] took us to a room where she already had the bed wheeled out and a mattress and bean-bag installed as we had planned. I reckoned that, even if the labour was painful, being high up on a bed wouldn't make it any easier, and at least Jim and I would be able to get at each other.* *

Relaxation   It is well established that fear of labour can create tension, which in turn can make birth more painful than it need be. There are several ways of preventing this fear-tension-pain syndrome from occurring. Finding out all you can about what can happen in labour can remove fear of the unknown, and finding out about what the obstetricians and midwives can do can remove fear of the unexpected. Learning about the way your body will work in labour so that you can visualize your cervix opening up and your baby descending in your pelvis is an important way of using your labour positively and helping yourself cope with contractions.

Sometimes a woman is not actually afraid of labour as such, but finds herself tensing up automatically as the pain of contractions builds up; the more tense she becomes, the greater the pain becomes: a downward spiral is set in motion. By being as relaxed as possible, by encouraging your body to release tension, to relax into your contractions, you need only experience the actual pain of labour, which is a positive pain. Remembering that the pain is positive — the only positive pain the human body experiences — is helpful too.

By being as relaxed as possible between contractions, you will be conserving your energy and will feel ready to take on the next contraction. It is also important for your labour partner to remain relaxed during labour; tense partners can make mothers tense too!

PRACTISING RELAXATION Any relaxation technique you know can usually be adapted to labour. The relaxation exercise on page 85 is suitable for coping with contractions. Practise relaxing for a few minutes each day in one of the positions for labour described above. Once you are in the position, think down your body, checking that each part of it is relaxed. If any part feels tense (neck and shoulders are often the first to grow tense), concentrate on breathing out and using your out-breaths to let any tension flow away from that part until you recognize that it feels relaxed. Keeping your mouth loose and relaxed will help your pelvic floor and vagina stay relaxed; this is useful throughout labour, but particularly so in second stage. Music may help you relax; some people find relaxation and yoga tapes useful, but this is a matter of personal preference. Visualizing a peaceful, relaxing scene may also help you relax — use your mind to imagine a favourite landscape, such as a beach or piece of countryside. Imagine yourself in a relaxing place where you feel safe — your own bedroom at home, a warm bath, your garden.

DARKNESS You may find it difficult to relax in a brightly lit hospital room, preferring to concentrate on your labour in darker conditions. Darkness can be achieved by closing your eyes, switching off and dimming lights, and closing curtains and blinds.

When you are in labour, you can use each contraction as a time for focusing on your body and your baby, greeting the challenge of contractions with your strength and resilience. Thinking of each contraction as one step nearer the birth of your baby can help you remember what they are actually for! It is better to try and take each contraction as it comes; deal with one at a time, neither looking back nor anticipating. Most women also find that working in short time spans helps, particularly as time can come to mean very little during labour. Try saying to yourself and your partner: 'I'll just see how the next ten minutes/half-hour/hour goes, then see how I feel.'

DISTRACTION TECHNIQUES Although you may prefer to concentrate intently on your contractions, letting your body go with each contraction, some women do find it helpful at times to use some form of distraction technique until the contraction is at an end, such as:

o   **COUNTING — IN THREES, OR BACKWARDS FROM 100**
o   **SINGING**
o   **FOCUSING ON A SPECIFIC OBJECT OR PERSON, WITH EYE TO EYE CONTACT**
o   **IMAGINING SOMETHING OR SOMEWHERE OUTSIDE THE PRESENT EXPERIENCE**

Using water as a relaxation aid For many women, enjoying a warm bath or shower helps them to relax and may encourage a slow labour to speed up. Most hospitals have bathing facilities on the labour ward, and some now have special facilities for water births, with a pool kept full of warm water, where you can relax into a comfortable yet upright position. If you are at home and decide you would like a bath, make sure you have someone else in the house, and do not lock yourself into the bathroom!

• I eventually took to my bath for some hours, as that was the only place I felt remotely comfortable. •

• I was getting contractions about every seven minutes, but just relaxing and breathing deeply through them. I was shaking like a leaf in between them with nerves and excitement. •

• I was getting my husband to take me off for a shower about every hour — it was wonderful in there; warm, relaxing, and refreshing. •

Breathing   The pregnancy hormones enable a woman to achieve a more efficient exchange of oxygen and carbon dioxide than in her non-pregnant state; by breathing normally during labour you will ensure you and your baby obtain sufficient oxygen, and maintain good energy levels. Often a person's instant reaction to pain is to tense and hold the breath — watch yourself next time you knock into something or experience a twinge of pain. Some women do this in labour too, the result being that they experience more pain than they need to and run the risk of themselves and their baby becoming tired through lack of oxygen.

A technique for overcoming this reaction to pain and helping maintain a state of relaxation during contractions, is to do the opposite. When you feel a contraction coming, you immediately breathe out slowly through your mouth, concentrating on keeping your shoulders loose and your mouth relaxed. Once your lungs are fully emptied, they will automatically refill, so if, during a contraction, you concentrate on emptying your lungs slowly and fully, the in-breaths will take care of themselves and you and your baby will have a good supply of oxygen.

Practising breathing The following exercise will show you the importance of out-breaths:

> ○ **BREATHE OUT GENTLY, EMPTYING YOUR LUNGS AS THOR-OUGHLY AS YOU CAN.**

○ WATCH AND WAIT — YOU WILL NOTICE A SLIGHT PAUSE
   BEFORE YOUR LUNGS BEGIN TO REFILL.
○ NOTICE HOW YOUR LUNGS AUTOMATICALLY FILL UP AGAIN,
   WITHOUT ANY EFFORT ON YOUR PART.

Now try the opposite:

○ TAKE A DEEP BREATH IN AND WATCH AND WAIT: YOU WILL
   PROBABLY FIND THAT YOUR SHOULDERS TENSE UP AND
   THAT YOU HAVE TO MAKE A CONSCIOUS EFFORT TO
   BREATHE OUT AGAIN.

This is why concentrating on your out-breaths is so effective. One important advantage of using this breathing technique in labour is that it is simple to practise in everyday life: practised regularly, relaxed breathing will become second nature for you and easy to use in labour. Try practising it every time you feel a pain or feel tense. It is excellent for driving, especially in traffic jams or on long journeys, or for preparing for a difficult meeting at work, an important telephone call, or an interview. It works equally well when coping with a fractious toddler or an argumentative child. If you become aware of the Braxton Hicks contractions (see page 68) towards the end of pregnancy, these offer an ideal opportunity for practising the technique for labour contractions, since they can feel quite powerful at times.

It is important that your labour partner understands and practises this breathing technique with you too, so that he can help you with it in labour. It is quite possible for a woman to forget to breathe in labour, perhaps if she is deeply relaxed between contractions, tired, or sleepy from pethidine. By breathing out loudly enough for a labouring woman to hear, or gently asking her to breathe out, a labour companion can remind her to keep up her oxygen supply while remaining relaxed.

HYPERVENTILATION Occasionally a woman in labour hyperventilates, or overbreathes, because she has become tense. Breathing at an abnormally rapid rate results in an increased loss of carbon dioxide.

If this happens to you, you may begin to feel dizzy or notice that your fingers and toes feel tingly. The remedy for this is to breathe in and out into your hands cupped around your nose and mouth. In this way, you redress the balance in your bloodstream by breathing back your own exhaled carbon dioxide.

It is even better to avoid hyperventilation in the first place by using your gentle slow out-breaths to release tension.

' I found that concentrating on breathing to help me relax was all I needed to get me through. '

' I had to remind Mark to keep his breathing slow and calm as well, because he was getting so excited, he was affecting me too. '

Touch and massage

Many women find touch of some sort helpful in labour, but it may ultimately depend on how they feel about being touched in general, and how they react during labour. Touch can be helpful both as a way of helping you cope with strong pain and as a channel of communication. A strong contraction lasting a good minute can be a lonely time for a woman; being touched with sensitivity by her partner may remind her that she is not alone. Equally, there may be

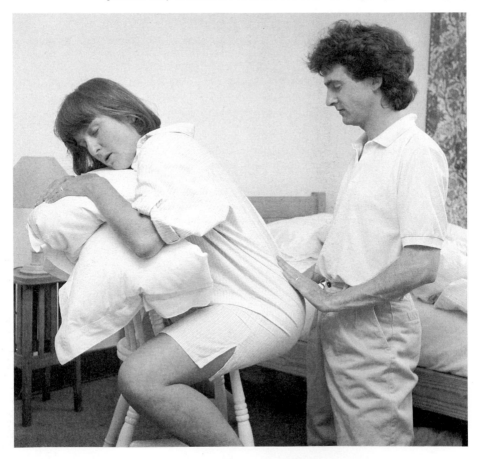

times in labour when a woman does not want to be touched, for instance during transition. There are no rules; if it feels good and you enjoy it, it is well worth trying.

Some women find they themselves want to hold, stroke, or rub the place that is hurting; others like their partner to do it. Some of the positions for labour require the woman to be held or supported; often this degree of touch is sufficient for comfort and reassurance and as an aid to relaxation. Sometimes a woman will want to be actively massaged in a particular way. There may be times when light, gentle strokes feel best; at other times, a deep, firm massage will best relieve pain and help relaxation.

If you and your partner massage each other during your pregnancy and find out what sort of touching and massage you really like, you will communicate easily during your labour and your partner will be able to respond quickly to your needs.

PRACTISING MASSAGE Your partner could begin by massaging your back and shoulders, while you kneel forward on to a chair or pile of cushions, your knees apart. You will probably find that massage works best when it is done on to your bare skin, but your partner will need to use oil or cream to prevent your skin becoming sore from the rubbing. (It is better to avoid any strong-smelling oils or powders in labour, as labouring women are often particularly sensitive to powerful scents.)

○ YOUR PARTNER CAN GENTLY KNEAD THE TOP OF YOUR SHOULDERS AND BACK OF YOUR NECK. IF HE FINDS ANY SPOTS OF TENSION, HE CAN CONCENTRATE ON THOSE FOR SOME MOMENTS.

○ MAKE SURE YOU GIVE YOUR PARTNER PLENTY OF FEEDBACK ABOUT WHAT FEELS GOOD FOR YOU. YOU CAN THEN ASK HIM TO DO IT HARDER, SOFTER, MORE SLOWLY, FURTHER DOWN, OR WHATEVER SUITS YOU.

○ HE CAN THEN TRY LONG STROKES RIGHT DOWN YOUR SPINE WITH ALTERNATE HANDS, MAINTAINING CONTACT ALL THE TIME.

○ FROM HERE HE CAN DO LONG STROKES ROUND YOUR HIPS AND DOWN YOUR THIGHS — YOUR PARTNER MAY HAVE SOME MORE IDEAS, OR YOU CAN SIMPLY USE YOUR IMAGINATIONS.

○ IF YOU HAVE PREGNANCY BACKACHE, IT IS NICE TO GET INTO THE ALL-FOURS POSITION, AND THEN ASK YOUR PARTNER TO MASSAGE THE PART THAT HURTS.

○ MANY WOMEN FIND THAT HAVING THEIR BUTTOCKS KNEADED (JUST LIKE KNEADING BREAD DOUGH) IS BOTH WONDERFULLY RELAXING AND USEFUL IN PROVIDING A COUNTER-PRESSURE TO A BACKACHE. IT WILL BE LESS TIRING FOR YOUR PARTNER TO USE HIS FIST RATHER THAN HIS FINGERS TO MASSAGE A PARTICULARLY PAINFUL SPOT.

To massage your back yourself, lean firmly against a wall behind you, place a tennis ball between you and the wall just where your back hurts, and rub yourself hard against it.

Because providing constant massage in labour is extremely tiring for the labour companion, it might be worth investing in one of the massage aids now available. Most chemists and cosmetics shops sell wooden rollers for massage, which are particularly good for backs, but work well on thighs or anywhere else.

• I just rocked my bottom about and thought of John's hands on my back, rocking into them. •

• My midwife spent hours massaging her hands and thumbs into the small of my back — she managed to find exactly the right place every time and kept it up throughout every contraction. •

• I'd thought I would enjoy being massaged in labour as I really liked it when I was pregnant, but when it came to the point I couldn't bear anyone near me. •

Putting the techniques together

As well as practising the four main techniques described above separately, many women find it helpful to combine them in practice contractions, both in antenatal classes and at home. Ideally, it is nice to have a third person timing a practice contraction for you; timing a minute and drawing your attention to the peak of intensity in the middle; this then leaves you and your partner free to concentrate on imagining the contraction and using positions, relaxation, breathing, and touch to deal with the imagined sensations. If this is not possible, however, your partner can time a contraction, or you can do it for yourself if there are times when you want to practise on your own. An alternative would be to record a tape of practice contractions.

PRACTISING CONTRACTIONS When the practice contraction starts, or when your labour contractions begin, greet them with a breath out, making sure your lungs are emptied, and mentally using the time to check that your body is well relaxed, particularly your shoulders and mouth. As the contraction continues, reaches its peak, and fades away again, concentrate on the out-breaths; emptying your lungs thoroughly each time, relaxing, and letting your lungs breathe in new air as they are ready. Your partner may help you by holding or massaging, as you wish, and drawing attention (tactfully!) to any parts of your body that are not relaxed — often just an aware touch is enough to remind you. When the contraction comes to an end, greet its end with an out-breath and relax fully. Smiling with your 'resting breath' relaxes the sides of your face and stimulates the circulation to those muscles, making you feel less tired.

Reading Chapter 16, Pain Relief in Labour, will suggest further ideas for how you might respond to contractions in labour. For many women and their companions, simply maintaining a positive attitude throughout will help them find their own ways of coping in labour, though it has to be recognized that not every labour is as easily coped with.

You can use the respite between contractions to rest and relax, to change your position, or to use one of your labour aids (see below) to refresh you.

TRANSITION

If you have a noticeable transition, you may need some extra techniques to help you cope. Making sure you move into an upright position if you are not in one already, or changing your position, will help to speed the dilatation of the cervix.

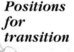

Positions for transition

Positions for transition:
a. The knee – chest position
b. On all-fours

○ A KNEE—CHEST POSITION, PAR-
TICULARLY IF THERE IS A
PREMATURE URGE TO PUSH
○ A POSITION IN WHICH YOU
KNEEL AND LEAN FORWARDS
OR BACKWARDS IF YOU HAVE
AN ANTERIOR OR POSTERIOR
LIP
○ ANY UPRIGHT POSITION WHICH
WILL ENCOURAGE THE CERVIX
TO DILATE MORE SWIFTLY
WILL BE HELPFUL

If you have a premature urge to push, you may find it helpful to blow out briskly (like blowing hair out of your eyes), remembering to pause between breaths, until your midwife gives you the go-ahead to push. You could blow on each out-breath, or perhaps on every third or fourth out-breath, to slow the rhythm.

Your partner might find he needs to comfort and reassure you a great deal at this stage. He might talk to you, reminding you that you are nearly there, or help you with your breathing by breathing out with you for a while. It can help to maintain eye contact or discover distraction techniques like singing a song. Encouraging you to make a noise as you breathe out, if this helps, and being ready to accept and understand tears and moods at what can be a very confusing time, are also useful ways of supporting you through transition.

● *I nagged at him [husband] and the doctor and kept saying that I couldn't go on and that I didn't want the baby. I think the gas and air had made me a bit woozy as I don't remember this very well.* '

' *Although the pain was making my eyes water, so to speak, I kept thinking — I will breathe through just one more before thinking about accepting any drugs. My biggest problem actually was feeling sick; that I hadn't bargained for.* '

' *Steve was agitated and I was irritable. The drive to the hospital was pretty awful. It was 12.30 a.m. and Steve drove fast and I wanted to push. I could feel my waters trickling with each contraction.* '

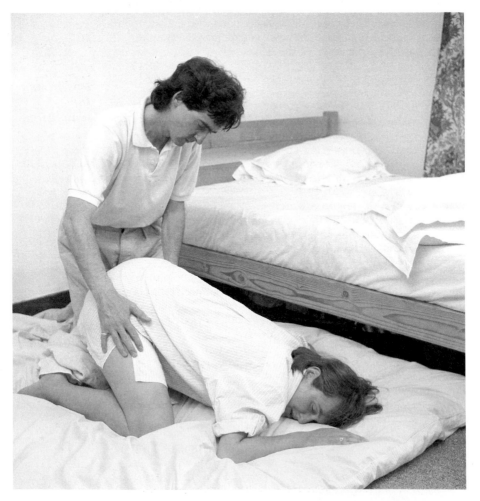

THE SECOND STAGE

Women often experience second-stage contractions as being quite different from those of the first stage; once the cervix is fully dilated and the contractions change to expulsive ones, the quality and location of the pain may alter and the contractions become shorter and further apart than those at the end of the first stage. This fact, and possibly the hormones affecting these changes, often give women their new lease of energy.

You may want to get into a more upright position and you may feel absolutely normal between contractions, cheerfully waiting for the next one to come.

Positions

Positions for second stage

○ A SEMI-SQUAT, SUPPORTED BY TWO PEOPLE
○ A SEMI-SQUAT, SUPPORTED BY A SMALL STOOL OR TODDLER'S STEP
○ A SEMI-SQUAT, SUPPORTED BY YOUR PARTNER SITTING BEHIND YOU
○ SITTING ON A BIRTHING-CHAIR OR STOOL OR CUSHION (AVAILABLE IN SOME HOSPITALS)
○ SITTING ON A BUCKET THE RIGHT WAY UP (DIFFICULT TO BELIEVE UNTIL YOU TRY IT!)
○ SITTING IN YOUR PARTNER'S LAP
○ STANDING WITH KNEES BENT, HOLDING ON TO YOUR PARTNER IN FRONT OF YOU
○ STANDING WITH KNEES BENT, YOUR ARMS TUCKED AROUND TWO PEOPLE STANDING EITHER SIDE OF YOU, THEIR KNEES TUCKED BEHIND YOURS TO HELP BEAR THE WEIGHT
○ STANDING, KNEES BENT, YOUR PARTNER SUPPORTING YOU FROM BEHIND, HOLDING HIS ARMS UNDER YOURS
○ KNEELING UPRIGHT, LEANING ON TO A BEDRAIL OR PARTNER
○ KNEELING UPRIGHT, SUPPORTING YOUR OWN WEIGHT WITH YOUR ARMS, OR LEANING ON TO A BEAN-BAG
○ HALF-KNEELING, ONE KNEE ON THE FLOOR, THE OTHER BENT IN FRONT OF YOU
○ KNEELING ON ALL-FOURS (SOME WOMEN FIND THEY NEED SOMEONE TO PUSH AGAINST THEIR KNEES TO BE ABLE TO PUSH EFFECTIVELY IN THIS POSITION)
○ RECLINING ON ONE BUTTOCK (IF YOU SIT SQUARELY ON BOTH BUTTOCKS, THE BASE OF YOUR SPINE CANNOT MOVE BACK AND YOU LOSE ABOUT ONE-THIRD OF THE POTENTIAL SPACE FOR THE BABY TO COME OUT)

Among all the positions suggested for second stage, you may have noticed the absence of the supine position. This position, in which a woman lies on the bed, often with her feet against the

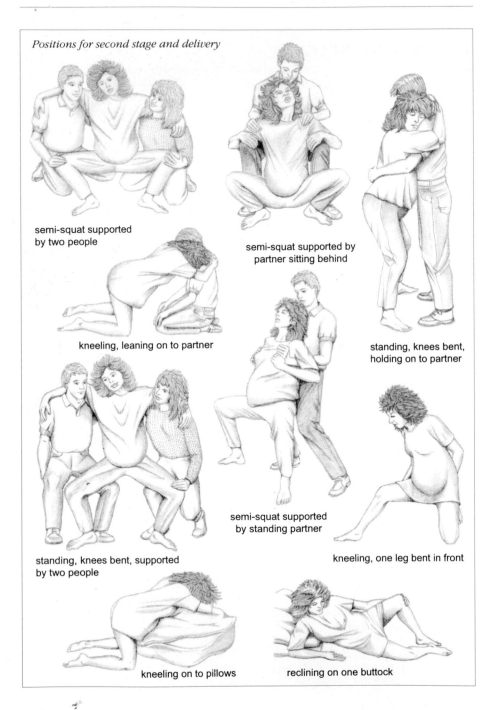

Positions for second stage and delivery

semi-squat supported
by two people

semi-squat supported by
partner sitting behind

kneeling, leaning on to partner

standing, knees bent,
holding on to partner

semi-squat supported
by standing partner

standing, knees bent, supported
by two people

kneeling, one leg bent in front

kneeling on to pillows

reclining on one buttock

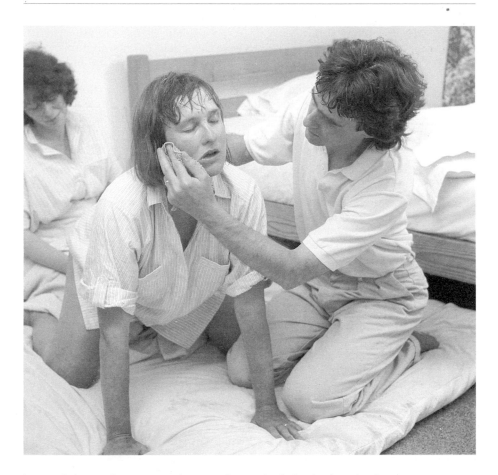

hips of the midwives standing at the end of the bed, is both uncomfortable for many women and an ineffective position for second-stage expulsive contractions. If you are lying down, the amount of space within your pelvis will be greatly limited, you will be pushing your baby uphill, and you may find it difficult to feel where you should be pushing without the benefit of gravity helping the baby's descent. A great deal of energy will also be going into your legs and the midwives' hips rather than into your abdomen.

It is also important to remember that, if you choose a position in which you are squatting, you should make sure that this is a semi-squat rather than a full squat where your buttocks are right down on the floor or mattress, as a full squat exerts too great a pressure on the pelvic floor, and means the baby has to be born uphill. Any position where your legs are held firmly apart stretches your pelvic floor so far sideways that it is bound to tear as the baby's head emerges. This could happen in a full squat, or reclining with your hands holding your legs up and out.

Second-stage contractions

As long as you do not have an urge to push, you can cope with contractions in the same way as for first stage, concentrating on your out-breaths and ensuring that you are completely relaxed, particularly your vagina and pelvic floor. When you do have an urge to push, your body will tell you where to push, and you need push only as hard or as long as your body wants to. As before, greet each new contraction with a slow, steadying out-breath to relax yourself. As you feel the need to push or bear down, you might let your breath out as you bear down.

Some women prefer to hold their breath while pushing; it is important to remember not to hold your breath for more than about six seconds to make sure the baby does not go short of oxygen. Keeping a relaxed, steady rhythm is a more efficient use of your energy than trying to force your baby down the birth canal too fast.

Practising second-stage contractions

You can practise breathing and relaxing through a one-minute second-stage contraction in one of the positions suggested for second stage when you have no desire to push. There is no peak, so greet it with an out-breath and concentrate on emptying your lungs fully, breathing regularly, keeping your mouth and pelvic floor as relaxed as possible, and visualizing your baby moving down. When it is over, breathe out again and relax as fully as you can.

Now try another position and practise pushing. While you are practising and not actually in labour, it is wise not to push hard, but just enough to feel where you will be directing your energies when the time comes.

○ **GREET THE CONTRACTION WITH AN OUT-BREATH, THEN BREATHE IN, HOLD YOUR BREATH AND BEAR DOWN FOR NO MORE THAN SIX SECONDS.**
○ **BREATHE OUT FULLY.**
○ **WHEN YOU ARE READY, BREATHE IN, HOLD YOUR BREATH, AND PUSH FOR NO MORE THAN SIX SECONDS, THEN BREATHE OUT.**
○ **REPEAT THIS UNTIL THE CONTRACTION IS OVER.**

In a second-stage contraction you may have three or four urges to bear down during the minute or so that the contraction will last. When the contraction is over, greet its end with a breath out and relax completely to gather your energies for the next one. If it feels more comfortable for you, do not hold your breath at all but push down on your out-breath for no more than six seconds at a time. After a few practice contractions you should find yourself getting into a rhythm: this is an excellent aid for coping with labour. Remember that the uterus is doing most of the work: when you get an urge to push, your body is just asking you to help.

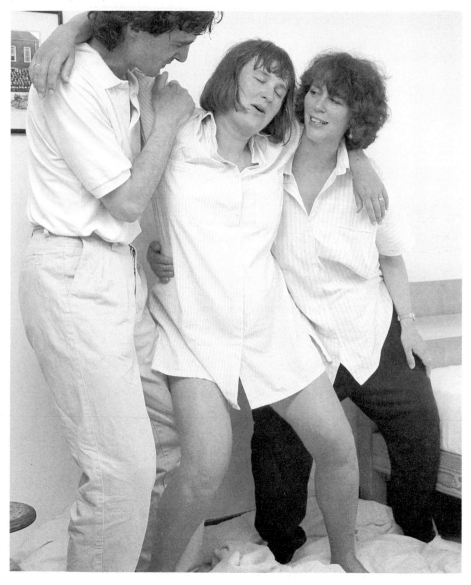

In labour, some women find it difficult to push in the right direction, wasting energy by pushing hard ineffectively. If you can, it helps to:

○ VISUALIZE PRECISELY WHERE YOUR BABY WILL BE COMING FROM AND HOW IT IS TRAVELLING ROUND A CURVE — INTO YOUR BOTTOM AND ROUND TOWARDS YOUR KNEES.
○ REMAIN IN AN UPRIGHT POSITION SO THAT GRAVITY WILL HELP YOU.
○ RELAX FULLY.
○ REMEMBER TO KEEP YOUR EFFORTS AS GENTLE AS POSSIBLE.

In this way you should then be able to bear down effectively without straining. Touching your baby's head after it is born stimulates your hormones to make another contraction quickly to free your baby's chest so that it can breathe easily. Smiling to welcome your baby ensures that your pelvic floor stretches easily as the shoulders are born.

She asked me where I wanted to deliver, and I said "Right here, standing."

Prior to going in to labour I had thought that the all-fours position seemed to be the best one for second stage, but when it came to the point I was so confused and exhausted that I didn't really know what I was doing.

The sister eventually suggested I sat on the bean-bag, leaning slightly back — she was quite positive that in this position the baby would be born quickly, and she was right!

I felt intense pressure and said I wanted to push — instinctively I put my knees into a semi-squat to try to ease the pressure.

I could feel the head coming down, and as I'd been warned, it felt at first as if it was coming out of the back passage.

DELIVERY

Positions   Positions in which you might like to deliver your baby will include most of the positions for second stage, but your midwife will need to be able to see the baby and to carry out some medical procedures.

Breathing   The actual delivery of your baby is a time when you may be asked by your midwife not to push, so that she can deliver your baby's head gently and carefully, as well as checking that the cord is not wrapped round your baby's neck. Any breathing technique which stops you holding your breath is helpful. Many midwives will ask you to 'pant' in this situation. Practise this by breathing out, allowing your lungs to fill up, and then panting the breath out, making a noise if it helps.

❛ It felt as though I was absolutely full of baby. ❜

❛ After about three or four contractions into second stage, I began to feel as though I had a melon in my bottom, and I was getting a tearing feeling in my vagina. I reminded myself that that feeling meant I hadn't torn. ❜

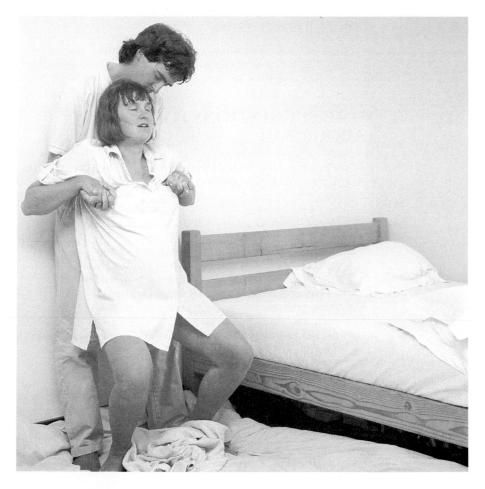

I wondered who was making that extraordinary noise, like a bellowing camel, and realized it must be me!

I felt a burning, splitting sensation and it felt as though the student midwife was pushing the perineum down around the head, so I got cross and said, "What is this woman doing?" The midwife smiled and said, "She's just supporting the baby's head — do you want to look?" I couldn't move, but put my hand down and felt an enormous spongy mass — the baby's head.

The next thing I knew was them saying, "It's a girl", Lorna on my stomach, and Peter and me in tears.

I heard the magic words, "pant, pant". No one told me "pant" was the best word in the English language.

I could not believe the direct gaze of this little thing with large, dark eyes who had determinedly brought herself into the world without any help until the last minute.

SOME SUGGESTIONS FOR YOUR LABOUR BAG

Keeping a separate carrier bag of all the things you think you will find useful in labour will mean you will not have to rummage through your entire suitcase to find the items that you want. You might take with you:

- ☑ WARM, LONG SOCKS — FEET AND LEGS ARE OFTEN CHILLY IN LABOUR
- ☑ A BAGGY T-SHIRT, OLD SHIRT OF YOUR PARTNER'S — WHATEVER YOU WANT TO WEAR IN LABOUR (YOU DO NOT HAVE TO WEAR A HOSPITAL GOWN IF YOU WOULD RATHER NOT; YOU DO NOT HAVE TO WEAR ANYTHING)
- ☑ FOOD SUPPLIES FOR YOU AND YOUR PARTNER — SANDWICHES, FRUIT, BISCUITS, ETC.
- ☑ DRINKS FOR YOU AND YOUR PARTNER — FRUIT DRINKS OR A THERMOS OF TEA/COFFEE; MANY HOSPITALS WILL PROVIDE DRINKS, BUT POSSIBLY NOT IN THE DELIVERY ROOM
- ☑ SMALL, NATURAL SPONGES FOR WIPING YOUR FACE AND FOR SUCKING WATER
- ☑ SMALL SPRAY BOTTLE OF COOL WATER TO REFRESH YOUR FACE (FIZZY WATER IS MORE REFRESHING THAN STILL WATER BECAUSE OF THE BUBBLES BURSTING)
- ☑ OIL OR CREAM FOR MASSAGE

☑   **ROLLER FOR MASSAGE**

☑   **CASSETTES, PLUS RECORDER IF ONE IS NOT AVAILABLE; TRY CASSETTES OF BOOKS TOO**

☑   **A GAME FOR YOU AND YOUR PARTNER TO PLAY IF IT IS SLOW GOING AND YOU CAN CONCENTRATE**

☑   **THERMOS FULL OF CRUSHED ICE-CUBES TO SUCK (TIP THEM INTO A CLEAN TEA-TOWEL AND BANG THEM ON THE FLOOR TO BREAK THEM)**

☑   **BENDY STRAW FOR TAKING SIPS OF DRINK WITH MINIMUM EFFORT**

☑   **HOT-WATER BOTTLE — FOR RELIEVING BACKACHE**

☑   **ICE-PACKS, ALSO FOR RELIEVING BACKACHE — THE SOFT SORT YOU USE IN A FREEZER AND COOL-BAG ARE VERY GOOD (NCT MATERNITY SALES SELLS A JOINTED ICE-PACK)**

☑   **SOMETHING TO REMIND YOU OF HOME OR OTHER PLEASANT MEMORY — A PICTURE OR PHOTO; SOME SMALL REMINDER THAT COMFORTS YOU**

A SUMMARY OF SELF-HELP METHODS FOR COPING WITH LABOUR

You may find yourself adding to the list for your labour bag as you read this section!

- **Positions**: Familiarize your body and your labour partner with as many of these as possible during pregnancy, and remember to change position from time to time during your labour.
- **Movement**: Moving or rocking yourself within a position is also useful.
- **Relaxation**: Relaxation is for both you and your partner. You may find different techniques help at different times in labour.
- **Touch and massage**: You can use different techniques at different times and sometimes none at all. Often a woman prefers to massage herself.
- **Breathing**: The aim is to breathe as normally as possible. If you get lost in some of the strong contractions, do not worry, just make the most of the lulls in between.
- **Darkness**: You may prefer darkness. Do not forget to darken the room again if lights have been put on for a vaginal examination.
- **Eye contact**: Eye contact can help a woman concentrate on difficult contractions. If you wear glasses or

contact lenses, you may prefer to wear them or to leave them off. Some women welcome the world being slightly out of focus; others hate it!

o **Sips**: Sipping water, broth, or non-acidic fruit juice or sucking on crushed ice-cubes from your Thermos are refreshing. You might prefer spoonfuls of honey or glucose tablets.

o **Sponging**: This can be bliss for the brow and face, or anywhere else that feels hot. Dipping a sponge in cold water first is deliciously soothing. Alternatively, your partner can hold a sponge for you to suck, if drinking is too much effort.

o **Hot-water bottle or ice-pack**: These can provide relief from backache, although, as the labour progresses, cold is more likely to be soothing than heat.

o **Music**: Take a cassette recorder and a selection of tapes so you can choose music to suit your mood. Many midwives and doctors welcome it too!

o **Warm bath or shower**: Water is marvellous for relaxation. A bath will not be an option in hospital if your waters have broken, because of the risk of infection.

o **Making a noise**: Some women moan, groan, shout, sing, or make other noises in labour as instinctive ways of coping with the pain. It is sometimes difficult for partners and medical staff to remember that a woman making a lot of noise may be really 'into' her labour and coping very well, even if it does not sound like it.

o **Positive encouragement**: A labouring woman can never have too much encouragement. Her partner should spontaneously tell her how well she is doing and respond to any negative statements, such as 'I can't go on', with positive ones, like 'Yes you can, you're managing marvellously'. During difficult moments her response may be rather unpredictable! Always remind yourself that a cervix strong enough to retain the uterus and its contents for nine months needs strong contractions to dilate it.

o **Visualizing**: Imagine how labour might be feeling for your baby. Visualizing the cervix dilating or the baby moving down in second stage can help you feel more in tune with your body and your uterus and help you relax into your labour.

> ○ **Labour partner**: He or she may not think of him/ herself as a form of pain relief in labour, but it is true!

All of these methods can be used on their own in labour or at times when artificial pain relief is not available or is inappropriate. The beauty of learning the relaxation, breathing, and touch techniques is that, however you use them in your labour, you (and your labour partner) will have acquired skills invaluable for coping with breastfeeding your baby, life with young children, and life in general.

COPING WITH EMERGENCY CHILDBIRTH

Expectant parents are often concerned that their baby will arrive precipitately, at home or elsewhere, and that they will not know what to do. In fact it is highly unlikely that this will happen; most women get ample warning that their baby is on the way. There is not a vast amount either you or a companion can actually do beyond remaining as calm as possible, and you will probably find that you do the right things instinctively, using your common sense, but here are some guidelines that you may find useful just in case!

If you realize that the baby is coming faster than you had anticipated:　*Preparation*

○ RING A FRIEND OR NEIGHBOUR TO BE WITH YOU UNTIL MEDICAL HELP ARRIVES IF YOU ARE ON YOUR OWN.

○ RING FOR YOUR COMMUNITY MIDWIFE OR YOUR GP OR BOTH — WHOEVER YOU THINK WILL GET THERE FIRST.

○ RING FOR AN AMBULANCE IN CASE YOU NEED TO BE TRANSFERRED TO HOSPITAL.

○ MOVE TO A COMFORTABLE ROOM IF YOU CAN AND, IF THERE IS TIME, COVER ANY VULNERABLE SURFACES WITH SOME OLD SHEETS OR TOWELS — WHATEVER IS HANDY.

○ GET A TOWEL READY TO WRAP YOUR BABY IN TO KEEP HER WARM.

○ TRY TO MAKE SURE THE ROOM WILL BE WARM TO RECEIVE THE BABY, IF YOU HAVE TIME.

○ TRY TO DELAY THE ACTUAL BIRTH BY MOVING INTO A KNEELING POSITION WITH YOUR HEAD ON YOUR FORE-ARMS AND YOUR BOTTOM AS HIGH IN THE AIR AS YOU CAN GET IT. THIS MAY BE ESPECIALLY USEFUL IF YOU ARE IN THE CAR ON YOUR WAY TO HOSPITAL, BUT IT DOES WORK BETTER IN THE BACK SEAT!

○ TRY TO BREATHE SLOWLY AND DEEPLY AND TO RESIST
ACTUALLY PUSHING OR BEARING DOWN FOR AS LONG AS
POSSIBLE.

Delivery

If, despite everyone's best efforts, this baby has decided to arrive anyway, your companion or occasionally a mother alone, will have to deliver the baby.

○ IT WILL BE POSSIBLE FOR A COMPANION TO SEE THAT THE
HEAD IS ABOUT TO BE BORN BY THE BULGING PERINEUM,
OR BY ACTUALLY SEEING THE HEAD EMERGE! A MOTHER
WILL NOT SEE THIS, BUT WILL BE ABLE TO FEEL THE HEAD
FOR HERSELF.

○ THE MOTHER CAN BE ENCOURAGED TO GET HERSELF INTO A
COMFORTABLE POSITION AS DISCUSSED EARLIER — SHE IS
UNLIKELY TO CHOOSE LYING-DOWN AS AN OPTION.

○ LET THE HEAD SLIDE OUT GRADUALLY, IN ITS OWN TIME —
A MOTHER SHOULD TRY NOT TO PUSH AS THE HEAD IS
CROWNING.

○ ONCE THE HEAD HAS BEEN BORN, FEEL AROUND THE
BABY'S NECK FOR THE CORD, IF POSSIBLE. IF NECESSARY,
LOOP IT OVER THE HEAD, OUT OF THE WAY.

○ WIPE AWAY ANY TRACES OF MUCUS FROM THE BABY'S FACE
WITH A CLEAN FINGER — OR ANYTHING ELSE AS LONG AS
IT IS CLEAN.

○ GENTLY HOLD THE BABY SO THAT THE SHOULDERS AND THE
BODY CAN BE DELIVERED SAFELY; DO NOT PULL THE BABY
AT ALL, JUST GUIDE HER OUT.

○ WRAP THE BABY UP IMMEDIATELY TO KEEP HER WARM —
THE VERY WARMEST PLACE IS IN BETWEEN HER MOTHER'S
BREASTS. A NEW-BORN BABY CAN RAPIDLY LOSE HEAT
FROM HER HEAD, SO IT IS IMPORTANT TO REMEMBER TO
KEEP THE HEAD WELL COVERED TOO.

○ LET THE BABY FIND HER WAY ON TO THE BREAST TO
STIMULATE CONTRACTIONS FOR THE THIRD STAGE. AN
UPRIGHT POSITION WILL ENCOURAGE THE DELIVERY OF
THE PLACENTA.

○ LEAVE THE CORD ALONE; THERE IS NO NEED AT ALL TO CUT
OR TIE IT.

○ IT IS MORE THAN LIKELY THAT THE BABY WILL BREATHE
SPONTANEOUSLY AND IMMEDIATELY. IF NOT, MAKE SURE
YOU HAVE WIPED AWAY ANY MUCUS. IF YOU HAVE A
DRINKING-STRAW HANDY, YOU CAN *VERY GENTLY* PUT
THIS INTO THE BABY'S MOUTH, AND THEN SUCK TO CLEAR
ANY MUCUS FROM THE THROAT AND MOUTH. IF YOU DO
NOT HAVE A DRINKING-STRAW, SIMPLY WIPE HER MOUTH

WITH YOUR CLEAN FINGER AND THEN *EXTREMELY GENTLY*
BREATHE INTO HER MOUTH A FEW TIMES, USING ONLY
THE AIR YOU CAN HOLD IN YOUR CHEEKS. THIS SHOULD
BE ENOUGH TO STIMULATE HER TO BREATHE FOR HER-
SELF.

○ IF THE PLACENTA IS DELIVERED BEFORE MEDICAL HELP
ARRIVES, PUT IT IN A BOWL OR WRAP IT IN A SEPARATE
TOWEL OR CLOTH AND LEAVE IT ALONE.

○ MAKE SURE THE MOTHER IS WARM ENOUGH AND REASON-
ABLY COMFORTABLE. SHE WILL NEED A SANITARY TOWEL
OR WHATEVER ELSE YOU CAN FIND TO PUT BETWEEN HER
LEGS.

○ ONCE THE PLACENTA IS DELIVERED, MAKE HER A CUP OF
TEA IF SHE FANCIES IT. UNTIL MEDICAL HELP ARRIVES, SHE
MAY WELL PREFER NOT TO BE LEFT ALONE, HOWEVER, SO
YOU MAY HAVE TO WAIT FOR YOUR OWN SUSTENANCE!

○ PUT ANY SOILED TOWELS, SHEETS, OR CLOTHES INTO COLD,
SALTED WATER TO SOAK.

○ ADMIRE AND ENJOY THIS NEW BABY.

15 MEDICAL PROCEDURES

Medical procedures and the use of modern technology are undoubtedly useful in complicated labours but, just as some couples decide to have their babies in hospital 'in case anything happens', so some medical procedures are carried out in labour with a view to *possible* complications rather than because they are necessary for the safe outcome of a normal labour. Some of these procedures have become 'routine', though unfortunately they may give rise to their own complications.

The care given by midwives and obstetricians to a woman and her baby in labour is governed in each hospital by a series of policy documents, updated as necessary. In the event of something going wrong in a labour, failure to adhere to these procedures may result in disciplinary proceedings for the birth attendant. This is why, if you should decide to decline a routine procedure, your refusal will be written in your notes. You may even be asked to sign a declaration that you have chosen not to have a particular procedure. Notes are written in labour to record what happens, and to inform new attendants after a change of shift and senior staff should complications arise. It can be useful to ask an obstetrician to go through these with you after the birth, especially if something happened in labour that you have not understood. It is often also extremely helpful for both obstetricians and midwives to discuss births when there has been some complication, not only with their colleagues, but also with the woman who has given birth. You can find out at your antenatal appointments and hospital antenatal classes what the hospital policies are, if there are particular procedures you would prefer to avoid or if you are thinking of writing your birth plan (see Chapter 11, Communicating with Health Professionals).

Procedures vary somewhat between hospitals and will be different if you have booked a home birth or domino delivery; check with your community midwife what policies apply to her which could affect your delivery.

MONITORING THE HEALTH OF THE MOTHER

General procedures

On admission to the labour ward, the midwife will read your notes, then take your temperature, pulse, and blood pressure. These will be checked periodically throughout your labour. She will possibly also give you a vaginal examination to see if your cervix is dilating and, if so, how far.

VAGINAL EXAMINATIONS Vaginal examinations are usually repeated every two to four hours, depending on your hospital's procedure, and should always be carried out before any artificial pain relief is administered. If done too frequently, vaginal examinations increase the risk of infection and may be discouraging for a woman whose labour is considered to be progressing slowly. Done at the right time, however, they can encourage her about her rate of progress and reduce her need for artificial pain relief. Many experienced midwives perform few, if any, vaginal examinations, relying instead on their understanding of women in labour to assess progress.

SHAVE AND ENEMAS It is fortunately extremely unusual now for women to have their pubic hair shaved or to be given enemas, as there is no value in either of these procedures. If you are seriously constipated, however, you might prefer to opt for an enema or suppository to prevent a rectum full of hard faecal matter delaying your baby's birth. You may find you involuntarily open your bowels during the second stage of labour. An enema will not actually prevent this happening and it is not a problem for either the midwife or your baby.

FOOD IN LABOUR Until recently, most hospitals maintained a policy of not allowing women to eat or drink once they were in labour, which included even those women who had gone into hospital for an induction of labour. The concern was that the woman's stomach should be empty just in case a general anaesthetic should prove necessary. Now, however, with fewer general anaesthetics being performed, and with better anaesthetic techniques, many hospitals are well aware that any benefits of starving women for long periods during early labour are largely outweighed by the risks. Fasting during labour does not ensure an empty stomach, nor does it lower the acidity of the stomach contents. Although the digestive system does slow down to a virtual standstill once labour is properly under way, some women do become hungry during labour, and find it most distressing if they are allowed neither to eat nor to drink. Starving a woman throughout her labour may indeed change a normal labour into a problem one.

It is important for your own and your baby's well-being that your blood-sugar levels do not fall so low that you become ketotic (see Chapter 3, Antenatal Medical Care), especially if your labour begins slowly, whether spontaneous or induced. Making sure that you continue to eat regular, light meals at home will help to keep your strength up, and leave you far better equipped for coping through the hours of your labour. Remembering to drink when you feel thirsty will help to prevent dehydration too.

The usual recommendation is to try and keep to low-fat meals and drinks which will not stay in the stomach for too long. Some suggestions for suitable foods and drinks are:

○ **CLEAR SOUPS**
○ **COOKED FRUITS**
○ **CRISP TOAST AND BUTTER WITH HONEY, JAM, OR YEAST EXTRACT SPREAD FOR FLAVOURING**
○ **LOW-FAT YOGHURTS OR *FROMAGE FRAIS***
○ **LIGHTLY COOKED EGGS**
○ **CEREALS WITH SKIMMED MILK**
○ **SEMI-SWEET BISCUITS**
○ **LOW-FAT, READYMADE CUSTARDS**
○ **FRUIT JUICES**
○ **TEA, OR HERBAL TEAS**
○ **LOW-FAT INSTANT BEDTIME DRINKS**

Some women, however, prefer to have very high-calorie snacks and drinks. Others find they are happy to eat and drink normal meals while in very early labour, but then have no need for anything more than sips of water or fruit juices once labour is under way.

Should a general anaesthetic become necessary at any stage, any stomach contents can be neutralized with an alkaline solution, and the anaesthetic very carefully monitored to avoid any danger of inhalation.

EMPTYING YOUR BLADDER You may be reminded to empty your bladder regularly during your labour, since a full bladder can impede progress. If you find you cannot because of the pressure of the baby's head on your bladder, you may have to be catheterized. This involves a fine tube being inserted into the urethra to drain away any urine from the bladder. Catheterization is worth avoiding if possible, because of the potential risk of infection and the unpleasantness of the procedure.

• The midwife told me that vaginal examinations weren't supposed to be painful. I couldn't help that — they jolly well were! •

• I ate a chocolate bar about half-way through. It was delicious, staved off the hunger pangs, and kept me going. •

• Geoff made me a cup of tea and offered me a sandwich, but I didn't fancy anything, partly, I think, because I was too excited. •

MONITORING THE HEALTH OF THE BABY

The baby's condition and how it is reacting to labour can be assessed in two ways. Both can show whether or not the baby is receiving sufficient oxygen; when a baby becomes short of oxygen, the condition is termed fetal distress.

ASSESSING AMNIOTIC FLUID When appropriate or feasible, the amniotic fluid can be examined. If your waters broke before you went into hospital, you will be asked what colour they were. A baby in distress may pass meconium, so if, instead of being pale or colourless, the amniotic fluid is stained with meconium, it is possible that the baby is finding labour difficult and intervention may be necessary.

MEASURING FETAL HEART RATE The baby's heart rate varies from about 120 to 160 beats per minute. It can be counted using either a fetal stethoscope or an electronic fetal monitor (EFM) or Sonicaid. The term 'fetal distress' is normally used when the baby's heart rate rises above 160, or falls below 100–120 beats per minute, or when the heartbeat is irregular.

Electronic fetal monitoring

The EFM is a computer which gives a continuous print-out of both the baby's heartbeat and the strength of contractions of the uterus. Both can be measured using a belt monitor, or an internal monitor. A belt monitor is a circular machine, about 15 cm. in diameter, mounted on a webbing belt and fastened round the woman's abdomen so that it is positioned over the baby's heart. It measures the heart rate by ultrasound, and the strength of contractions using a pressure-sensitive gauge. It is linked to the monitor by wires long enough for the woman to be able to shift position with a little help. A woman must stay in one position, sitting up or lying down or kneeling while the belt monitor is being used.

Sometimes the baby's heart is difficult to locate or the baby moves away from the belt monitor. In such cases, the staff might want the baby's heart rate to be picked up by a fetal scalp electrode, fastened to the baby's head by a little hook, and connected to the monitor by wires. It can only be used if the waters have broken; if the waters have not broken spontaneously, the staff may wish to break them artificially.

Whether the belt or electrode is used, your mobility will be greatly reduced and the scalp electrode can leave a wound on the baby, which occasionally becomes infected, resulting in a small bald patch.

When using the fetal scalp electrode, the staff may also prefer (if the equipment is available) to measure the strength of contractions

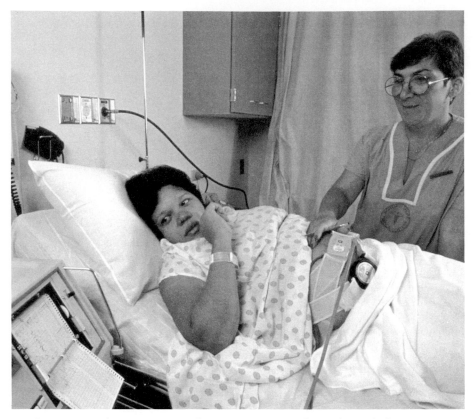

*An electronic
fetal heart
monitor in use
during labour*

by inserting an electronic uterine catheter through the cervix, past the baby's head, into the uterus; this is connected to a second machine with a separate print-out and digital display. It will thus be possible to see, side by side, your contractions and the baby's heart rate in reaction to the contractions.

STRIP-MONITORING It is policy in many hospitals for most women to be monitored routinely on admission, for twenty minutes. This is known as 'strip-monitoring', and is considered sufficient time to give a reliable read-out of the baby's reactions to labour. It is also required by some hospitals' insurance policies. The woman is then monitored at intervals during labour if it is thought necessary. If the baby is considered to be at risk (if, for example, the initial read-out was unsatisfactory, or if the woman has a medical problem such as raised blood pressure), she will normally be monitored continuously.

Some women (and their partners) find the continual print-out, visual display, and bleep of the baby's heart provided by the monitor rather comforting. Many midwives like to have the continuous print-out as a tool in managing a woman's labour; it also means that a midwife does not have to be with a woman all the time, but can look at the print-out periodically and come in if the monitor sounds its alarm. Other women, however, are distressed at being linked up to a machine, particularly if they feel the attention of their partner and/ or their medical carers shifts from themselves to the machine. Sometimes a monitor or other equipment is faulty, giving read-outs which look as if the baby is distressed; this can be unnecessarily frightening. Conversely, they may fail to give the right information if the baby is distressed.

Current research shows that the continuous use of an EFM alone in labour does not guarantee a safe outcome. It is thought that the reduction to the woman's mobility may itself give rise to problems, interfering as it does with the normal course of a labour. There is also a greater likelihood of further intervention for a labouring woman who is receiving continuous fetal monitoring. Some hospitals do have 'telemetric' monitoring equipment, which allows a woman to walk around while being monitored. Electronic fetal monitoring is an effective tool only in the hands of skilled operators, and if backed up by fetal blood sampling as a more accurate assessment of fetal distress.

Fetal blood sampling

Fetal blood sampling is carried out so that the amount of oxygen in the baby's blood can be measured if there is uncertainty or concern about its condition. A little blood is obtained from the baby's scalp by passing a special knife up a tube placed in the mother's vagina: the woman has to lie on her back, with her legs apart. A machine analyses the blood and gives a result very quickly. If the baby's condition is found to be normal, further intervention will be unnecessary, but further samples might be taken every two or three hours if there is still some concern.

● *The doctor was rummaging around inside me for what felt like hours, trying to get the monitor on the baby's head. In the end, the midwife offered to do it. Even if he'd been more competent, I'd still have resented him doing it — he was somehow out of place in that room.* ●

ACCELERATION OR AUGMENTATION OF LABOUR

In most hospitals it is thought to be better for the woman and her baby if labour does not last beyond a certain length of time, with this period varying from hospital to hospital.

Artificial rupture of the membranes Routine breaking of the waters or artificial rupture of the membranes (ARM) is one method used to speed up labour. The membranes are ruptured using an amnihook — an instrument which looks rather like a long metal crochet hook. The procedure is normally painless provided the cervix has softened and begun to dilate.

Once the waters have broken, whether spontaneously or artificially, labour contractions become stronger. This is because the baby's head now presses directly on to the cervix during contractions, making the sensation of the cervix being dilated more intense and increasing the production of oxytocin. This usually means that contractions become noticeably more painful for the woman. Whether or not, and if so by how much, ARM speeds up labour is less clear. In a case where perhaps the baby's head has been pressing unevenly on the cervix and dilation has been proceeding very slowly, once the cushion of waters is removed by ARM labour may change gear dramatically and progress very rapidly. It is very tempting to extrapolate from this that the earlier ARM is performed, the shorter labour will be. Research suggests, however, that ARM shortens labour only by an hour, on average. Therefore ARM, performed early on in the first stage, say at 3 cm., may reduce the length of the first stage from twelve hours to eleven hours, but the woman may spend more of it in extra discomfort and be more inclined to resort to artificial pain relief. It can also cause swelling on the baby's head because of the direct pressure on the cervix. ARM offered later on, however, perhaps at 7 or 8 cm., may reduce its length at a time when the woman and baby have become accustomed to intense contractions and have benefited from the cushion of waters for most of the first stage of labour.

Syntocinon drip Another method of accelerating or augmenting labour, especially if the waters have broken spontaneously, but labour is progressing slowly, is to administer synthetic oxytocin, Syntocinon, in a drip. The dosage is normally built up gradually over several hours, until it has made the contractions strong enough to dilate the cervix more quickly. The baby is usually monitored continuously, since the artificial strengthening of the contractions may affect its condition. Syntocinon can shorten labour, but many women find the sudden intensity of contractions hard to bear without the normal, gradual build-up. Most women find that the nature of synthetic contractions differs from those of a spontaneous labour, describing them as 'mean' or 'spiteful'. Some women feel rather cheated at not being able to have the same degree of control over their own labours, though others welcome the speeding-up because they want to get on with their baby's birth.

Research has, however, shown there to be little difference in the length of labours between women who have been encouraged to remain upright and mobile throughout labour, and those where labour has been artificially accelerated. Of those women who had received the hormone drip, 80 per cent found it unpleasant and would prefer not to have it for a subsequent labour.

ACTIVE MANAGEMENT OF LABOUR

In some hospitals, nulliparous women, that is those expecting their first babies, are assessed more frequently than is usual once established labour has been diagnosed, and labour is augmented if little or no progress is being made. Early intervention by ARM and/or Syntocinon is believed to lower the rate of Caesarean section and instrumental delivery, and proponents of this method believe it lowers the rate of artificial pain relief because no woman has to labour for longer than twelve hours. Theoretically, therefore, the woman is in less distress because of the shorter labour, and the uterus does not become overtired and is helped to work more efficiently. Women themselves, however, often prefer not to have their labours managed and find that the increased strength of the contractions managed in this way is more likely to make them resort to artificial pain relief.

This procedure is not the same as induction of labour, being used only once a woman is in established labour but not progressing at a rate previously determined by the obstetrician.

Units where active management of labour is not practised use other means of helping a slow labour speed up which are less arduous and do not involve such invasive procedures, leaving the woman with a greater degree of control. Many small maternity units where the emphasis is on the individual and her carers rather than technology also tend to have significantly lower rates of Caesarean section, instrumental delivery, and artificial pain relief than there are among similarly low-risk women in larger hospitals.

My cervix didn't happen to be dilating at 1 cm. an hour and I was made to feel I was letting the side down, being a naughty girl! I felt immensely pressurized into accepting intervention so that my labour would be over and done with quickly.

It was nice to know that they wouldn't let me carry on in strong labour hour after hour; that there was a definite time by which my baby would be born. I was disappointed by not having been in charge of my own labour though.

EPISIOTOMY

In many hospitals, episiotomy is still routinely performed on mothers at the end of the second stage, either to speed it up if the time limit set by the hospital has run out, or to prevent the woman's perineum tearing. An episiotomy is a cut made with scissors (women and their partners are sometimes alarmed by the size of the scissors and the sound of the 'snip'), to enlarge the vaginal opening so the baby's head can be born more quickly and easily. It is a sterile, surgical procedure performed by either a midwife or an obstetrician. The cut is made during a contraction when the baby's head has already distended the perineum. Although the perineum is already numb when it is stretched by the baby's head, hospitals do give a local anaesthetic; you can ask for one if there is time for it to take effect. Episiotomies are currently performed on between 50 and 90 per cent of women having their first babies in hospital. You might like to find out what the episiotomy rates are in your area before deciding where to have your baby.

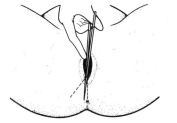

Without an episiotomy, many women have tears in the skin and superficial muscles round the vaginal opening, but these are often less extensive than episiotomies, whose size and position is determined by judgement rather than need. Whilst some obstetricians prefer to sew a neat episiotomy rather than an uneven tear, others have taken notice of the fact that women find even second-degree tears (when both the skin and superficial muscles are torn) less painful afterwards than episiotomies, and they also heal more swiftly. Moreover, as with all surgical procedures, episiotomies do carry a number of risks, including excessive blood loss and infection.

An episiotomy incision might be performed either at the midline, or medio-lateral

Many women also find their sex lives affected for months or even years by episiotomies which may remain uncomfortable long after the wound has healed. An episiotomy may feel like an assault on a particularly precious and tender part of your body.

AVOIDING AN EPISIOTOMY   There are, of course, cases where episiotomy is necessary (see Chapter 17, Complications in Labour), but in other cases it is possible for a woman to choose for herself whether or not she is prepared to have a routine episiotomy. A woman who has prepared for the birth and is able to relax her perineum during the second stage in an upright or semi-upright position, and can work with her midwife to deliver the baby in a gentle, controlled way, is less likely to tear badly or to require an episiotomy. A good midwife will also be very anxious to avoid performing an episiotomy unless it becomes absolutely essential and will encourage a woman to deliver in ways which will reduce the likelihood of stress on the perineum.

Ways in which you can prepare for the birth to try to avoid an episiotomy include perineal massage (see Chapter 6, Looking After Yourself) and pelvic-floor exercises.

Taking the homoeopathic remedy Arnica 30 or 200 before and after delivery will help any bruising and encourage healing whilst discouraging infection. It also protects the baby from shock if taken during labour in the 30th potency.

You will find information about the care of any stitches as the result of an episiotomy or tear in Chapter 22, Early Days.

SYNTOMETRINE AND THE THIRD STAGE

The essentials of the two ways of dealing with third stage are summarized in the table:

Physiological third stage	*Managed third stage*
1 No drugs in labour	1 Syntometrine
2 No time limit	2 7-minute time limit
3 No intervention	3 Clamp and cut cord
4 Upright position	4 Pressure on the uterus
5 Hold (and suckle) baby	5 Controlled cord traction
6 Observation by midwife	6 Observation by midwife

Physiological third stage

In a physiological third stage, no drugs are given, and it is preferable that the woman has received neither drugs nor medical intervention during her labour, so that the normal physiological process has in no way been interfered with. The baby is delivered and given to the mother to hold; physical contact encourages the woman's body to produce the right hormones for third stage; allowing the baby to suckle, if it wants to, increases the amount of oxytocin produced by the mother. The cord is left intact. The uterus is left alone; touching it can set up irregular contractions which could interfere with the natural process. The woman is encouraged to stay upright, either sitting, kneeling up, or standing, whichever is most comfortable. The midwife stands by observing the woman. After a time, the cord stops pulsating, indicating that the baby has no more need of the placenta. Then, as the placenta peels away and lies at the bottom of the uterus, the midwife usually sees the cord lengthen (more difficult with no clamp) and a little gush of blood from the placental site. The uterus expels the placenta with the next contraction; if not, the midwife will encourage the woman to push out the placenta with the following contraction — this is not painful, since the placenta is smaller and softer than a baby's head. The cord is then cut. The physiological third stage can last anything from a few minutes to two hours, but tends to occur sooner rather than later. Sometimes the placenta is just waiting to be pushed out, but the midwife has not observed the signs that it is ready.

Managed third stage

It is almost universal policy in UK hospitals for the placenta to be delivered with the help of Syntometrine, unless a woman has specifically requested a physiological third stage if possible. Syntometrine is a mixture of two drugs: Syntocinon and Ergometrine.

EFFECTS OF SYNTOMETRINE The Syntocinon causes the upper part of the uterus to contract down quickly after the birth of the baby, and the Ergometrine closes the cervix by inducing strong uterine contractions; using the combination drug is thought to reduce blood loss after the birth by rapidly reducing the site of the placenta so that the blood vessels are sealed more quickly. It does, in a way, replicate the natural surge of oxytocin that many women have at delivery. The use of Syntometrine is thought by many obstetricians to reduce the risk of post-partum haemorrhage (see Chapter 17, Complications in Labour), but this is currently the subject of some controversy; it is no cast-iron guarantee against post-partum haemorrhage and may occasionally give rise to complications of its own. If it takes effect before the placenta is delivered, the placenta can be trapped and need to be removed manually under general anaesthetic. Many women feel nauseous after Syntometrine; it can lead to a rise in blood pressure and it has been suggested that its use delays the production of breast milk. A further disadvantage of Syntometrine given routinely is the potential danger to an undiagnosed second

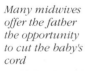

Many midwives offer the father the opportunity to cut the baby's cord

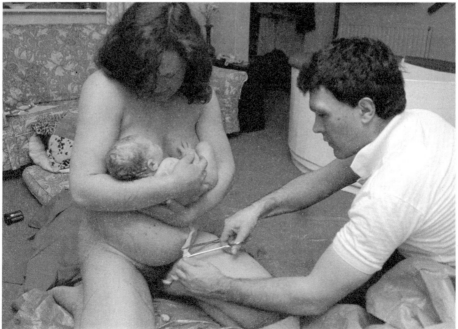

baby. Such an occurrence, though rare, would lead to the second twin becoming trapped by the contracting uterus, with generally unfavourable prospects.

ADMINISTRATION OF SYNTOMETRINE The midwife administers Syntometrine into the woman's thigh intramuscularly, immediately after delivery of the baby's first or 'anterior' shoulder. The midwife then has seven minutes in which to deliver the placenta, before the drug takes full effect and closes the cervix. Immediately the baby is born, the umbilical cord will be clamped and cut and the midwife rubs the uterus through the woman's abdomen to encourage contractions, so the uterus reduces in size and the placenta peels away from the inner wall. When she sees or feels the cord lengthen (the clamp on the cord is a marker) and, perhaps, a little gush of blood from the placental site, she knows the placenta is lying in the lower part of the uterus and will deliver the placenta by gentle pulling on the cord, at the same time pressing on the woman's abdomen to steady the uterus ('controlled cord traction'). The drug, when it takes effect, clamps down the uterus into a hard ball. The procedure is quick and rather uncomfortable when the midwife puts pressure on the uterus, but usually the woman is so absorbed in her new baby that she does not notice much of what is going on. Many women are aware of the placenta as a large, soft lump descending into the vagina.

Is there a choice?

It is important that the elements of these two procedures are not mixed up. Some women, when writing their birth plans, think it would be nice to leave the cord intact at delivery so that they or their partner can cut it themselves to symbolize the baby's independence, or they would simply like to leave it to stop pulsating while the baby receives all the blood it would naturally. If, however, Syntometrine is given, it is necessary for the cord to be clamped and cut to prevent the baby becoming over-transfused by blood being pushed down the cord as the uterus contracts sharply. Other women would like to have a natural third stage but would also like to use an epidural for pain relief in the first stage, in which case the effects of the drug might interfere with the physiological process of third stage and prevent it being totally straightforward.

So, the physiological third stage is something to be chosen by a woman who has a drug-free labour, when the third stage is the culmination of this natural process of birth.

Once the placenta has been delivered, the midwife examines the placenta and membranes carefully, to ensure they are complete. If you like, you can ask to see your placenta and to have it explained by your midwife. It will resemble a large piece of very shiny, raw liver.

* *We had agreed that third stage would be completed without Syntometrine if possible, and it was a further half-hour before I pushed the placenta out, with the help of Laura sucking at the breast to stimulate my uterus.* '

* *I expect I did have the injection for third stage, but I didn't notice it. I don't really remember much about the third stage at all.* '

PROCEDURES FOR THE BABY AT DELIVERY

THE CORD Immediately the baby's head is born, and before the next contraction, the midwife feels for the cord around the baby's neck. If it is wound round once, she slips it over the baby's head (sometimes a baby has a little bruise or a slightly bloodshot eye as a result of this); if it is wound round more than once or it feels tight, she will clamp and cut it so the baby does not pull on the placenta when its body is born.

MUCUS EXTRACTION At this point a mucus extractor may be used to suck out the baby's nose and mouth so that there is no impediment to breathing. The extractor is operated by the midwife sucking or, occasionally, by a machine. Some doctors and midwives prefer to let any mucus drain out of the baby naturally. A baby's tissues are extremely delicate and easily damaged, so many parents dislike the idea of a rubber tube being pushed down their new baby's mouth and throat unless it is absolutely essential.

RESUSCITATION Every delivery room is equipped with a Resuscitair, which has an oxygen mask and a heater for the few babies who need help in starting to breathe. New babies lose heat rapidly, so they are wrapped up in a blanket for holding after delivery before being dressed in a nappy and nightgown. The very warmest and most comfortable place for a new baby is, of course, cuddled up with its mother. The temperature of your breasts can rise as much as 4 degrees with a baby snuggled between them.

VITAMIN K Before leaving the delivery room, nearly every baby in the United Kingdom is given vitamin K either orally or by intra-muscular injection. This is done to counteract a potential deficiency which could lead to problems with blood-clotting.

There has been some controversy about this practice in recent years, mainly because one study suggested a possible link between injected vitamin K and childhood cancer. This link has not, in fact, been substantiated by any further studies, but some units now offer parents the choice of one single large dose of vitamin K administered by injection, or a lower dose given orally, which needs a follow-up dose later on. There is a further complication in that oral vitamin K has yet to be licensed for use in the United Kingdom, and some units do not offer this choice.

Recent research has shown that a woman's colostrum is rich in vitamin K, thus offering the baby some degree of natural protection. Formula milks also have a higher added vitamin K content. Much of the research into vitamin-K deficiency was carried out many years ago, when it was normal practice to separate mothers and babies in the early days after birth, and to restrict the early feeds, which meant that very few babies received all the available colostrum with its valuable vitamin K.

If you are at all worried about the possible effects of your baby receiving a high dose of vitamin K soon after birth, you may like to discuss this with a paediatrician at the hospital during the antenatal period. This will offer you an opportunity to discover what your hospital's policy about the administration of vitamin K is, and to talk over your concerns with a specialist, so that you can come to an informed decision about the most appropriate course of action for your baby.

MAKING YOUR DECISIONS

As with all procedures, discussions with the medical staff at your hospital can help you understand what is performed in your unit and why, as well as helping you to clarify your own ideas about how you would like your labour and delivery to proceed. Nobody is under any obligation to accept any medical procedure she does not feel is right for her at that time, but it is important that any decisions you make are based on information, freely and honestly offered by the medical staff. If you need to know more in order to make your choices, or if you feel you are being pressed into something more swiftly than you feel happy about, keep on asking questions until you get satisfactory answers which do help you to make up your mind about what you want for yourself and your baby.

16 Pain Relief in Labour

• It wasn't anything like as painful as I had expected it to be. •

• No one prepared me for quite how painful it was. •

• No one could have told me how painful it would be — I wouldn't have understood before. But it was never so painful that it was unbearable, and I shall certainly do it again. •

In the majority of situations, pain is the body's way of informing the brain that something is wrong — a bruised shin, a cut finger, an ear infection. In labour, however, it performs a different function: pain informs the brain what the body is doing so that the woman in labour can react to the pain signals and use her body appropriately for her labour. It is asking rather a lot of anyone to forget her lifetime's learned response to pain as a warning signal, but understanding that pain in labour is different — 'pain with a purpose' or 'constructive pain', even 'good pain' — will help her to feel more relaxed about labour and more aware of what is actually happening with her body. Women who have in some way pushed their bodies to the limit of physical and mental endurance when running, swimming, or cycling long distances, for example, or in climbing mountains; women who have coped well with period pains at some time, will understand something of the possibilities of a positive mental attitude towards pain, and may already accept that pain can be used by the body in constructive ways.

Many women do stress the positive aspect of pain in labour, saying that it is unlike any other pain, because they were able to feel their bodies working with them and vice versa. Some women will view any pain as 'necessary', an essential part of the rite of passage for this baby's birth. Other women, however, find that they feel diminished or humiliated by the pain they experience in labour. Each labour is entirely unique, but so is each woman's individual reaction to each labour. Pain is highly subjective — one woman's perception of labour as 'intense discomfort' may be another's unbearable pain. One woman from an antenatal class may describe her labour as having been much less painful than she had expected, whereas another from the same group may say that she felt unprepared for just how painful it would be. Some women will gladly accept any pain-relieving drugs, deciding that the relative freedom from pain they can offer outweighs any possible side-effects for mother and baby. Conversely, some women feel that accepting any form of pain relief in labour that is not naturally available would somehow indicate a failure on their parts. These women may be sadly disappointed both by labour and themselves should drugs eventually prove necessary.

You may already have firm ideas about how you hope to handle your labour and any pain you experience, and making a decision about what you would like to do is a useful tool in helping you cope with your labour. It may be that your labour turns out rather differently from what you had imagined, so finding out about the methods of pain relief that are available, discussing them and your feelings with your labour companion and your midwife, if possible, and, above all, retaining a fairly flexible attitude will ensure that whatever decisions you make are ones that you can feel positive and happy about.

AVAILABLE METHODS OF PAIN RELIEF

There are three main areas of relieving pain in labour:

- NATURAL METHODS WHICH DO NOT RELY ON DRUGS, BUT ON SELF-HELP AND YOUR LABOURING ENVIRONMENT (INCLUDING YOUR CARERS)
- METHODS WHICH DO NOT RELY ON DRUGS BUT ON SPECIAL-IST EQUIPMENT OR EXPERTISE
- METHODS WHICH RELY ON DRUGS

Each of these groups contains a variety of methods, and what matters is the reaction of the individual to any of these methods. You may wish to use a combination of methods appropriate for different moments during your labour. A basic understanding of the methods allows you to make the right choices for your labour and the degree of discomfort or pain you are experiencing.

NATURAL METHODS OF PAIN RELIEF

Natural methods of pain relief have been described in detail in Chapter 14, Preparing for Labour, and they include movement, position, relaxation, and touch. Because they are many and varied, it can be easy to underestimate the value of each, but used with understanding and support they are an invaluable aid to coping with labour, and many women need nothing further to help them through labour. It can help to remind yourself of why these natural methods work. Labour pain, as previously discussed, is not felt directly by the uterus, but any pain is caused by the reduction of the blood supply to the abdominal tissues surrounding the uterus, and pressure of the baby against your pelvis or spine. Any method which helps to reduce the effects of this decreased blood supply will reduce pain. Movement works by improving your circulation, reducing pain; relaxation makes the whole body less tense, also reducing pain. Touch both improves circulation and helps relaxation as well as being soothing in itself. A positive mental attitude helps you to welcome the stronger (and therefore more painful) contractions, knowing they are shortening your labour.

Using your labour companion and the support and interest of your midwife; your relaxation techniques; breathing to aid relaxation; moving around as much as you can; choosing positions which are comforting and upright to speed labour, as well as using any methods of touch or massage which make you more comfortable and/or relieve pain, are all acceptable and vital methods of pain relief. These are skills and resources that you have and can use whenever and however you wish, as your sole methods of pain relief or in conjunction with other forms of relief.

PAIN RELIEF FROM SPECIALIST EQUIPMENT OR EXPERTISE

Transcutaneous electrical nerve stimulation

How TENS works TENS is a method of pain relief in which four electrode pads which discharge a variable electrical stimulus are placed on your back. You control the amount of electrical input for yourself with a hand-held control, varying its strength by using the boost and choosing whether the stimulus is constant or pulsating.

The technique aims to 'interfere' with the passage of pain signals to the brain by sending tingling sensations across the skin, thereby blocking the 'gateways' through which these messages normally pass. It is thought that the technique may also release the body's own pain-killing hormones — the endorphins — in the same way that relaxation techniques do.

EFFECTS ON THE MOTHER The feeling produced by the electrical input is usually described by mothers as tingling or buzzing or like a 'very mild shock'. Many mothers find it extremely useful and a good distraction technique too, something to rely on and hold their concentration, using it during the whole labour, right through to delivery. To gain maximum effect, it is suggested that it be used from very early on in labour. Some women have found it ineffective; either totally, or once contractions have passed a certain intensity. It may also be an irritant, as the pads and wires may come to feel a nuisance once labour is well established and you do not want to have to concentrate on anything other than yourself and your contractions. Visiting the lavatory can be a complex manœuvre, and you do, of course, have to remove the machine each time you want to have a bath or shower. The advantage TENS has over some methods which rely on drugs, however, is that, if you find you do not like it, you can simply remove it.

Most hospitals have several TENS machines for use in labour, and some units encourage women to come into the hospital in early labour to collect a machine for use at home. You may wish to hire your own machine so that you can use it at home for backache in pregnancy as well as for early labour. This can be done through Spembly Medical (you will find the address listed at the back of this book).

EFFECTS ON THE BABY There is no known adverse effect on the baby.

* *A TENS machine was fitted, but provided absolutely no relief at all — I was despondent as it was to have been my lifeline. Another machine did work, and pretty soon it was being used at mark 10.*

* *I was hoping for minimum intervention as Pethidine hadn't agreed with me last time. TENS worked fairly well I thought, and at least I knew I could take it off if I didn't like it.*

* *Towards the end of first stage, the TENS machine got on my nerves, so I got rid of it, along with my clothes.*

HOW HYPNOSIS WORKS Hypnosis is occasionally used by women in labour.

Hypnosis

The hypnotist, through suggestibility, can induce you to believe that pain can be abolished. It is also possible to achieve this through auto-suggestion, and in fact the majority of hypnotherapists prefer women to learn to induce the pain-relieving technique for themselves.

The aim is that, by training in deep progressive relaxation, it becomes possible for you to rely on the removal of anxiety and fear and so concentrate on the joy of giving birth.

EFFECTS ON THE MOTHER With a trained hypnotist, some women do experience a 'pain-free' labour. Others combine it with other methods, including drugs.

Some hospitals, however, will not permit you to bring in more than one labour companion, and some will not permit any alternative practitioner such as a hypnotherapist at all. In such a case, if you were hoping to rely on external help with your pain-relieving technique, you may need to negotiate with your hospital to work out how your wishes can be accommodated. You could try speaking with the Director of Midwifery Services in the first instance, or discuss the matter with your consultant obstetrician.

EFFECTS ON THE BABY There are no adverse effects on the baby as far as is known. Indeed, there may be beneficial effects as maternal stress is virtually eliminated when it is working well.

Acupuncture

HOW ACUPUNCTURE WORKS The process of acupuncture involves the insertion of fine needles which stimulate special points in the body. The acupuncturist is present throughout your labour.

The needles stimulate acupuncture points in energy flow 'meridians', and natural endorphins are released.

EFFECTS ON THE MOTHER Those with previous acupuncture experience can find this method very effective in relieving pain. Others have found it has not worked at all.

As with hypnosis, some hospitals will not permit an extra person or alternative practitioner to attend you in labour.

Acupuncture may not be a cheap option, as your acupuncturist may have to be on call for some weeks, and in attendance for several hours.

EFFECTS ON THE BABY There is no known adverse effect on the baby.

PAIN RELIEF FROM DRUGS

Entonox (gas and oxygen)

HOW ENTONOX WORKS Entonox is a form of inhalation analgesia, a mixture of 50 per cent nitrous oxide (laughing gas) and 50 per cent oxygen, stored in cylinders, usually mounted on a wheeled carrier which is easy to move to where you want to use it. It is sometimes contained in a wall unit instead.

To use Entonox, you breathe in through either a mouthpiece or a mask, which you hold yourself. The gas is allowed to flow by a demand valve and therefore flows only when you inhale. It has a delayed effect, so you need to begin inhaling immediately you sense a contraction starting. The Entonox will then be effective as your contraction reaches its peak. It is essential that you take only four or five breaths, or the effect continues between contractions, and you may miss the onset of the next one. It works by altering your perception of the pain rather than anaesthetizing the actual pain.

EFFECTS ON THE MOTHER The effect varies from woman to woman.

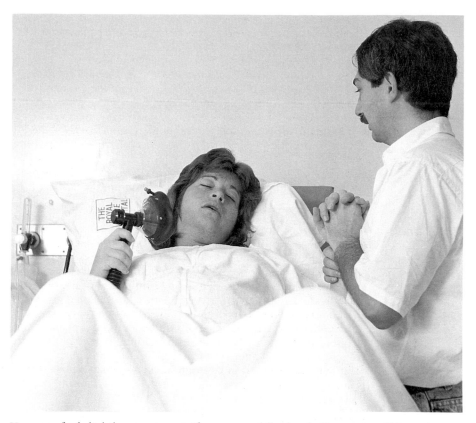

You may feel slightly woozy or as if you are mildly drunk. You may feel sleepy. Some women find they feel nauseous. You may find it makes it much easier to relax and cope with your contractions, but some women find the wooziness makes it harder for them to concentrate on and cope with contractions. The effects are not cumulative, so once you put the mask or mouthpiece down, and breathe normally, its effects will cease.

Using entonox (gas and air) during labour

Some midwives will allow Entonox to be used only when labour is well established and towards the end of first stage, to avoid the unpleasant effects of any nausea building up over longer periods.

If you do not like it, you can simply let the mask or mouthpiece go; you administer it yourself, therefore you control what goes in. You may need to remember to ask for it yourself; staff may not realize that you would like to try it, so may not actually suggest it.

EFFECTS ON THE BABY The baby clears any effect from its system with its first breath. It has no adverse effect.

• *I took one sniff of the mask and decided I didn't like the smell, and anyway, if I was almost there I might as well manage without.* ,

• *I had thought it wasn't really doing much. Then I went to the loo and had a couple of contractions without the gas and air and realized just how effective it was.* ,

• *It didn't do all that much for me, but was quite useful while I was waiting for the epidural to take effect.* ,

• *I used it when I was being stitched up afterwards. It made me feel I didn't mind about the stitching after all.* ,

Pethidine

HOW PETHIDINE WORKS Pethidine is a synthetic, narcotic, analgesic drug derived from morphine, with a powerful action, usually administered by intramuscular injection, in varying doses between 50 mg. and 150 mg. It normally takes effect within twenty minutes, and lasts about 2–4 hours, depending on the size of the dose and the individual's reaction to the drug. In most hospitals it is given with an antihistamine or other drug to prevent nausea.

Pethidine acts as a muscle relaxant and a mood-enhancer (like alcohol). Pethidine is *not* an anaesthetic drug, so will not take the pain away, but will affect your perception of the pain.

It may also be used in labour to relax a woman whose tension is apparently affecting the dilation of the cervix, causing contractions to be powerful but ineffective.

The size of the dose of Pethidine needs to be discussed with your midwife — smaller doses can be given and any dose should be related to your own body weight. Pethidine should, if possible, not be given within 1–4 hours of delivery, to avoid effects on you during delivery and on the baby afterwards; the actual time of delivery is, of course, very difficult to assess, and you may need to make sure that your midwife checks the dilation of your cervix before administering Pethidine.

EFFECTS ON THE MOTHER As it is a mood-enhancer, reactions to Pethidine are very mixed: some women find it makes them feel euphoric, 'outside' their bodies, as if they were floating above themselves, looking down on the pain; others find it disorientating and frightening, as they find themselves feeling out of control and unable to communicate. Some women feel as though they were unpleasantly drunk. It commonly makes mothers feel very nauseous and, as it increases the length of time undigested food remains in the stomach, this could create problems should a general anaesthetic become necessary. It may make you feel rather sleepy, or you may even fall asleep. This can be difficult if you then find you are waking up only at the peak of strong contractions. You could try asking your partner to feel for contractions, so that you can be roused sufficiently to cope with them when they come.

Given too late in labour, the lack of awareness of your surroundings and your body may mean that you are unable to bear down effectively during the second stage. You may find that you forget all that happened during the time that the Pethidine was effective, thus erasing great chunks of your labour from your memory. If your baby's birth falls during this period, you may be unable to remember giving birth afterwards, which you may find extremely distressing. You will normally need to be kept in bed once Pethidine has been administered, so will be unable to benefit from mobility and upright positions which would help your labour to progress.

You may be able to relax much better once the Pethidine takes effect, thus improving the progress of labour by reducing some of the more harmful side-effects of stress such as hyperventilation.

EFFECTS ON THE BABY Pethidine readily crosses the placenta and may have a marked effect on the baby both before and after birth. Side-effects are more likely after large or repeated doses or when given 1–4 hours before delivery.

It can cause delay in breathing at birth because of its depressive action on the baby's respiratory centre. An antidote can be injected into the umbilical vein at birth if necessary, to stimulate the baby's breathing.

Many babies are very sleepy after Pethidine, which can interfere with the normal alert period of getting to know each other at birth. This drowsiness may persist for several days.

Pethidine can also suppress the normally strong sucking reflex. This may make early feeds very difficult and possibly frustrating. Mothers will find that their milk still 'comes in' between the third and the fifth day after delivery, but may suffer severe engorgement if the baby is unable to keep up with the supply.

Subtle changes in new-born behaviour have been studied by many researchers; such changes may continue for weeks or months. Babies born after 50–100 mg. of Pethidine have been given in labour have been found to be:

○ **SLEEPY**
○ **LESS ALERT**
○ **EASILY STARTLED**
○ **FRETFUL OR DIFFICULT TO COMFORT**
○ **SLOW TO RESPOND TO FACES AND SOUNDS**

Such effects may sound trivial, but a sleepy, unresponsive baby who cries a lot, who may not feed well, or cannot be comforted can cause a new mother to lose confidence in herself and find the early days with her new baby less rewarding than she had hoped.

If you have had Pethidine during labour, you will need to be aware of any possible side-effects, and give your baby extra attention if necessary.

* *I wouldn't say I liked the feeling when I had the Pethidine, but it did give me a very pleasant couple of hours' rest.* *

* *It made me feel totally disorientated — horrible, like being really drunk and not able to control yourself.* *

* *I had Pethidine in both my labours and thought it was great; it just took the edge off the pain.* *

* *I didn't really want any drugs. I felt I was coping rather well; but my midwife kept coming in and suggesting that I might like some pain relief. In the end I gave in — I didn't have the confidence in myself to carry on without drugs when the experienced midwife clearly believed I couldn't do it. This time I feel certain I shall be able to manage.* *

Epidural anaesthesia

HOW AN EPIDURAL WORKS This is an injection of an anaesthetizing drug given through a catheter (a fine tube) inserted between two of the spinal vertebrae. The drug used is the same as those used to anaesthetize your jaw by your dentist. The catheter, once in place, is taped into position and the phial for administering the anaesthetic taped over one shoulder. The anaesthetic can then be topped up as required. Some hospitals now also use a system whereby the anaesthetic is pumped in continuously, using minimal amounts of the drug. This alleviates the problem of an epidural wearing off and then having to be topped up. It is, however, an extremely expensive piece of equipment, so is not readily available everywhere. A number of units also use so-called 'mobile' epidurals, where the amount of anaesthetic is very carefully regulated so that pain is relieved, but the woman retains sufficient feeling to change her position, possibly even to walk around.

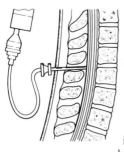

The site of an epidural anaesthetic

The nerves carrying sensations from the uterus/cervix/vagina to the brain are numbed by the anaesthetic effect of the drug. The lower half of your body will usually also be numbed. You will usually be put on to an electronic fetal monitor (EFM) to assess the baby's reactions to the labour, and possibly a drip to counteract the effect of the epidural in lowering blood pressure. You may also have a catheter inserted to drain your bladder, as all sensation in your lower abdomen will have been lost. An epidural will have the effect

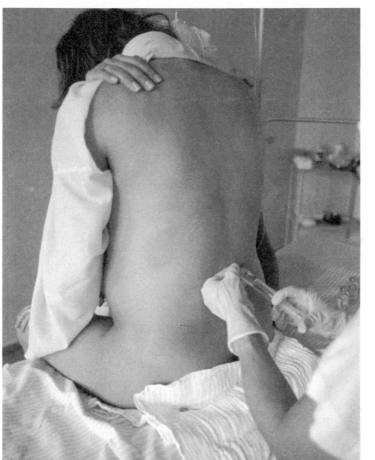

Setting up an epidural anaesthetic

of slowing down your labour once normal sensations have been numbed.

Epidurals can be used for clinical reasons as well as for pain relief, for example, to lower blood pressure or for certain medical conditions in a mother.

Epidurals are not always available on demand round the clock at every hospital; do check local policy before aiming to rely on this option.

Effects on the mother An effective epidural anaesthetic will remove pain from the lower half of your body, though you may be aware of contractions as tightenings, whilst feeling no pain. You may only realize you are having a contraction because you can see it recorded on the computer print-out.

If your blood pressure drops, you may feel sick and/or dizzy.

Some women experience severe headaches and/or backache for several days afterwards. Some women find their backache lasts several months. Occasionally a dural tap is performed by mistake, when a small amount of spinal fluid leaks out; this will cause very severe headaches indeed, so that a woman thus affected will have to lie quite still on her back for forty-eight hours or more.

Some women find that their legs are affected for several days after delivery, so it is some while before they are able to walk properly. There may also be bladder problems for a day or two after delivery.

Many women report feeling pleased at the pain-relieving aspects of an epidural but still feel rather disappointed emotionally, as though they have missed out on something. Women may also feel rather disappointed if they have chosen to have a mobile epidural, but then find their legs are still too wobbly or lacking in sensation for them to walk freely. True mobility is still uncommon once an epidural is in place, and any epidural will mean that a labour will become a much more clinical, managed affair, which may not quite match up to what you had been hoping for.

If the epidural has not been allowed to wear off sufficiently before you are asked to start pushing in second stage, you may be unable to feel where or how to push, as the sensations from the pelvic floor are lost. If this happens, the baby may have to be delivered by forceps or vacuum extractor. This loss of feeling also delays the normal reflex responses for the descent of the baby's head, which will slow labour down and may increase the chances of an instrumental delivery. Instrumental deliveries are more common in women who have had an epidural, however competently given and monitored.

You will need to make sure you have had an examination before an epidural is administered; it may be too close to the second stage of labour to be a sensible option.

An epidural takes about twenty minutes or more to set up, and you will have to remain extremely still whilst it is being administered, which may be most uncomfortable while you are coping with contractions.

Epidurals do not always work, or may work on one side only, which can be depressing if you had been relying on an epidural for pain relief.

Effects on the baby As with Pethidine, an epidural anaesthetic will cross the placenta. Some babies seem very jumpy and 'on edge' after an epidural anaesthetic; others are sleepy and difficult to feed for a week or so after delivery. Research has shown feeding problems frequently lasting for about three days only, but the baby crying for about six weeks.

• *Suddenly my mind unclouded and it seemed to me that an epidural would be the answer. Removing the discomfort would mean that I wouldn't have to worry about what was going to happen to me — I might even be able to enjoy the actual birth. An epidural had never been part of my birth plan, but I was sure of my decision.* •

• *The pain relief was excellent, but actually I'd rather not have an epidural next time I have a baby because it wasn't really what I wanted. I felt a bit cheated and didn't like either the side-effects or the way everything became a very clinical business after it was administered.* •

MAKING YOUR DECISIONS

Labour pains are highly individual and mothers will react in very different ways, so there is no way of knowing beforehand how you will choose to manage your labour. Being aware of all the information available about all the options, both pros and cons, will help you remain flexible and help you make a positive decision when the time comes.

There is no ideal analgesia for labour. The use of any drug is ultimately a compromise between benefits for the mother and possible risks for herself and her baby.

17 COMPLICATIONS IN LABOUR

About 85 per cent of labours are totally straightforward. Even where women or their babies are classified as 'high risk', most of those labours are normal. As well as approaching labour in a positive frame of mind, it is as well to know what to expect should complications arise.

It is also worth taking the time (unless of course, it is an emergency) to find out:

- ○ **WHAT IS HAPPENING**
- ○ **WHAT THE ACTUAL RISKS ARE**
- ○ **WHY THE SUGGESTED PROCEDURE IS BEING PROPOSED**

Having done this, then you can, if necessary, ask for a second opinion. It is a good idea to take time to get used to the idea of any proposed action before making your final decision.

After the birth, you can ask your obstetrician to go through your labour notes with you, which will help you understand exactly what was done, why, and what the implications are, if any, for a future birth. If you have any unresolved feelings about the birth, and many women do, try to find an opportunity (or several) to talk in detail about what happened and how it felt for you; your partner may well need to do the same.

LABOURS WHICH DO NOT START OR DO NOT PROGRESS

INDUCTION OF LABOUR

Reasons for induction

There are several reasons for an induction to be performed. As with any obstetric procedure, you may wish to question whether an induction is being proposed on sound clinical grounds in your situation or whether it is being done as a matter of routine at your hospital.

'OVERDUE' An induction may be performed if a woman is 'overdue', that is, if she does not go into labour spontaneously by about 42 or

43 weeks. Hospitals vary in the time that they will allow a woman before they advise induction, but most women, provided they and the baby are well, will be left until at least 42 weeks, though a few hospitals do have a policy of inducing so-called 'older' mothers earlier than this. The main concern is that, by this stage of pregnancy, the placenta could be beginning to function less efficiently and therefore be conveying less oxygen and food to the baby.

Depending on the medical indications, therefore, extra check-ups and special tests may be carried out. Many hospitals now have a fetal assessment unit, so that a woman can visit on a daily basis if necessary, to check that her baby is growing well and that there is no reason to risk an unnecessary induction. If it is thought that the baby is at risk from a failing placenta, an induction may be performed earlier than 42 weeks.

When women are unhappy about a suggested induction, many manage to negotiate very successfully with their obstetricians, who may then allow them further time if all is well. They may take the length of their actual menstrual cycles into account or simply allow them to remain at home for an extra night if they prefer. Although many women dislike the idea of being induced, the decision to induce may also be met with some relief, as it means that there is a known date for the baby's arrival and the end of pregnancy.

OTHER REASONS Labour may also be induced for the following reasons:

- O **DIABETES (A WOMAN IS USUALLY INDUCED AT 37 WEEKS TO PREVENT THE BABY GROWING TOO LARGE)**
- O **RAISED BLOOD PRESSURE**
- O **PRE-ECLAMPSIA**
- O **RHESUS INCOMPATIBILITY**
- O **TWINS**
- O **BLEEDING IN LATE PREGNANCY**

Methods of induction

Shortly before induction is to take place, a woman is given a vaginal examination to assess the 'ripeness', or readiness for dilation, of her cervix. If it is unripe, it is hard, long, and closed; if it is ripe, it is soft, effaced, or partly effaced, and sometimes a finger can be inserted. An unripe cervix feels like the tip of your nose, rather hard and gristly, whereas a ripe cervix feels soft, like the inside of your mouth.

CERVICAL 'SWEEP' ('SWEEPING' OR 'STRIPPING' THE MEMBRANES)

The examination to assess your cervix can be quite painful, particularly if you are given a 'sweep': a finger is inserted through the cervix and then swept around between the membranes and uterus. If your cervix is ripe and your body is ready for labour, a cervical sweep may be enough to induce your labour.

Induction consists of three steps, which may be taken at intervals determined by the condition of the woman and baby and by the obstetrician's judgement.

PESSARIES The first step is usually to insert prostaglandin pessaries into the woman's vagina, either last thing at night or first thing in the morning. Prostaglandin is a naturally occurring hormone which acts as the trigger to start labour. The dose may be repeated once or twice. The pessaries soften and also irritate the cervix, which can stimulate contractions.

ARTIFICIAL RUPTURE OF THE MEMBRANES (ARM) Depending on the effect of the pessaries, ARM (see Chapter 15, Medical Procedures) may be performed. This can either initiate or strengthen contractions.

SYNTOCINON DRIP Again, depending on the effect of the pessaries and ARM, the next step is to give the woman a Syntocinon drip. The dosage of Syntocinon is increased from two drops a minute to a level sufficient to produce effective contractions; this is normally done fairly gradually, to give the woman's body time to become accustomed to the hormone and the stronger contractions. Most women find the strong, induced contractions both painful and less easy to cope with. Once the drip has been put up, the baby will usually be monitored continuously (see Chapter 15, Medical Procedures), since the strong artificial contractions caused by Syntocinon may have an adverse effect on the baby's reactions to labour.

There may be cases where the three possible steps for induction are not all necessary, depending on how the woman's body responds, but ARM is normally effective only when used in conjunction with a hormone drip.

Once a Syntocinon drip has been set up, it will remain in place until after the placenta has been delivered, as the woman's body will stop producing any of its own hormones once artificial hormones have been introduced.

❛ *I really didn't want to be induced — it somehow seemed to take away all the excitement of going into spontaneous labour, and I was worried that the whole event would become very clinical. In the event, I managed to start off by myself the night before the induction was due.* ❜

● *It was a disappointment having to be induced, but I was jolly glad to be seeing the end of this pregnancy.* ●

● *The induced labour was noticeably more painful and harder to feel in control of than either of my spontaneous labours.* ●

ACCELERATION OR AUGMENTATION OF LABOUR

An acceleration or augmentation of labour is performed when the obstetrician believes that labour is not progressing fast enough. If the waters have broken spontaneously but contractions are absent or ineffective, a woman may be given pessaries and a Syntocinon drip, or just the drip. If contractions are ineffective and the waters are intact, ARM may be performed, followed by a Syntocinon drip if necessary. If labour is progressing slowly, but you feel comfortable and all is well with the baby, you may prefer to let things proceed at their own pace without any intervention. (See also the section on 'Active Management of Labour', Chapter 15, Medical Procedures.)

ENCOURAGING YOUR OWN LABOUR

There are ways and means of helping your labour start without necessarily resorting to medical intervention. Possibly the most interesting way is for you and your partner to have sex, with full penetration, as often as you can manage it. The stimulation to the cervix — pressure as well as the hormonal effect of the semen — may be enough to nudge your body into starting labour, but unfortunately this method will only work if your body is about ready to go into labour anyway. Cuddling someone else's small baby can also encourage your hormone production, as may looking at baby photos, or hearing a baby cry.

If you dislike the idea of going into hospital for an induction, perhaps you could ask your community midwife, whom you should have met by this stage, to come and give you an internal examination to assess your cervix at home. Many community midwives are only too happy to help out in this way, and you may well feel happier starting off in your own home, in familiar surroundings, than in the hospital.

A slow labour can be encouraged in all sorts of ways too. Often just a change of scenery, a walk around, or a relaxing bath will be enough to get contractions going again if they are somewhat recalcitrant. You might also try ways of stimulating your own oxytocin production: try some intimate kissing and cuddling with your partner (your midwife will understand and leave you in peace if you explain to her what you want to do). Nipple stimulation is an extremely effective way of encouraging production of oxytocin too; you can do it for yourself or — more fun — ask your partner to do it for you.

If your baby is to be born in hospital, it is worth remembering that labour often does slow down or come to a complete standstill for as much as two hours once you leave home and enter the unfamiliar, clinical surroundings of the hospital. You may like to sit in your own car or walk around the grounds before you go in, to help your contractions to get going again.

CAESAREAN SECTION

A Caesarean section will have to be performed if a woman's body does not respond either to induction or to acceleration — i.e. the cervix fails to dilate, or stops dilating before 10 cm. is reached (see Chapter 18, Caesarean Section).

POSITIONS OF THE BABY NOT IDEAL FOR LABOUR

BREECH PRESENTATION

Between 30 and 34 weeks, most babies settle into a position head down. Three per cent of babies remain the other way up and are born bottom or feet first. This is called a breech presentation, and may occur:

○ **IN A TWIN PREGNANCY — IT IS GENERALLY THE SECOND TWIN THAT IS THE BREECH**

○ **IF THE PLACENTA HAPPENS TO BE LYING SO LOW IN THE UTERUS THAT THERE IS NOT ENOUGH ROOM FOR THE BABY'S HEAD**

○ **FOR NO APPARENT REASON — A BABY MAY SIMPLY FEEL MORE COMFORTABLE IN THE UTERUS LIKE THIS**

DISADVANTAGES FOR THE MOTHER The main disadvantage for the mother is that, unless the baby's bottom fits very snugly on to the cervix and presses down on it in labour, just as the baby's head normally would, labour can take longer than normal, making both the woman and the baby tired. A mother may also be aware that her chances of having an instrumental or Caesarean delivery are increased.

DISADVANTAGES FOR THE BABY The disadvantages for the baby are in second stage. The legs and trunk of the baby are usually delivered easily, but the head, the largest part of the baby, has to be delivered

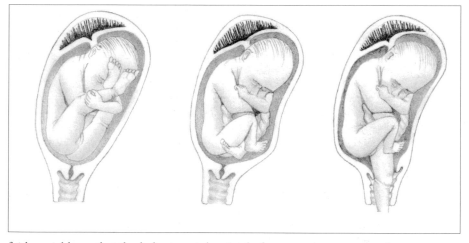

fairly quickly so that the baby is not deprived of oxygen, but not so quickly that the baby suffers brain damage. This is without the benefits of the gradual moulding and subsequent decrease in size of the baby's head which would occur in normal labour.

Common breech positions

This can cause problems if:

○ **THE BABY'S HEAD IS LARGER THAN NORMAL**
○ **THE NECK IS NOT SUFFICIENTLY FLEXED**
○ **THE BABY IS FACING THE WRONG WAY**
○ **THE WOMAN'S PELVIS IS SMALLER THAN AVERAGE OR AN ABNORMAL SHAPE**

Each case of breech presentation is treated on its own merits and, since opinions on how to manage breech births vary widely between different hospitals and obstetricians, it is important for you to discuss the facts and the options carefully with your obstetrician, asking for a second opinion if necessary.

Turning a breech baby

Some obstetricians try to turn the baby into the right position during the last month of pregnancy (external cephalic version), sometimes using ultrasound to guide them, but others say that this is successful only with babies who would have turned anyway. Some babies refuse to be turned, whilst others simply turn themselves back again! Fewer obstetricians will now perform external cephalic version than in the past, since the procedure is not without risk.

SELF-HELP Some women find that spending two or three fifteen-minute periods every day in the knee–chest position encourages the baby to turn of its own accord.

Another method of persuading a baby to turn is to spend at least half an hour a day crawling on all-fours.

Many women have had their babies turned by osteopaths, acupuncturists, or homoeopaths — worth a try if other methods have proved unsuccessful.

Assessing your situation

In the last month of pregnancy the baby's head and the woman's pelvis may be measured using ultrasound and X-rays to assess whether the baby's head will be able to pass through the pelvic outlet. The obstetrician uses this information to advise you on the safest method of delivery in his opinion.

Sometimes it is clear from the measurements and/or other indications that the baby would be in difficulty; in such a case a woman would usually be recommended to have an elective Caesarean section. In other cases, where there is a good chance of a vaginal delivery, it is a matter of choice for the woman and her obstetrician. Some obstetricians prefer to deliver all breech babies by Caesarean section, and some women would prefer to have an elective Caesarean rather than risk a difficult labour, possibly culminating in an emergency Caesarean section. Other women and their obstetricians would rather avoid a Caesarean as far as possible and give nature a chance.

Management of breech deliveries

FIRST STAGE Some obstetricians think that the best management for the first stage of labour is to give the woman an epidural in case the labour is long and painful; others believe that the woman remaining mobile and frequently changing into whatever is the most comfortable position encourages and allows the baby to move into the optimum position for birth, just as it would in a normal delivery. Another argument for having an epidural in place for a breech birth is that, should an emergency Caesarean prove necessary, the woman could avoid a general anaesthetic, and her partner could be present for the birth. On the other hand, it could be argued that administering an epidural 'just in case' could become a self-fulfilling prophecy. Nor is there any guarantee that, in an emergency situation, you could have an epidural anaesthetic for the Caesarean, as a top-up dose of anaesthetic might take too long to take effect.

SECOND STAGE During the second stage the woman is often asked not to push, but to allow the uterus to push the baby out on its own; this gives some time for the baby's head to descend and mould a little. (Unassisted progress of the baby also gives good indications for a vaginal delivery.) Some obstetricians would prefer this slow descent of the baby's head to be achieved by having an epidural anaesthetic in place, but this is another controversial area, with obstetricians having very different opinions.

Once the baby's body has been born, safe and speedy delivery of the head can be helped in two ways. An episiotomy on its own may be sufficient. If further help is considered necessary, forceps or a vacuum extractor (Ventouse) may be used to turn or pull or merely protect the baby's head.

Breech babies are sometimes born with swelling of the genitals from pressure during the birth; this goes down rapidly within a few days.

* *My breech baby decided to turn at 36 weeks and it was extremely uncomfortable. I was sitting through an evening at the cinema with this painful heaving and turning going on inside me. I was glad the baby wasn't breech any more though.* *

TRANSVERSE LIE

Transverse lie affects about 0.5 per cent of pregnancies; it may be the result of there being a large amount of amniotic fluid, of the woman having slack abdominal walls and uterus (perhaps after many pregnancies), or, more rarely, of fibroids or a cyst. If the baby does not respond to external cephalic version at the beginning of labour, it will have to be delivered by Caesarean section.

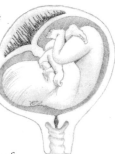

A transverse lie, across the uterus

UNSTABLE LIE

Some babies constantly change their position right up to the start of labour. This might indicate an obstruction to the birth canal, which would require special treatment. Sometimes when the waters break with a baby in this situation, a prolapse of the cord occurs, when the cord slips between the baby's head and the cervix, cutting off the oxygen supply. For this reason, women with an unstable lie often have to spend the last few weeks of pregnancy in hospital so that any complications can be dealt with immediately. In hospital or not, an unstable lie is an exceptionally frustrating situation for a pregnant woman, who may also be feeling rather anxious about the birth.

ABNORMAL POSITIONS OF THE BABY'S HEAD

Usually, the baby begins labour upside down, facing towards the mother's spine, with the back of its head lying towards the abdomen — occipito-anterior position (see Chapter 3, Antenatal Medical Care). Its chin is tucked well into its chest (flexed), so that the

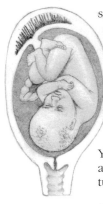

smallest part of the head, the top of the back part or vertex, is the part which leads the way down the birth canal.

OCCIPITO-POSTERIOR POSITION In an occipito-posterior position, the baby begins labour with the back of its head pointing either to the mother's spine or to one side, so that it faces towards her abdomen. For the woman, this often means a prolonged labour, with backache and irregular contractions. The waters may break early,. adding to the strength of the contractions. Many women find being in an all-fours position (see Chapter 6, Looking After Yourself) very helpful for the backache; this position also encourages the baby to turn into a better position. In fact many babies do turn to face the mother's spine and are delivered normally.

A posterior lie, the baby's back to the mother's back

PERSISTENT POSTERIOR When the baby remains in the posterior position — persistent posterior — facing directly forwards, for the second stage, it can be delivered normally. This is called a 'face to pubes' delivery.

DEEP TRANSVERSE ARREST More serious is when the baby's head partially rotates and descends into the pelvic outlet facing to one side: in this position it gets stuck and cannot move its head either to the back or to the front, so is unable to negotiate the pelvic outlet. This is deep transverse arrest, for which delivery by either forceps, vacuum extractor, or Caesarean section is necessary. Deep transverse arrest is caused by forceful, commanded pushing, inappropriate to the mother's or baby's needs.

Problems of head flexion

If the head is not tucked well down into the baby's chest, the leading part will not be as small as it could be, and labour may be prolonged, particularly in the second stage. Sometimes 'deflexion' occurs with a posterior position or deep transverse arrest, which can be corrected with forceps. If the neck is bent backwards so the face is the leading part of the head, 'face presentation', the baby can be delivered quite normally, but its face may be swollen for a few days. This soon returns to normal. If the baby's head is deflexed so the brow is the leading part, 'brow presentation', the baby's head cannot negotiate the pelvic outlet and the baby must be delivered by Caesarean section; this is, however, a very rare complication of labour.

CEPHALO-PELVIC DISPROPORTION

Cephalo-pelvic disproportion occurs when the baby's head is too big to pass easily through the woman's bony pelvis, either because the head is relatively large, or because the woman's pelvis is relatively small. If disproportion is suspected before labour begins, measurements are taken using ultrasound and X-rays.

TRIAL OF LABOUR If pelvic disproportion is not absolutely certain, a woman may be given a trial of labour to see if the baby can pass through the pelvic outlet. If satisfactory progress is not made during labour, or pelvic disproportion is diagnosed before labour, delivery will be by Caesarean section.

ASSISTED DELIVERY

There are four forms of assisted delivery available when the baby needs help in coming down the birth canal, or needs to be turned. The options are:

- ○ **EPISIOTOMY**
- ○ **FORCEPS DELIVERY**
- ○ **VACUUM EXTRACTION (VENTOUSE)**
- ○ **CAESAREAN SECTION**

EPISIOTOMY

Episiotomy is used to speed up delivery when second stage has gone on for too long in the obstetrician's view, and the woman and baby are growing tired. Sometimes a woman's vaginal opening will not stretch on its own to accommodate a large baby and needs to be enlarged.

Episiotomy is sometimes used during delivery of pre-term babies to protect their heads, which are softer than those of full-term babies, but this is a controversial issue and should be discussed with the obstetrician. Episiotomies are performed by midwives as well as obstetricians. (See Chapter 15, Medical Procedures, and also Chapter 22, Early Days, for suggestions on care of episiotomy stitches.)

* *I'd specifically asked not to have an episiotomy, but, when it came to the point, my midwife said she had no option. It was just as sore afterwards as I'd expected. Probably worse.* *

* *Peter nearly passed out when he saw the episiotomy scissors brought out.* *

* *In the end it was a relief to have the episiotomy, because, after all that pushing, she came slithering out immediately.* *

FORCEPS DELIVERY

This is a surgical instrument which comes in two halves which are locked together in use, rather like a pair of metal salad servers. There are various kinds, capable of different forms of assistance, varying in shape and size. People sometimes talk of 'high', 'mid-cavity', or 'low' forceps. High forceps are used when the baby is still relatively high in the pelvis, and assisted delivery using these is now much less frequent than in the past, since delivery by Caesarean section is nowadays normally a safer option. The majority of babies born by forceps delivery are 'lift-out' forceps, where the baby is almost delivered by the mother's efforts, and only needs a little help in the very last stages.

Procedure for forceps delivery

A forceps delivery is carried out with the woman lying in the lithotomy position, on her back with her legs in stirrups. Some form of anaesthesia will be necessary, which might be:

- AN EPIDURAL IF ONE IS ALREADY IN PLACE
- A GENERAL ANAESTHETIC
- A PUDENDAL OR SPINAL BLOCK

PUDENDAL BLOCK A pudendal block is an injection of local anaesthetic given high in the vagina, using a long needle, to deaden the pudendal nerves serving the vagina and vulva.

SPINAL BLOCK A spinal block is an injection of local anaesthetic administered at the base of the spine, numbing the lower abdomen. You will find further information about spinal anaesthesia in Chapter 18, Caesarean Section.

The woman is also given an episiotomy to make room for both the forceps and the baby's head. When the anaesthetic has taken effect, the forceps are inserted into the woman's vagina and fitted round the sides of the baby's head, one by one, and then locked together. The obstetrician uses the forceps to pull and/or turn the baby. This is done during contractions and the woman may be asked to push with the doctor. Sometimes very little help is needed; at other times, women and their partners may be alarmed by the amount of sheer force necessary. A woman's partner is usually allowed to stay for a forceps delivery, unless it has to be performed under general anaesthetic.

After a forceps delivery, the baby is often left with small red marks or bruises on its head, but these will soon disappear.

' *I was amazed when the doctor suggested she would have to use forceps. I suppose it was obvious things weren't going too smoothly, but I hadn't a clue that's what they were all hinting at.* '

● *It was horrible waiting while they got the forceps and everything ready. We just sort of sat, or rather lay, there, while the doctors and midwives wrote up notes and chatted amongst themselves. I felt frightened yet resigned and relieved all at the same time.* ●

VENTOUSE DELIVERY

The Ventouse or vacuum extractor is an alternative to forceps: the choice depends on the judgement and preference of the obstetrician. Local anaesthesia is given and the woman usually lies in the lithotomy position. A suction cap is connected to a machine by a tube. The cap is then fitted to the baby's head (or possibly its bottom) using vacuum extraction. The obstetrician holds the cap with one hand and pulls on the connecting tube with the other. Episiotomy may or may not be necessary and the baby is born with a little raised area on its head where the suction cap was applied. Ventouse is now used more frequently in the United Kingdom than in the past, although it has been in common use in other countries for many years. Women tend to find it a far less invasive procedure than forceps and the outcome for the baby is equally good. It does, however, take longer than a forceps delivery, so may not be suitable for use in an emergency.

CAESAREAN SECTION

See Chapter 18 for details of delivery by Caesarean section.

PRE-TERM BIRTH

A baby who is born before 37 weeks is considered to be pre-term, or premature. For parents who have been anticipating several more weeks of pregnancy, followed by delivery of a full-term baby, both labour and the arrival of this tiny, early baby come as a tremendous shock. Some women are aware in advance that their babies will probably have to be delivered prematurely because of problems with the pregnancy or the mother's medical condition; others are surprised by the onset of labour, unprepared for it, and may even fail to recognize that they are indeed in labour.

You might be given drugs to attempt to slow down or stop your labour, particularly if the baby is less than 34 weeks. These do not always work; some babies are quite determined to be born, but you may have some anxious or depressing days on the antenatal ward hoping your baby will manage to hang on for just a little longer! Although labour itself will be similar to a full-term labour, premature babies are usually delivered by forceps as a means of protecting the immature skull from the pressure of birth. There is,

The labour

however, some degree of controversy about an instrumental delivery for pre-term birth, and the management of the actual delivery is something you may wish to discuss with your obstetrician if you have time.

You may find it more difficult to cope with your labour if you are feeling worried that your baby may be beginning life with more problems than you had bargained for, but it is nevertheless important to try and relax during labour, as this will be more beneficial for both you and your baby. It may also seem rather frightening to have your delivery room fill with medical staff ready for the delivery, preparing to give your baby life-saving treatment as soon as she is born.

Once your baby is delivered, you may have a chance to hold her, or at least see her, before she is taken to the Special Care Baby Unit. Many hospitals do also take photographs of the new baby so parents can think about her in the hours before they are ready to visit her in Special Care.

You will find further information in Chapter 29, Babies in Special Care.

TWIN OR MULTIPLE BIRTHS

A birth of twins or more babies may well be more of a highly supervised medical event, with possibly twice as many medical personnel in the delivery room as for a singleton birth. There are, however, many twin births that start of their own accord and proceed naturally and normally, with both babies born vaginally. Occasionally twins can remain undetected until the second one puts in an appearance.

Mothers expecting twins may find they have a good deal of pressure put on them to accept medical intervention, but there is no reason why the same procedures need not apply to a multiple birth as to a single birth. Many twin and triplet births are entirely straightforward, as well as being extremely exciting events. As with any birth, ask questions and query medical procedures until you feel happy that the course being taken is the right one for your babies' births.

Two factors are particularly crucial to a twin birth:

○ **THE MATURITY OF THE BABIES (MANY BIRTHS OF TWINS OR MORE OCCUR PREMATURELY)**
○ **THE POSITIONS OF THE BABIES**

PRE-TERM TWINS If they are very small and premature, the birth may not be long and arduous for the mother, but great care must be taken and the birth made as gentle as possible for the babies. This often means an epidural anaesthetic may be administered so that the babies are not pushed too forcefully into the world, and forceps may be used.

DIFFICULT POSITIONS It is not as easy for twins as for a baby on its own to get into a good position for the birth. It is true that the most usual position for twins is with both of them head down, or cephalic, which is also the most favourable position. This accounts for only a half of all twin births, however. The next most common presentation is where one twin is cephalic and the other breech — the cephalic baby often comes first. Both babies can be born safely by vaginal delivery if there are no other complications.

Somewhat more unusual is for both babies to be in a breech position, and most twins in this situation end up being delivered by Caesarean section. Occasionally one or both babies is in a transverse position. If both are transverse, they will certainly need a Caesarean section to find their way into the world, but if only one is in that position and the other head down, the latter is born first vaginally and the transverse twin can then be turned by the doctor to follow its sibling along the same route. If it cannot be turned, then this second twin has to have a Caesarean birth. This can also happen if the second twin (whatever its position) becomes distressed and the heartbeat falters.

PROBLEMS FOR A SECOND TWIN Birth always presents more of a hazard for the second twin than for the first. For a start, it has to experience the strong expulsive contractions twice over, which may be a particular strain for a small, pre-term baby. Secondly, the uterus is smaller and the placenta more compressed once the first baby has been delivered. Thirdly, the second baby is often in a less favourable position for birth.

Births of supertwins

Triplets and larger multiples are more likely to be born by Caesarean section, but, again, a sizeable proportion of larger multiple births are perfectly straightforward. Since a Caesarean is always a possibility with more babies, this is something you can take the time to prepare yourself for. If you end up having to have a Caesarean, but would like to be conscious during the birth, an epidural can usually be arranged (see Chapter 18, Caesarean Section, for more information). When an epidural is successfully administered, parents find the births of their babies immensely moving, exciting events, with the doctors, midwives, and paediatricians in attendance sharing the joy of the birth.

BLEEDING IN LABOUR
Whilst it is usual to lose a little blood with the plug of mucus from the cervix at the beginning of labour, or whenever the show occurs, fresh bleeding during labour is not normal. There may not be any reason for serious concern, but it could indicate a

problem with the placenta; if this is the case, delivery by Caesarean section might be necessary.

MANUAL REMOVAL OF THE PLACENTA

If the placenta fails to come away during the third stage, or if it becomes trapped after the administration of Syntometrine, it will have to be removed manually under general anaesthetic, or epidural anaesthetic, if there is one already in place. The obstetrician passes a hand along the vagina and into the uterus to separate the placenta with his fingers and then removes it.

Sometimes, the placenta is delivered incomplete, in which case the same procedure is followed to remove the remaining part or parts. Retained placenta can give rise to bleeding and infection, so it is important that all traces are removed.

REACTIONS TO THE POSSIBILITY OF PROBLEMS IN LABOUR

After reading about all these complications, you may find that you dismiss all thought of potential difficulties, imagining it will never happen to you. You may, however, begin to imagine that, with all these potential problems, birth is a far more hazardous process than you hitherto realized. Either of these reactions is entirely normal and understandable, but it may help to share any fears you have with friends, an NCT teacher, or your midwife in your antenatal classes.

If you bear in mind that the vast majority of labours proceed normally, presenting no occasion for concern, this will help you put the possibility of complications into perspective. Even if you feel unable to imagine that anything could go awry with your pregnancy or labour, reading this chapter will give you a good indication about questions you might wish to ask should any problems arise.

Caesarean Section   18

This book devotes a whole chapter to delivery by Caesarean section, partly because there is a fair amount to say about its various aspects, but also because every woman having a baby in the United Kingdom in the 1990s has at least a one in ten chance of having her baby delivered by Caesarean section, and in many areas a considerably greater chance. However normal your pregnancy and however healthy you feel, it is worth reading this chapter, so that you know what to expect should a Caesarean section prove necessary.

Sometimes the reasons given by obstetricians for advising a Caesarean are clear cut, and in certain emergencies only delivery by Caesarean section will save the life of the mother or the baby. In other cases, however, the reasons for the advice are less clear cut, and Caesarean section is being recommended in preference to other options, sometimes because of hospital policy and sometimes because of an obstetrician's personal preference. Occasionally Caesareans are performed because it is the quick, easy course of action, when there is a good chance that the woman might have delivered her baby herself, or with another form of assistance.

A Caesarean section is a major abdominal operation, performed at a time when you are going to be working harder than ever before in your life (usually with interrupted nights). It is important, therefore, to determine the exact reasons for the recommendation of a Caesarean, and to take an active part in the decision-making. Whilst you may be relieved after a Caesarean and able to take the experience in your stride, you or your partner may find yourselves angry, depressed, or disappointed, perhaps feeling the birth could have gone differently, and you may be unable to resolve these feelings. Sometimes, these feelings do not emerge until a subsequent pregnancy. If you feel like this, do find an opportunity to talk at length about the experience, either to your GP or to someone from the groups listed at the end of this book. In any case, use your stay in hospital to go through your notes with an obstetrician, so at least you know what happened and why a Caesarean was considered necessary. If you are already at home, make an appointment to go back and discuss the birth. Some people find it therapeutic to write down what happened (which also makes interesting reading for the child in years to come!). Parents should feel able to regard delivery by Caesarean section as a positive event rather than a failure on anyone's part.

REASONS FOR CAESAREAN SECTION

FETAL DISTRESS Of the many reasons for a Caesarean section being performed, one of the most common is a lack of oxygen for the baby. This condition is known as fetal distress, and may be caused by:

○ THE STRESSES OF LABOUR
○ THE PARTIAL OR COMPLETE COMPRESSION OF THE CORD
○ PLACENTAL INSUFFICIENCY
○ THE SEPARATION OF THE PLACENTA FROM THE UTERINE WALL (*PLACENTA ABRUPTIO*)

INEFFICIENT CONTRACTIONS The contractions may be inefficient and perhaps irregular, so the cervix dilates only a little or not at all. This is known as cervical dystocia.

CEPHALO-PELVIC DISPROPORTION Cephalo-pelvic disproportion (see Chapter 17, Complications in Labour) is another of the more common reasons for a Caesarean section being considered necessary.

ABNORMAL PRESENTATION A breech presentation where the baby is in an abnormal position and cannot be delivered vaginally, a transverse lie, deep transverse arrest or brow presentation may all make a Caesarean section the preferred option.

PLACENTA PRAEVIA A Caesarean section will be performed if the placenta is low-lying (*placenta praevia*), but usually only when the placenta is lying right over the cervical opening.

MATERNAL MEDICAL CONDITION A serious medical condition in the mother — such as diabetes, very high blood pressure, or pre-eclampsia — may make a Caesarean a sensible option.

GENITAL HERPES A Caesarean will be performed if there is active genital herpes in the mother, to avoid the infection being passed to the baby.

(See also Chapter 17, Complications in Labour, for other possible reasons for a Caesarean section.)

ELECTIVE AND EMERGENCY CAESAREANS

A planned or 'elective' Caesarean is performed when the reason for its necessity is apparent before labour; an 'emergency' Caesarean is performed when a reason becomes apparent once labour has begun, such as fetal distress or undiagnosed cephalo-pelvic dispro-portion. Few Caesarean sections are true 'emergencies' in the normal understanding of the term. Unless there is sudden fetal distress or haemorrhaging in the mother, there is usually plenty of warning that all is not progressing smoothly.

TRIAL OF LABOUR Sometimes, when cephalo-pelvic dispropor-tion is suspected rather than definitely diagnosed, or when there is a breech presentation which might be delivered vaginally, a woman is given a 'trial of labour'. This means that she is allowed to go into labour spontaneously, or is induced, and her progress is carefully monitored. If the labour does not progress satisfactorily, she is then given an emergency Caesar-ean. Some women like to feel they have done all they can to give birth vaginally in such a situation, even should an emergency Caesarean prove necessary; others prefer to pre-pare themselves mentally for an elective Caesarean rather than risk 'the worst of both worlds' by having a disappointing trial of labour culminating in an emergency Caesarean. This is a matter of choice for the woman after having discussed all the options and possibilities with her obstetrician and her partner.

REGIONAL OR GENERAL ANAESTHETIC

Regional anaesthesia such as an epidural or spinal anaesthetic is increasingly available for Caesarean section, and there are several advantages in choosing this method:

- ○ YOU WILL BE AWAKE FOR THE OPERATION AND CAN SEE YOUR BABY BEING BORN.
- ○ YOUR PARTNER CAN BE PRESENT.
- ○ NEITHER YOU NOR YOUR BABY WILL HAVE TO RECOVER FROM THE EFFECTS OF A GENERAL ANAESTHETIC.
- ○ IF YOU HAVE AN EPIDURAL, YOU WILL HAVE THE BENEFIT OF CONTINUED PAIN RELIEF AFTER THE BIRTH.
- ○ THERE ARE FEWER MEDICAL RISKS IN A REGIONAL THAN A GENERAL ANAESTHETIC.

An epidural takes about thirty minutes to administer, and there is not always sufficient time if the need for a Caesarean becomes apparent during labour; in an emergency, a general anaesthetic can be administered and the Caesarean section performed within ten minutes.

Other reasons for a regional anaesthetic not being possible are:

○ THE NON-AVAILABILITY OF A SUITABLY QUALIFIED ANAES-
THETIST
○ LOW BLOOD PRESSURE IN THE MOTHER
○ INFECTION AT THE SITE OF INSERTION
○ INJURY TO THE LOWER BACK, OR OTHER BACK PROBLEMS
○ GROSS OBESITY
○ BLOOD-CLOTTING PROBLEMS (SOMETIMES ASSOCIATED WITH
SEVERE PRE-ECLAMPSIA)

Sometimes a woman will prefer not to be awake for a Caesarean or perhaps dislikes the idea of a spinal injection, and will opt for a general anaesthetic even if a regional anaesthetic is available. Modern general anaesthesia has fewer side-effects on the woman and her baby than in the past. It is also important that a woman chooses the experience that she feels will be best for her, emotionally as well as physically.

PROCEDURES FOR CAESAREAN SECTION

Before the operation

If there is time, the pubic hair is shaved, so it does not get in the way of the incision, and you may be given an enema or suppository. You can discuss with the anaesthetist and the obstetrician the choice of anaesthetic and the location of the scar; the incision nowadays is usually horizontal, below the line of the pubic hair. This is discreet and is also less likely to give rise to problems during a subsequent pregnancy or labour as the scar tissue will be most resilient here. Occasionally a 'classical' or vertical incision is necessary for medical reasons, or in cases of obesity where sweating between layers of abdomen could prevent the wound from healing. If you are having an elective Caesarean, the anaesthetist will visit you beforehand to discuss the most appropriate form of anaesthesia for you, and to let you know what each of the different methods entails. This can be an excellent opportunity for you to talk about any worries you may have about the operation and its possible effects on you and your baby.

General anaesthetic

If the operation is planned and you are having a general anaesthetic you will be asked not to eat for at least six hours before the operation. You may be given a 'pre-med', which makes you feel drowsy and your mouth dry, but this is seldom given nowadays. An antacid drink is usually given to neutralize stomach acidity, and sometimes a tube may be passed through the nose into the stomach to ensure it is emptied. A catheter will be inserted to keep the bladder emptied and this may be left in place after the operation. The anaesthetic is given by intravenous injection in the arm and you will drift off to sleep within two minutes.

The baby is often given to the father as soon as she is born, and he can then show her to you in the recovery room after the operation. Partners are not usually allowed to be present during a general anaesthetic, but will be asked to wait nearby. If you have not been told that your baby will be handed to the father immediately after birth, do check that the hospital will be doing this, providing all is well.

Epidural anaesthetic

An epidural anaesthetic is administered in the usual way (see Chapter 16, Pain Relief in Labour), though it may take up to one and a half hours beforehand in the anaesthetic room to set the epidural up. You will then lie on the operating table, unable to see your abdomen because of the small screen positioned over your diaphragm (this is actually to protect you from the cathiodermy used to seal the blood vessels cut during the operation). Your partner may stay with you if you want and can watch as much or as little of the procedure as he wishes. It is generally the case that the medical staff do all they can to explain what is happening and make the birth a positive experience. You will not feel any pain, but many women do mention feeling stretching sensations, as if they are being 'pulled about'. Sometimes, the obstetrician will ask you to push to help your baby out — psychologically, a lovely idea. Both you and your partner can see your baby being born and hear the first cry, which is an important bonus. Once your baby has been checked, you and/or your partner can hold your baby until the operation is over.

Spinal anaesthetic

A spinal anaesthetic, or spinal block, is used in some hospitals in preference to an epidural for both Caesarean section and for instrumental delivery. It is administered as a single injection at the base of the spine, directly into the fluid surrounding the spinal cord. It takes effect much more rapidly than an epidural, and wears off much more quickly too. No top-up dose is given, which is why it is really only suitable for short-term pain relief. One advantage of a spinal anaesthetic is that it affects a much more specific area than an epidural, though some women do still find that they have some degree of paralysis in their legs. In some hospitals, the anaesthetist prefers to use both an epidural and a spinal anaesthetic simultaneously for speed with effective pain relief plus the benefits of pain relief after the operation is over.

Spinal blocks used to be associated with a markedly higher incidence of dural taps (see the section on epidurals in Chapter 16,

Pain Relief in Labour), but the recent introduction of better needles has lessened this likelihood considerably, so that in experienced hands there is about the same risk from a spinal anaesthetic as from an epidural.

The
operation

You will have an intravenous drip in your arm, which remains in place until after the operation, and you may be given oxygen through a mask so that the baby can get as much as it needs. The operation is performed by an obstetrician. An incision is made in the abdominal wall and then in the uterus; its length depends on the size and position of the baby. A machine is used to suck out the amniotic fluid and any blood loss. The obstetrician then puts his hand into the uterus and delivers the baby through the incision. Sometimes forceps are used to deliver the baby. The cord is clamped and cut and the baby is handed to a paediatrician to be checked over carefully and given any necessary assistance with breathing. The obstetrician removes the placenta and membranes manually and checks that they are complete. The incisions in the uterus and the abdomen are then sewn, layer by layer. The birth itself takes less than ten minutes, but the sewing may take up to forty-five minutes, depending on the length of the incision. Various techniques are used to close the incision in the abdomen, aimed at achieving a scar which is both discreet and strong; sometimes clips rather than stitches are used, according to the obstetrician's preference. Syntometrine is administered in the usual way once the operation is over.

MEDICAL CARE AFTER THE OPERATION

For the
mother

If you have a Caesarean section, you will have a drip, which may be left in place for a few hours, as well as drains to take away any blood loss from the wound. The wound will be covered with a small dressing, plastic tape, or spray dressing. The wound is extremely painful, so the most important part of the aftercare is adequate pain relief. If you have had an epidural, this may be left in place for a few hours, but after this, or if you have had a general anaesthetic, pain-relieving drugs are administered either by injection or orally, depending on your needs. Drugs which do not affect your baby will be chosen if you are breastfeeding. Most women remain in hospital for five days, until the stitches are taken out, but you can stay longer if necessary either for yourself or for your baby. The drip in your arm is removed as soon as you are able to drink adequate amounts — after twelve to twenty-four hours. The wound will be inspected daily, and your temperature and blood pressure taken frequently to check for any signs of infection. The lochia is discharged just as after a normal birth, and this and the size of your uterus will be checked in the usual way.

Babies born by Caesarean section are more likely to need resuscitation immediately after birth, as they have not had the physiological benefits of a vaginal birth to help stimulate their own respiratory systems. If the initial reason for the Caesarean was fetal distress, then the baby may need resuscitation because of this too. Sometimes babies have to spend time in an incubator or in Special Care, depending on their condition. (You will find further information in Chapter 29, Babies in Special Care.) *For the baby*

COPING AFTER A CAESAREAN

The golden rule is: accept all the help that is offered and ask for more help if it is needed.

As a result of the operation, many women experience rumblings in their abdomen, and may pass a lot of wind for a few days; this is painful as well as potentially embarrassing and it is as well to avoid fizzy drinks, including mineral water, during this time. Drinking peppermint water, which should be available from the hospital, will help lessen the discomfort. If you have trouble opening your bowels after two to three days, you may be offered a laxative or suppositories. *Comfort*

Anything which rubs the wound is most uncomfortable, so waist-high pants to hold the sanitary pads in place are better than sanitary belts. The pants sold by NCT Maternity Sales Ltd. are excellent for this purpose.

You might also consider taking homoeopathic or herbal remedies for any abdominal pain or other problems following your Caesarean.

Although it may seem cruel at the time, you will be encouraged to get out of bed as soon as possible and to do as much as you can for your baby, because mobility improves circulation and aids recovery. You will also have a better chance to get to know your new baby. *Mobility*

While you are in bed, wriggling your toes and moving your feet around keeps the circulation going. A physiotherapist is always available to help with breathing and to demonstrate how to support your scar when coughing, sneezing, or laughing, all of which will be painful for the first few days. Many women find it helpful to accept pain-killers (or sleeping tablets) at night, but try to do without or with very few in the daytime, so that they can move about more safely.

This can be a painful experience in the early days. If your hospital bed is one that can be lowered, so much the better. You can make it easier by pushing your palms into the bed close to *Getting out of bed*

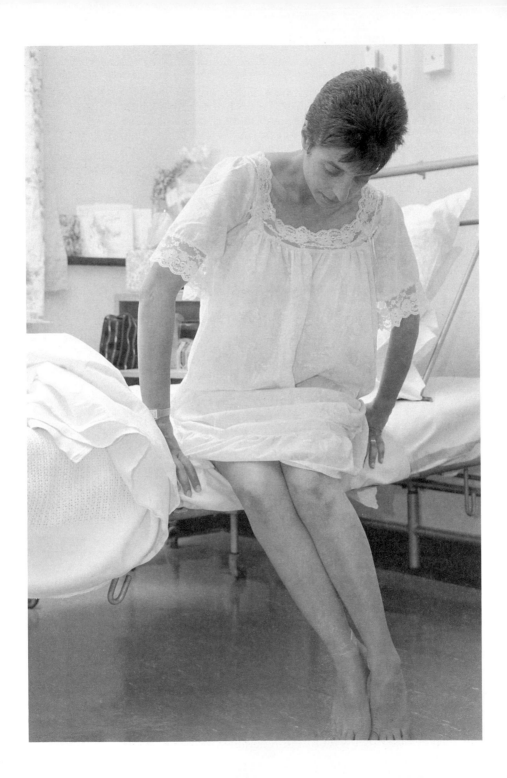

your sides and lifting your bottom. Now repeat this shuffling movement until you reach the left side of the bed and, with both hands, lift your left leg at the knee on to the footstool or floor. Then lift your right leg, so that you can ease yourself out of bed. You should not try lifting a whole leg from the hip; always move from the knee.

Alternatively, you could try shifting your legs to the side of the bed by shuffling one foot sideways and then the other, until both legs are together. Then, sit upright on the edge of the bed and swivel your body round.

In either case, take your time, breathe slowly and gently (use your relaxation techniques), and do everything yourself — a helper might pull or let go before you are properly balanced. The sooner you start moving, the sooner you will recover.

HORIZONTAL SCAR Sit well back on to the bed, with your back against the pillows, then slowly lift and slide your legs on to the bed, and lift your bottom into the pillows by pushing down with your palms.

VERTICAL SCAR Face the side of the bed, climb on to the footstool and then on to the bed on all-fours, turn and move your bottom backwards until your back is against the pillows. This is more comfortable than inching sideways.

After the first few days, if you slip down the pillows, pull yourself up by holding on to the bar above you, dig your heels into the bed and tuck your bottom against the pillows.

Stand up as straight as possible, so that gravity does not pull your abdominal organs against the scar. It is quite normal, if frightening, to feel as though your entire abdominal contents are going to drop out through your stitches. Support your abdomen, use the breathing techniques you learned for labour, and move from bed to chair as though this were a contraction. Breathing and relaxation techniques will help you not to become tense from abdominal pain.

Choose hard, upright chairs, if possible with arms to help take the strain. To sit down, put one leg behind the other, bend your knees, and sit. To get up, lean forward, putting one foot behind the other, and bend the knees. If an armchair is not available, sit on one buttock and edge back sideways.

You may be asked to use the lavatory on the first day. Use bent knees to take the strain and hold on to any rails. Relax your pelvic floor (remember to keep your face relaxed as well) to help the flow of urine. If you decide to use the bidet, do check the temperature first

(Opposite)
Take every precaution to avoid straining your abdomen in the first few days after your Caesarean section

Getting into bed

Walking

Sitting

Using the lavatory

— you will not be able to leap up if it is too hot! Bidets are also the most comfortable means of washing your feet. (See Chapter 22, Early Days, for information on avoiding postnatal infection, however.)

Breast-feeding

Breastfeeding after a Caesarean is perfectly possible, even if you and your baby are drowsy after a general anaesthetic. With frequent suckling the milk will come in, so, if you find lifting the baby uncomfortable, you should ask for help in picking her up each time she cries. A Caesarean wound does make it more difficult to find a comfortable position, but any position in which the baby is supported and not resting directly on your abdomen is helpful. Breathing and relaxation techniques which you learned for labour are also excellent for breastfeeding.

You will also need to think carefully about feeding positions which are really comfortable.

HORIZONTAL-SCAR POSITIONS

- SITTING UP, WITH PILLOWS LAID HORIZONTALLY ACROSS THE STOMACH
- LAYING YOUR BABY ON A PILLOW ON TOP OF THE MEAL TABLE WHICH FITS OVER THE BED
- LYING ON YOUR SIDE, WITH YOUR BABY FACING YOU

VERTICAL-SCAR POSITIONS

- SITTING UP WITH A PILLOW ON EITHER SIDE OF YOU, THE BABY'S HEAD ON ONE OF THE PILLOWS AND HER FEET OVER YOUR THIGHS
- LAYING YOUR BABY ON A PILLOW, HER HEAD FACING YOUR BREAST AND HER BODY UNDER YOUR ARM (THIS LEAVES BOTH HANDS FREE TO SUPPORT YOUR BABY'S NECK AND SHOULDERS)
- LAYING YOUR BABY OVER THE MEAL TABLE, AS ABOVE

GETTING BACK TO NORMAL

Although you might have felt quite fit and well in hospital, do not be surprised if you feel a bit 'wobbly' when you get home. This happens to women who have had vaginal deliveries too. You have had a major operation as well as the emotional experience of giving birth, and it may be particularly hard if your Caesarean was preceded by a long, difficult labour. Concentrate on looking after your baby and getting to know her, leaving *everything* else undone or to someone else.

Heavy lifting needs to be avoided for at least six weeks, so if you have to lift something (toddlers do not always understand about Caesareans and may need extra attention themselves at this time!), remember to bend your knees, keep your back straight, and directly face the object to be lifted.

It may take you as long as a month to recover. It is important not to compare your recovery with that of friends who have had vaginal deliveries, and it may be now that the support of other women who have had Caesareans may be especially valuable: contact your local NCT teacher or branch for details. If you feel low or are having problems relating to your baby, talk to your partner and seek help from your GP, midwife, or health visitor. Many women find that getting out of the house, seeing friends, and joining a local NCT postnatal support group can be enough to help them cope at what may be a difficult time. One of the most irritating after-effects of a Caesarean is that you will be advised not to drive for six weeks, in case you risk damaging the scar in an emergency stop. If you are normally dependent on a car, you may feel rather 'trapped', or embarrassed by having to ask friends to transport you or your other

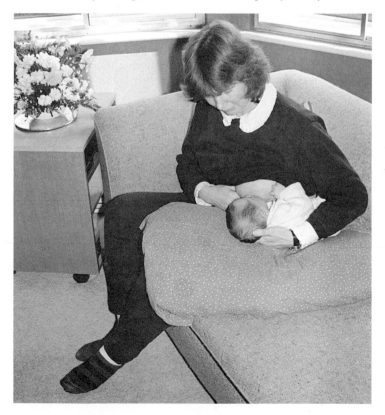

Feeding the baby 'under-arm' avoids pressure on a Caesarean scar

children for a while. You could, of course, look upon this as a bonus of extra rest at a time when you have plenty of recuperation to get through. Try not to feel shy about asking friends and other mothers for lifts if you want to go out — most people are only too happy to help out.

THE SCAR Your scar will gradually feel less sore and may then become itchy. It sometimes remains sensitive for a while, but its appearance will gradually fade from red to brown to white. Larger pants that come up to your waist are more comfortable initially and loose clothes are essential.

If you have had your pubic hair shaved, this will also be horribly itchy as it regrows.

RESUMING LOVE-MAKING You and your partner can resume love-making whenever you feel ready, though you might need to experiment with positions that do not put pressure on your scar. You will not be able to have a coil fitted for three months (instead of the usual eight weeks), so discuss some other form of contraception before leaving hospital if you wish. Some women feel worried about the effect their changed appearance will have on their attractiveness to their partner, or are concerned that they may seem less 'womanly', not having achieved a vaginal birth. Sharing these feelings and worries with your partner can help to resolve any anxieties.

FUTURE DELIVERIES

After a Caesarean section, future deliveries would normally take place in hospital, since there is some risk of the uterine scar tissue breaking down. There are women, however, who have had successful vaginal deliveries at home following a Caesarean birth, so this need not be an obstacle to a home birth in the future. It is certainly possible to have a vaginal delivery following a Caesarean, but much will depend on the reasons why a Caesarean was performed. 'One-off' reasons, for example, such as a breech baby, *placenta praevia*, or fetal distress would not prevent a future vaginal delivery if all else were well. A small or unusually shaped pelvis or uterus will, however, probably mean Caesarean sections for future births. It is a good idea to discuss these aspects before leaving hospital, and it is always feasible to arrange an X-ray at a future date if there is doubt about the possibility of future vaginal deliveries.

If a woman has had two Caesarean sections, an obstetrician would usually advise a Caesarean for subsequent deliveries, but this should be discussed in detail with your consultant.

• *I don't mind that I've had to have Caesars for all three of my babies. It was a bit disappointing initially, with the first, but I love having babies, however they are born.* •

• *It took me several weeks, maybe longer, to get over the feelings of disappointment, guilt, and failure at not being able to give birth to our son as I'd wanted. I had trusted my body and it had let me down.* •

• *I'll never forget the look on Stuart's face as he saw our baby being lifted from my abdomen, nor the delicious sensation of cuddling my own baby immediately after delivery. Unlike last time, when I had a general anaesthetic, I knew this baby was mine and I wasn't asleep for the first six hours of his life.* •

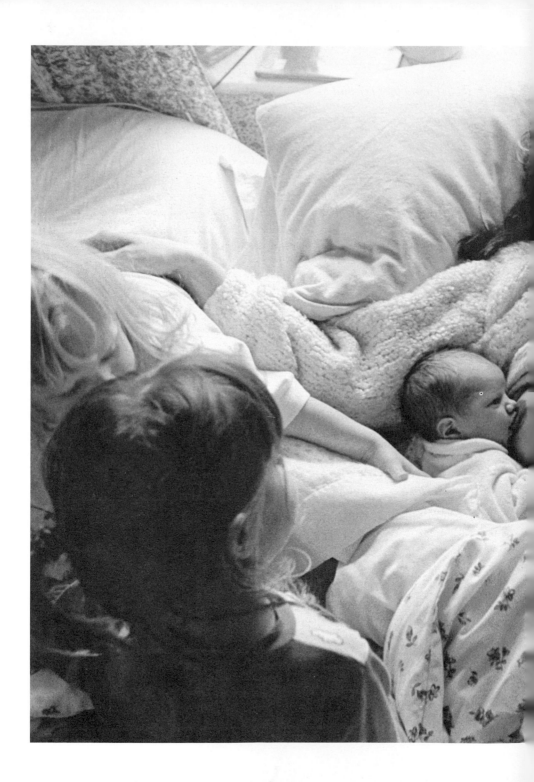

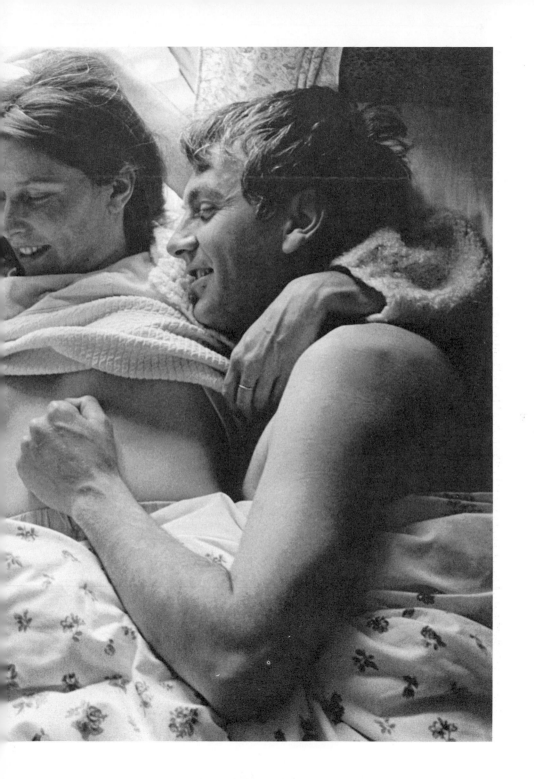

19 BIRTH AT HOME

Having her baby at home is not every woman's idea of bliss. There are, however, many women who feel that giving birth in their own home will be absolutely right for them and their families. Some of these women, having decided to opt for a home birth, find it relatively easy to organize. Others may have problems either in persuading medical attendants to deliver them at home, or in persuading those around them that they have indeed made sensible, responsible choices.

You may feel that you would very much like to have your baby at home, but are concerned that it might not be as safe, medically, as birth in a hospital unit. You may be worried that you will be expected to carry on as normal rather too soon after your baby's birth. You may not know anyone else in your area who has ever had a home birth. You may be unsure of your legal position. This chapter aims to help you sort out some of these issues, so that you can make your decision about where to have your baby, armed with all available information.

SAFETY

For most people, safety is the single most controversial area when considering home births. Opponents of home birth often claim that it is not a safe option, and you may well meet people who hold this view whilst you are considering what you would like to do.

There may indeed be complications in your labour and birth, and this is something which must be acknowledged. Few pregnant women choosing birth at home go into it without having given very careful thought to the safety aspect, recognizing that there are certain risks to be taken. These risks are not necessarily any greater than risks you might be taking by going into hospital, however, and ultimately the decision and the responsibility are yours.

PERSONAL SAFETY You can reassure yourself of your personal safety by checking what equipment is carried by your midwife or doctor.

○ **DO THEY HAVE A PORTABLE FETAL HEART MONITOR SUCH AS A SONICAID?**
○ **DO THEY HAVE FACILITIES FOR RESUSCITATING THE BABY?**

○ **DO THEY CARRY THE WHEREWITHAL FOR ADMINISTERING INTRAVENOUS FLUIDS?**

You may also wish to find out about the obstetric flying squad in your area; to know how easily it can be contacted, and how quickly it could be at your home, and how soon you could be in hospital if necessary.

It might also be worth considering how confident the doctor or midwife you are asking to attend you is about his or her willingness or ability to cope with a home birth. Some doctors or midwives may well cite safety reasons as arguments against your having a home birth, partly because they would prefer not to undertake the delivery themselves.

Studies in Britain and Holland now suggest that home birth may actually be safer for mother and baby than birth in hospital.

The statistics

Marjorie Tew, a statistician, looked at British studies and official still-birth figures. Her findings suggested that it is safer for most women to have a baby at home or in a GP unit than in hospital. Very high-risk women, however, are still safer in hospital.

In Holland researchers compared low-risk women delivered at home with low-risk women delivered in hospital. Low-risk women are those:

○ **EXPECTING A SECOND OR THIRD BABY**
○ **WITH NO HISTORY OF COMPLICATIONS IN PREVIOUS PREGNAN- CIES OR LABOURS**
○ **UNDER 35**
○ **OVER 5' 1" TALL**

They found that more complications arose amongst the women in hospital and concluded that, because emergency equipment is readily available there, it is used too often and too soon in perfectly normal labours. This study showed that it is a wholly responsible decision for a normal healthy woman to have her baby at home, given the right supervision.

Another study, comparing births in a GP unit with those in a hospital consultant unit, found that, although labours were longer in the GP unit, there were:

○ **FEWER EPIDURALS ADMINISTERED**
○ **LESS PETHIDINE ADMINISTERED**
○ **LESS ELECTRONIC FETAL MONITORING**
○ **LESS FETAL DISTRESS DIAGNOSED**
○ **FEWER BABIES REQUIRING RESUSCITATION**
○ **FEWER LOW APGAR SCORES AT ONE MINUTE THAN IN THE CONSULTANT UNIT**

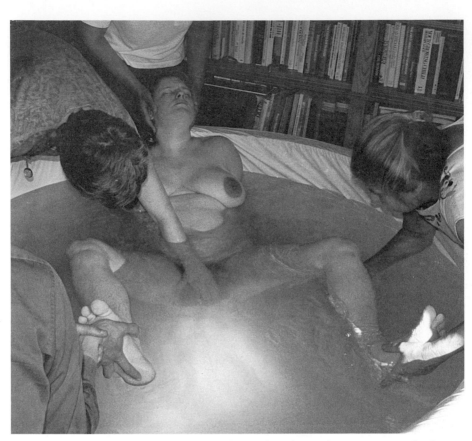

In your own home, the choices for the birth will be yours Their conclusion was that, when low-risk women gave birth in a consultant unit geared for high-risk, they too were liable to be treated as high-risk.

The risks

The main risks which cause anxiety are post-partum haemorrhage (PPH) in the mother, fetal distress, and failure of the baby to breathe at birth. These are rare complications, however.

POST-PARTUM HAEMORRHAGE Should a mother have a haemorrhage, the midwife would take precisely the same action as she would in hospital. She will carry all the necessary drugs, and administer them as appropriate. The flying squad would be called and you would be taken to hospital with your baby. PPH is associated with delivery of the placenta, and management of this is something you should discuss with your midwife.

There is some controversy surrounding just how often PPH occurs, and why it does, but a Dutch study showed that PPH happened to:

○   **0.3 PER CENT OF WOMEN GIVING BIRTH AT HOME**
○   **1.1 PER CENT OF WOMEN GIVING BIRTH IN HOSPITAL**

A woman's position and any medical intervention during labour will affect what happens in the third stage. This could explain why fewer women suffered a PPH at home.

FETAL DISTRESS Fetal distress can be indicated by a change in the baby's heart rate. If this were to happen in the first stage of labour, you would be transferred to hospital. If it occurred during second stage, your baby would be delivered as quickly as possible: you would probably be given an episiotomy, and, if a doctor were available, the baby might be delivered by forceps.

FAILURE OF BABY TO BREATHE Should your baby not breathe at birth, the midwife would give mouth-to-mouth resuscitation and oxygen to the baby. The flying squad would be called. If necessary, a tube would be inserted down the baby's throat into its windpipe.

Marjorie Tew studied figures for babies with breathing difficulties at birth. She found that more hospital-delivered babies than babies born at home:

○   **HAD BREATHING DIFFICULTIES AT BIRTH**
○   **WERE TRANSFERRED TO SPECIAL CARE BABY UNITS WITH BREATHING DIFFICULTIES**
○   **DIED BECAUSE OF BREATHING DIFFICULTIES**

PARTNERS

Your partner may have very strong feelings about the place of birth. Men are often rather apprehensive about the idea of their child being born at home; they may feel less confident than you do. It can help to look at the actual statistics and also to chat with other fathers whose babies have been born at home. Your partner could find he needs more opportunities to find out about labour — how he can help, and what sort of feelings and reactions he might experience.

After the birth, most partners are enthusiastic, even if they had doubts initially, and those whose previous children had been born in hospital, compared the home births very favourably.

If you are under some pressure from other members of your family, or from members of the medical profession, having your partner's support and encouragement is a great help.

It may be that your partner feels under a greater pressure to be with you for a home birth than he would for a hospital birth. He may prefer not to be with you during the labour, and this is something for the two of you to discuss. You might like to think about who else you might like to be with you to support you during labour if your partner has chosen not to be there.

Other children

If you have other children already, you might like to consider whether they will also wish to be present at the birth, and, if they do, how you both feel about this. It is worth discussing this with your midwife too, to see how she feels about the presence of others at the birth.

HOW TO GET A HOME-BIRTH BOOKING

It is a legal right for any woman to have her baby at home. This includes mothers expecting a first baby and those considered at high risk of complications during labour, and also those whose doctor refuses to book them for a home birth. If you wish to have your baby at home, you may legally do so.

If you decide you would like a home birth having already booked in for a hospital birth, you are perfectly entitled to change your mind and book for a home birth.

Once you have made your mind up about a home birth, you will need to visit your GP. He may accept your booking, or may recommend that you transfer to another doctor, from whom you will receive your maternity care. Some GPs are willing to undertake your ordinary medical care while you receive maternity care elsewhere; others ask you to transfer completely for the duration of your maternity care. For some women, obtaining a home-birth booking is fraught with difficulty, enough to put off all but the most determined. You may find you need great powers of determination to achieve what you have chosen.

If you cannot find a doctor to accept you

If your GP will not accept your booking, and you cannot find another GP in your area (your local Family Health Service Authority holds a list of obstetric GPs), you do not have to have a doctor at all. All your maternity care — antenatal, postnatal, and intrapartum (labour) can be obtained from your community midwives. Midwives are independent practitioners in their own right, who are trained to give women all the care they need throughout pregnancy, birth, and the postnatal period.

The way to obtain such care is by a letter to the Director of Nursing Services (Midwifery) at the local District Health Authority. She (or he) is responsible for organizing midwifery care for the women in that area. You can find her name from your local Community Health Council if you wish.

The following sample letter is based on one drafted by Margaret Whyte of the Society to Support Home Confinements:

Dear (name),

I am expecting a baby sometime in (month) and intend to give birth at home. My GP (give name and address) feels unable to offer me medical care for the birth.

I am therefore writing to ask you to make the necessary arrangements for a midwife to undertake my pregnancy and delivery care in my own home.

I accept full responsibility for my decision to give birth at home and I know that you will accept the responsibility of providing me with a competent midwife fully backed up by such facilities as are necessary to make the confinement as safe as possible. I look forward to your kind attention.

Yours sincerely,

This can be written as a joint letter signed by you and your husband or partner. You will need to keep a copy for yourself, and you should send copies to:

- O   **DISTRICT MEDICAL OFFICER**
- O   **CHAIRMAN, DISTRICT HEALTH AUTHORITY**
- O   **CHAIRMAN, COMMUNITY HEALTH COUNCIL**
- O   **YOUR MP**

Sending copies of the letter to these people keeps them informed of the demand for home births in your area.

Having done this, you should then be contacted by one of a team of midwives, who will come to your home to book you for your home confinement and arrange to provide the rest of your antenatal care there.

Once the arrangements have been made, you should not be expected to be under any further pressure to change your mind. It is possible though that you will still be expected to argue your case, particularly if you are not considered to be a low-risk case.

It will help you if you are well informed and can remain confident and assured in the knowledge that *you* are responsible for your decision and know that you have made the best choice for you.

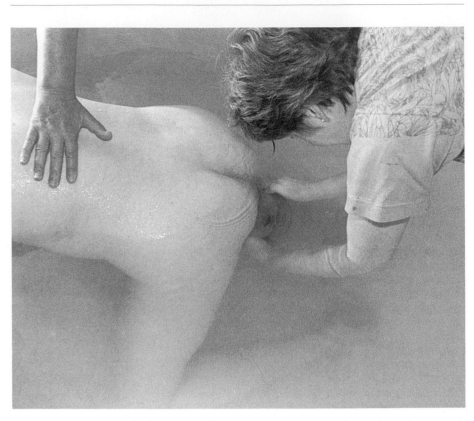

Ideally, you will be able to develop a relationship of trust with your midwife, so that you will be able to rely on her and accept her advice should she feel that you should be transferred to hospital care at any time. If your midwife appears to be opposed to your home delivery, or is not confident about her own role, then you can ask the Director of Midwifery Services to supply you with another midwife. You have a right to ask for a different midwife at any point; if you feel unhappy with your midwife and ask to change, it may well be that she will feel happier too.

The Association for Improvement in Maternity Services (AIMS) or the Society to Support Home Confinements will be able to help if you have real problems in obtaining a home birth. Both organizations have experience of helping women obtain the service they would like. (You will find the addresses listed at the back of this book.)

You might be asked to sign a form absolving the health authority from responsibility for your actions. This has no legal status and you can refuse to sign it without prejudicing your right to have your baby born at home.

ANTENATAL CARE

Antenatal care is normally provided at home, unless you are having shared care with your GP. In some areas, you might attend a local clinic. A midwife attending a woman at home has access to a consultant opinion and hospital facilities such as ultrasound through her midwifery supervisor. In an emergency, she can call on any doctor to assist her, and she is obliged, by her terms of service, to attend any woman in labour who calls on her.

Providing there are no problems, you will see your midwife at the usual intervals.

When you think you are in labour, you contact your midwife, or one of the team, who will call and assess the situation, and either leave, returning later, or stay with you, depending on your situation. The midwife is usually joined by another for the actual birth of the baby and they will stay with you until all is cleaned up and you are settled in bed with your baby beside you.

Preparing for the birth

At 36 weeks your midwife will bring round a delivery pack, which remains with you unopened, until you are in labour. She will also give you a list of things she would like you to have ready. You may wish to add to this some items of your own, such as a large shirt or T-shirt to wear in labour, a camera (plus film!), as well as any of the labour aids mentioned in Chapter 14. In many areas it is now also possible to hire a birthing-pool, so that you can have a water birth in your own living-room. (You will find details in the list of addresses at the back of this book.)

HELP AT HOME

It is essential that you should have adequate domestic help both during the birth and for at least ten days after the baby arrives. Aim to do as little as if you were in hospital. It is easy to feel so well after a home birth that you are tempted to get on with life as usual. (The same thing tends to apply to women who have had an early discharge from a hospital or GP unit.) Your body, however, still has to adjust from being pregnant to being a mother and has to establish breastfeeding. Allow yourself plenty of time to let these changes take place, and do not try to force the pace. This is your time to get to know your baby really well, in your own time and in your own home. It is difficult to enjoy this quiet time of adjustment if you are trying to run the household and your children as usual.

HOME HELPS Women have a right to have a home help supplied by the local Social Services Department in the ten-day period following the birth of a child. This service is means-tested to assess your ability to pay, but it can be a useful way of acquiring short-term help if nothing

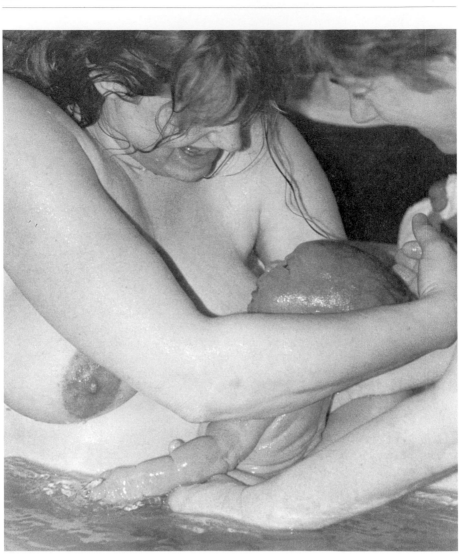

else is forthcoming. Some local authorities may be very discouraging if they have run down their home-help service, but it may be worth insisting on if you have no other firm offers of help.

THE BENEFITS

The reasons why you might decide to opt for a home birth will be entirely individual, but here are some of the many benefits women and their families have found:

○ YOU WILL BE ABLE TO GIVE BIRTH IN THE MOST FAMILIAR SURROUNDINGS, WHERE YOU FEEL COMFORTABLE.

○ YOU WILL HAVE NO NEED TO MAKE A DECISION ABOUT WHEN TO LEAVE FOR HOSPITAL.

○ YOU WILL AVOID HAVING TO TRAVEL TO HOSPITAL IN LABOUR.

○ YOU NEED NOT BE INHIBITED BY HOSPITAL ATMOSPHERE.

○ YOU WILL BE FREE FROM PRESSURE TO ACCEPT ACCELERATION OF LABOUR.

○ YOU WILL HAVE CONTINUITY OF CARE FROM A KNOWN AND TRUSTED MIDWIFE.

○ YOU WILL BE IN CONTROL OF THE CONDITIONS OF DELIVERY (WHICH IS LIKELY TO RESULT IN YOU REQUIRING FEWER DRUGS).

○ YOU WILL BE ABLE TO INVITE WHOEVER YOU CHOOSE TO BE PRESENT, INCLUDING YOUR CHILDREN.

○ YOU WILL WELCOME YOUR BIRTH ATTENDANTS AS GUESTS IN YOUR HOME, THUS MAKING A DIFFERENCE TO THE WAY YOU ARE TREATED.

Once your baby is born

○ YOU AND YOUR PARTNER WILL BE ABLE TO STAY TOGETHER WITH YOUR BABY.

○ YOU WILL NOT NEED TO MAKE ANY ADJUSTMENT FROM HOSPITAL TO HOME LIFE.

○ YOU WILL BE FREE FROM THE RESTRICTIONS AND ROUTINES OF HOSPITAL.

○ YOU WILL BE ABLE TO BREASTFEED YOUR BABY WHENEVER EITHER OF YOU WISHES.

○ YOU WILL BE ABLE TO EAT AND DRINK WHATEVER YOU WANT, AND AS MUCH AS YOU WISH.

○ YOU WILL NOT BE DISTURBED BY THE CRIES OF OTHER BABIES, OR OTHER PEOPLE'S VISITORS.

○ YOU WILL BE ABLE TO ENJOY YOUR OWN BABY, UNDISTRACTED AND UNINHIBITED BY THE PRESENCE OF OTHERS.

The most overwhelming feeling of all, and one which is hard to appreciate until you have had or been present at a home birth, is the sense of utter rightness and wholeness of a baby being born into its own family in its own home.

● *I found kneeling on all-fours over a bean-bag the best way to cope with strong contractions, and Gwen [the midwife] was quite happy to lie down on the floor to listen to the baby's heartbeat. (I do wish I'd found time to vacuum the carpet though!) As I changed position to cope with the contractions, so Brian massaged me and Gwen worked round us, stroking my arm and talking me through the really big contractions of the last hour or two. At home in the dimly-lit bedroom I felt quite able to wander round with an old cotton T-shirt on and nothing else, and to moan and groan as much as I wanted to. No one told me to be quiet or suggested I needed any drugs and between contractions I could cuddle Brian and chat to Gwen quite happily.*

Caitlin was born just after dawn, with the sunlight filtering through the curtains and the birds singing a welcome. She was delivered up on to me, still wet and warm, so Brian and I could stroke her and talk to her. I held her while the placenta was delivered and Brian sat on the bed next to me cuddling his new daughter while I was stitched where I had torn slightly. An hour later, four-year-old Sam woke and came and sat on the bed while Caitlin took her first bath. By nine o'clock, Gwen had left for some much-needed sleep, and Brian had crawled into bed beside me. I fell asleep watching Caitlin sleeping soundly beside me and listening to Sam playing in the garden. ♥

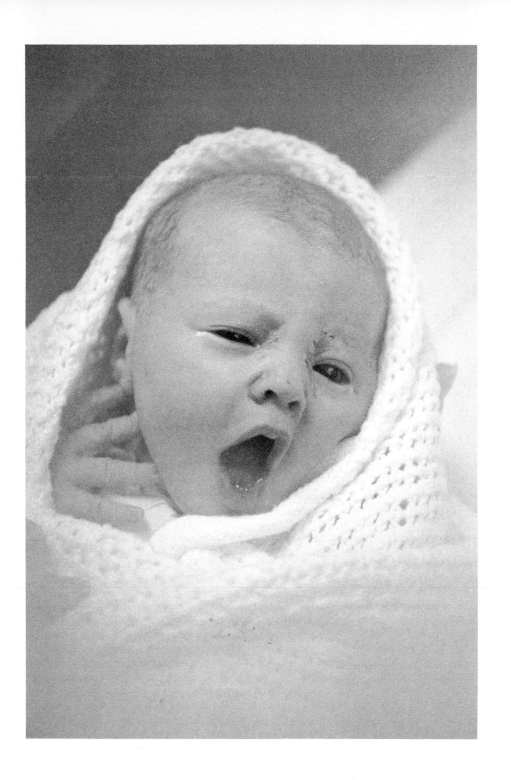

20 THE FIRST FEW HOURS

Your baby is born. Labour is over; the cord has been clamped; the placenta delivered; you have held your baby for the first time, and slowly everything shifts into a different gear. The sense of quiet concentration and bustle which was present during labour and delivery has been exchanged for a sense of peace and fulfilment. The baby may be crying; you may be feeling exhausted and drained, but you have the satisfaction of having just achieved something quite unique. Life with your new baby is just beginning.

YOUR NEW BABY

These early hours are a very special time for you and your baby. Most hospitals now deliver a baby into her mother's arms or on to her abdomen so that she can enjoy the first real look at her baby, the very first cuddle. If your baby has been delivered by forceps, or vacuum extractor (Ventouse), she will be thoroughly checked by a paediatrician before being handed back to you.

APGAR SCORE All babies are assessed at one and five minutes after the birth to check the condition of the following:

- O **HEART RATE**
- O **BREATHING**
- O **SKIN COLOUR**
- O **MUSCLE TONE**
- O **REFLEX RESPONSE**

These are measured on a chart, known as the Apgar score, with each of the five areas being allotted up to 2 points. A baby scoring 7 or more points is considered to be making satisfactory progress; a baby scoring fewer than 4 points will need to be resuscitated; those in between will be very carefully monitored, resuscitated if necessary, and treated according to individual circumstances.

It is unlikely you will actually notice this Apgar score being carried out, as it is usually a matter of your midwife running her experienced eye over the new baby and assessing her condition.

Sometimes a baby will need some help in starting to breathe easily, and will need to be resuscitated. Resuscitation involves first extracting any mucus from the baby's airways by means of a catheter, then using oxygen either to boost the baby's own supply, or to keep up oxygen levels until she is able to breathe of her own accord. It may seem like a lifetime if your baby has not begun to breathe yet, but in fact babies are able to survive undamaged without oxygen for many minutes longer than adults.

Resuscitation

Occasionally, a midwife will not have enough time to explain clearly what is happening, leaving you, the confused and frightened parents, wondering what is going on. Just when you were expecting to feel on top of the world, you may be left unsure and numb, uninformed and alone. Even if your carers communicate well with you, you may find it very difficult to take in what is happening anyway; the implications may not dawn on you until much later. It may be that your partner will be able to remember any hazy bits from these first few minutes and can fill any gaps in your memory when you discuss the birth later on.

If your baby has had an especially difficult start to life, she will be taken to the Special Care Baby Unit, where all the necessary equipment to look after new-borns needing extra help is available. (See Chapter 29, Babies in Special Care, for further information.)

COLOUR A new-born baby's colour can come as a tremendous shock if you were expecting her to be pink; in fact she is more likely to be a rather dull blue-ish grey. Partners particularly may be unaware of the appearance of new-born babies and feel frightened or disgusted when they first see theirs. You will notice your baby gradually become redder as the oxygenated air reaches every part of her body, though it is quite common for fingers and toes to remain grey-ish for a day or two. Sometimes people are concerned that their baby may be rather messy or covered with blood; occasionally a baby does have a few smears of maternal blood on her, but this can easily be wiped off if you wish.

Your baby's appearance

VERNIX Some babies are covered in vernix — the creamy-coloured substance which keeps the baby's skin protected in the uterus. It looks rather like cold-cream or cottage cheese, and tends to settle in the folds; you need not wash it off as it does prevent the skin drying out and flaking.

LANUGO Some babies are born with lanugo, or body hair like down, on the back, arms, and forehead in particular. This rubs off after a while and is also perfectly normal.

MOULDING If your baby has been born vaginally, she is liable to have moulding of the head from where she has been pushed down the

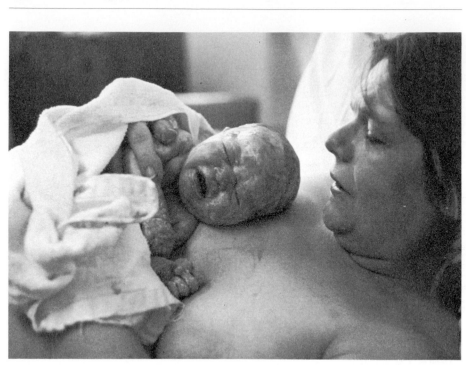

birth canal, and the skull has moulded to make her descent easier. Again, this will gradually disappear. Babies who have been born by Caesarean section have rather beautifully round heads from the beginning.

Getting to know your baby

Whether it is you or your partner holding the baby, it is nice to have time to yourselves after the birth to look at your baby, count fingers and toes, and search for any family resemblances, however unflattering, and quietly discover the child who has been born.

Your baby will feel, look, and smell quite different from any other baby; will be undeniably herself from the beginning. The personality with which a baby comes into the world can come as a surprise to many parents. For many months you have dreamed about and imagined this baby, and it may be a shock to realize that your baby is not the same as the imaginary baby. You may find you go through a period of mourning for the loss of your fantasy baby, which is particularly marked if you had been hoping for one sex and the baby has turned out to be the other. Even if you had not minded which sex you had, simply having made plans for either sex — naming, clothing, feeding, and, in imagination, playing with babies of both sexes in anticipation — may make you aware of missing the imaginary other. If this is not your first baby, you may have been expecting her to be identical in looks and character to your other child, and the fact that she is not may initially be disappointing; after all, you already know how to love your first child, and may be unsure if you will be able to love this new baby as much.

Most women who wish to breastfeed choose to breastfeed their babies straightaway, and this is generally encouraged by midwives. It has several advantages:

Feeding

○ **IT IS WHAT BABIES WANT TO DO; THEY ARE PRO-GRAMMED FOR IT AND IT WILL CALM AND COMFORT A BABY AFTER LABOUR.**

○ **IT WILL HELP WITH THE DELIVERY OF THE PLACENTA, AS THE OXYTOCIN RELEASED WHEN THE BABY FEEDS WILL HELP TO CONTRACT THE UTERUS TO EXPEL THE PLACENTA.**

○ **IF THE PLACENTA IS ALREADY DELIVERED, THE OXYTOCIN WILL HELP TO CONTRACT THE UTERUS DOWN FURTHER, HELPING TO PREVENT POST-PARTUM HAEMORRHAGE (PPH).**

○ **IF THE BABY IS ENCOURAGED TO SUCKLE, SHE WILL GRASP THE WHOLE IDEA OF SUCKLING AND FEEDING MUCH MORE QUICKLY THAN A BABY WHO HAS TO LEARN AT A LATER STAGE, AS THE SUCKLING REFLEX IS VERY POWERFUL IN THE FIRST FEW HOURS AFTER A NORMAL AND DRUG-FREE DELIVERY.**

Your baby may want to nuzzle, smell, or lick your nipple, or she may like to have a good, long feed. Whatever you and your baby decide to do, you do not have to force anything. This is a time for getting to know one another, and forcing the breast on an unwilling baby, at the wrong pace for her, will not help you to create the sort of atmosphere to give you both confidence in each other.

You will find suggestions on how to put your baby to the breast in Chapter 24, Feeding your Baby.

It is unusual for your birth attendants to do much with the baby at this stage, apart from checking that she is well and sufficiently warm, or helping you to breastfeed if you would like help. Your baby will be weighed fairly soon after delivery and wrapped up to keep her warm, but she will not need to be taken away to be bathed at this stage, so you and your partner can enjoy holding and watching her for as long as you wish. You may feel rather too exhausted, both physically and emotionally, by labour and birth to want to hold your baby for long at this stage. This is quite normal and you can make up for any lost time in the days and weeks to come.

Enjoying your new baby

THE NEW MOTHER

Although what you might fancy right now is a cup of tea and then a well-earned sleep, it may be a little while before you are ready to go on to the ward. If you are very tired, it is a good idea to use any periods of lull to rest as much as possible. Your midwife will have her notes to write up and various things to attend to before she can move you out of the delivery room.

Repairing a tear or episiotomy

If you have had an episiotomy, you will certainly need stitching, but if you have torn, things may not be quite so clear cut; a small tear will heal well without sutures, and your midwife will assess whether or not you need stitches.

In many units, midwives are now trained to do the suturing — something for which women are extremely grateful. Most women prefer the idea of having the woman who has attended them in labour being the one who also performs the suturing, rather than being attended by a doctor whom they have never met.

Suturing

Suturing is not much fun.

Depending on the number and depth of stitches required, you may or may not have to have your legs in lithotomy stirrups.

If you have had a relatively easy labour and birth, which you have managed to enjoy and feel good about, being stitched may be the most uncomfortable, not to mention inelegant, part of the whole proceeding. Suturing is usually carried out after you have spent some time enjoying your new baby, but before your tissues start to feel tender, normally about half-an-hour to an hour after the birth. You will be given a local anaesthetic for the suturing unless you already have an epidural anaesthetic in place.

Your doctor or midwife will have to pad the vagina and surrounding area with absorbent pads to remove any blood so that he or she can see what needs to be done; this can be extremely uncomfortable. Any internal tears in the vagina will be stitched first, followed by torn muscle; finally the external skin will be stitched. It is done very carefully and may take some time, which can seem very tedious, particularly if your legs start to feel shaky in the lithotomy stirrups. Soluble thread may be used for the stitching, so no removal is necessary, though any stitches which feel excessively tight after four days or so may be snipped.

This may all seem rather divorced from the excitement and pleasure you are otherwise feeling. It may seem unreasonably unpleasant after a good birth experience; after a long and difficult labour, it may feel like the last straw. (You will find information on the care of your stitches or tear in Chapter 22, Early Days.)

If you have to be sutured, you may find the following suggestions helpful:

Slightly more comfortable suturing

○ **IF THE STITCHING IS VERY PAINFUL, TELL YOUR DOCTOR OR MIDWIFE; HE OR SHE MAY NEED TO WAIT LONGER FOR THE LOCAL ANAESTHETIC TO TAKE EFFECT.**

○ **IF THE STITCHING BECOMES PAINFUL AFTER A WHILE, SAY SO; YOU MAY NEED A TOP-UP OF THE LOCAL ANAESTHETIC.**

○ **YOU CAN USE YOUR RELAXATION AND BREATHING TECHNIQUES TO HELP COPE WITH THE STITCHING.**

○ **YOU CAN ASK FOR THE GAS AND OXYGEN WHILE YOU ARE BEING STITCHED.**

○ **IF YOU ARE NOT ABLE TO HOLD YOUR BABY WHILE YOU ARE BEING STITCHED, YOUR PARTNER CAN HOLD HER NEAR YOU, SO THAT YOU WILL HAVE SOME FORM OF PLEASANT AND INTERESTING DISTRACTION.**

○ **MAKE SURE YOUR PARTNER HAS NOT GONE OFF HOME OR TO MAKE PHONE CALLS; HIS SUPPORT AND REASSURANCE WILL BE INVALUABLE.**

Emotions

Not every new mother, or indeed father, feels entirely delighted with her, or his, son or daughter. You may be feeling merely a sense of relief that it is all over at last, pleased to have your body to yourself after so long. You may be ravenously hungry. You may simply feel unbelievably exhausted, wanting only to close your eyes and sleep.

On the other hand, you may be feeling elated, on a 'high', unable to take in just how clever you have been, happily aware that no other couple in the world has ever been quite so wonderfully clever or so fortunate. Sleep may be the last thing on your mind as you stroke, cuddle, and watch your brand new child, relishing these early moments of her life when she is wakeful and alert.

You may feel a sense of anti-climax; you have been looking forward to this moment for so long, and now it has happened — so what? It may feel as though the pregnancy and labour you have just been through are totally unconnected with this baby you are holding and supposed to be enjoying. You may not even want to hold your baby, or feel too weary to take much notice of her. If your labour has been long and difficult, or not what you had been hoping for, it may be especially hard to feel very much for your baby at all.

Any or all of these reactions are normal, if bewildering to the mother and father. You may have been hoping or expecting to fall in love with your baby immediately, but this can take time. More often than not, love takes days and weeks to develop, as you gradually get to know each other. On the other hand, you may be almost overwhelmed by the sudden rush of emotion with which you greet your baby. However you feel, it is natural after you have been through the mentally and physically demanding experience of labour to want to spend some time looking after yourself now.

Time for yourselves

If you have not already had time alone, most hospitals allow parents to enjoy some uninterrupted time together before moving them out of the delivery room. Once you have had your cup of tea and a wash or bath, it is nice to have a while to reflect on the events just passed, and on the new, different life ahead. If your hospital does not normally allow for this, you could specifically request it when discussing your other preferences. If your baby has been born at home, there will not be the same need to make the most of whatever time you can grab for yourselves, since you will have as much as you wish once the midwife has gone. In any case, the need for privacy is not quite so striking in one's own home as in a busy hospital unit. These first moments alone together are a very precious time wherever you have delivered your baby and whatever your birth experience has been like. Whether you are elated, exhausted, or both, these will be unrepeatable moments.

MOVING ON

Once all the business in the delivery room is finished, you will be moved on to the ward. Some hospitals and units put newly delivered mothers into a side room for the first few hours, away from the bustle of the main ward. This will give you an opportunity to rest, though you may feel most unwilling to rest and may prefer to talk. If it is still night-time, moving into a side room does also cause the other mothers less disturbance, and you and your partner can spend more time together.

Even if you are tired, you may find it impossible to sleep, however long it is since you last slept, as you mull over all that has happened, as you lie watching your sleeping baby, or cuddle her and feel the awe of knowing she really is yours. You may find you doze then wake, believing you are still pregnant, unable to connect the baby beside you with your now flabby abdomen.

SOME PRACTICAL HINTS If you are exhausted but cannot get to sleep, check first that you are physically comfortable.

- O   **DOES YOUR SANITARY TOWEL NEED CHANGING?**
- O   **IS YOUR BLADDER UNCOMFORTABLY FULL?**
- O   **ARE YOU ABSOLUTELY RAVENOUS?**

You should have a buzzer to call a midwife for help, so do ask if you need anything or if something is worrying you.

FOOD Few hospitals these days have much food on tap outside meal-times, but someone may be able to rustle up some toast if you are starving. If you can, find out beforehand what the extra food situation is like in your hospital, and, if it is unreliable, take a few sandwiches in case, for a postnatal picnic.

EMPTYING YOUR BLADDER You may find it hard to pass urine after delivery. You will normally be expected to empty your bladder before leaving the delivery room, but this may not be easy. Your muscles and tissues may feel bruised and strange, like rather knobbly cotton-wool, and twice their normal size. You may find it absolutely impossible to use a bed-pan — not designed to be at all user-friendly. If you have problems with the bed-pan, ask if you can get up to use the lavatory. Many hospitals let mothers up within an hour after delivery anyway, to use the lavatory (or sit on the bed-pan on a chair) and have a proper bath, which is much more civilized. If you still have problems, or a bed-pan is insisted upon, try practising your pelvic-floor exercises; as you attempt to locate where you think your pelvic-floor muscles ought to be, you may find that you can empty your bladder as you relax them. In desperation, wait until you have a bath and relieve your bladder when your bath is finished. This is not an unhygienic practice. If you have had an epidural, you may find it takes several more hours, and maybe days, before you regain sufficient feeling to empty your bladder normally.

SLEEPING If you still cannot sleep but would like to, try going through your basic relaxation techniques; you will at least be well rested if not actually asleep. Above all, do not worry; it is quite usual to be too excited to sleep so soon after delivery.

Early discharge

If you have been delivered on a GP unit or under a community midwife domino scheme, you may have arranged with your community midwife to go home after six hours. This may turn out to be longer, depending on the availability of an ambulance to take you home. The waiting and the journey may be rather tiring, but the pleasure of being in your own home and bed again so soon, to be greeted by your family, far outweighs any minor discomfort. If you do decide to go home this early, a midwife will visit you soon after your arrival at home, then twice a day for the first three days, then daily until the tenth day, or longer if necessary. If you would like an early discharge, as with a home birth, it is wise to make sure you have plenty of help and support in the house. Trying to do too much too soon, or worrying about what is not being done, or being overwhelmed by interested but bouncy toddlers when you need to rest, is not the easiest way to start life with a new baby.

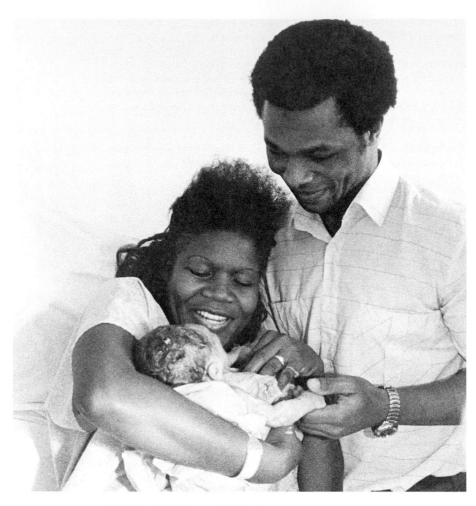

THE NEW FATHER

The birth is over, the new mother is safely tucked up in bed, and the new father may well be left to find his way home, alone. This can be a disheartening experience; arriving home, full of the birth, to a cold, empty house. If it is the middle of the night, he may feel reluctant to start phoning everyone with the good news. He may feel that he has abandoned you and your baby in a strange place. He may be feeling left out himself. If you have children already, it may be easier, but even then, if it is night-time, he will have to tiptoe in for fear of waking everyone, or they may be sleeping with friends or relatives; some hours may pass before they can be let in on the excitement.

Some fathers choose to go into work the next day, even after missing a night's sleep, so that they can share their elation, have some company, and generally keep themselves occupied until visiting-time.

Many hospitals are happy for fathers to stay as long as both partners wish, and arrange it so that other women will not be disturbed. This is something you could discuss at your hospital during an antenatal appointment. Once a partner does leave, however, you may find that either or both of you feel extremely lonely in these first hours of separation. If this is your first baby, it may be the first time you have really been apart at an important time. You will have been through a dramatic event together, and, right at the most exciting moment, you are thrust apart. You may have strange new feelings you would like to share, details of the labour you want to go over again, or worries you want to discuss; and the person you would most like to talk to is somewhere else!

• *I actually quite enjoyed my labour, except for the stitching up afterwards. That was undignified, painful, and a real anti-climax.* •

• *I simply couldn't equate the baby I could see lying beside me with the bump that had just come from inside me. I kept forgetting I wasn't pregnant any more.* •

• *I felt sore and leaky and a bit weepy, extremely tired, desperate to go to the loo, but immensely proud of myself and delighted with my baby. I couldn't believe it had all really happened.* •

21 STILLBIRTH

Stillbirth is perhaps the most difficult subject of all for any expectant parent to consider or acknowledge as a possibility. The very finality of a stillbirth; the crushing of hopes and dreams; the loss of the child you had hardly begun to know and love, is a frightening and terrible prospect. To have gone through a pregnancy yet have nothing to show for it seems unbearably cruel and you may feel that the subject will be too sad and awful for you even to contemplate reading this chapter. Women who have experienced a stillbirth or neonatal death, however, often express regret that they were not as well prepared as they were for other aspects of pregnancy and childbirth. They found they needed to make decisions from options they had not even had a chance to consider beforehand, at an extremely stressful time. To have read something, however little, at a time when your emotions are not in turmoil, thereby preparing yourself for any eventuality, could prove invaluable.

There is another good reason for reading this chapter: one day you may know someone who suffers the loss of a baby and who would be glad of any support and friendship you are able to offer. Reading this might help you to think about how you could be a sensitive and understanding friend to someone who needs all the support he or she can get.

WHAT IS STILLBIRTH?

Stillbirth refers to the death at or before birth of any baby who is more than 28 weeks. Neonatal death is the term used for babies who die within the first four weeks after birth; most neonatal deaths occur in the first week after birth. In this country about 1 in 100 babies is stillborn — not a high percentage, but certainly enough to make one think seriously about the possibility.

Why it may happen

There are many reasons for stillbirth and neonatal death; often no single reason is the cause, but several factors coincide with tragic consequences. The most common reasons are low birth-weight and congenital abnormality. Sometimes the placenta will fail towards the end of pregnancy or during labour. Sometimes the stress of labour itself is too great for the baby. Sometimes, rarely, something goes tragically wrong during labour, causing the baby's death.

It is natural for mothers and fathers whose babies are stillborn to want to know why it happened. If, sadly, you should lose a baby, you may ask whether there was anything you did, or failed to do, which could have caused it. 'Should I have taken more exercise?', 'Should I have avoided swimming so often?', 'Should I have known something was wrong?', 'If my antenatal appointment had been one day earlier, would my baby have been saved?' are typical of the sorts of questions parents ask themselves. It is exceptionally unlikely that anything you did or did not do will have caused your baby's death, though you will need to discuss all the questions you have with your doctor and midwife. It may well be that the reason for a baby's death remains unknown, and this too can be hard to come to terms with.

In your search for reasons and explanations, you may find hospital staff or your GP more or less open and honest. They may be very happy to share all the available information with you, but they may be rather reluctant to discuss it, especially if there is the possibility of litigation. It will be more helpful for you in coming to terms with your baby's death if you have been able to discuss everything freely with your medical carers. Speaking openly will also help you to feel less anxious during any subsequent pregnancy; sharing the knowledge, and understanding what went wrong as far as anyone knows, can make all the difference to how you approach a future pregnancy and birth.

You may find that you feel very angry with the doctors or midwives. It may be that a mistake has indeed been made, and, if this is clear, it may, for some people, actually be easier to deal with than if there is no obvious reason. Eventually, as you come to terms with your loss, you may feel easier in yourself, though for many parents there will always be a few 'what ifs . . .' to mull over.

AUTOPSY You will almost certainly be asked for your consent to an autopsy, or post-mortem examination, being performed on your baby, and possibly a chromosome analysis. You may feel under-standably upset at having to make such a painful decision, but the information gained from any examination could be extremely useful, particularly when considering a subsequent pregnancy.

Although an autopsy is unlikely to provide answers to all your questions, it may at least offer some guidance as to what happened. Should you find the autopsy results couched in unfamiliar or incomprehensible jargon, ask for an appointment with the relevant member of staff, who will be able to explain the results clearly to you.

IF YOUR BABY DIES BEFORE LABOUR BEGINS

If your baby has died before you go into labour, you may find out by becoming aware that any kicking movements have ceased or their pattern has altered dramatically. You may discover it at an antenatal check-up if a midwife or doctor cannot find the baby's heartbeat.

If no heartbeat can be heard, this may come as a tremendous shock to you, or may confirm a suspicion that all was not well. The baby's death can be confirmed by fetal heart monitoring and by an ultrasound scan. Very occasionally, although a baby has died before labour begins, no one realizes this until the baby is stillborn, which is perhaps the greatest shock of all.

The labour

INDUCTION Once the baby's death has been confirmed, you may be offered an induction of labour, but many hospitals ask mothers to wait for labour to start spontaneously. This is an exceptionally difficult time to have to live through and you may find it neither bearable nor acceptable. If your labour is to be induced straight away, you may however welcome a few hours in which to gather your thoughts, to spend a last evening at home saying goodbye to your pregnancy, informing family and friends, and creating a few special memories for yourselves, such as taking photographs of yourself while pregnant, and thinking about how you will manage during your labour.

CAESAREAN SECTION An initial reaction for some women is to think they would prefer to have the baby by Caesarean section. Others feel that going through the labour will help to build their bank of memories and help them to accept the reality of what has happened: that they really have had a baby and that it was stillborn. You may feel that you would like to do the same for your baby who has died as you would have done for her had she been alive. Physically, a normal birth will be better for you; a Caesarean section is still a major operation with all the attendant risks, and your body will recover better if you have actually been through labour and birth. Women who have laboured knowing their babies will be stillborn have said they have still felt a terrific sense of pride and achievement in the birth, and have even enjoyed it, despite the sadness.

Labour may take longer than usual if your baby has died, because the presenting part will be less firm and will not stimulate the cervix as efficiently. It is unusual for a mother to need an episiotomy as the baby's skull will be softer.

LABOUR COMPANIONS You may like to consider whether there is anyone else besides your partner you would like to share the labour with you, or to be there immediately after the birth — grandparents, siblings, close friends, or your antenatal teacher. It will be up to you to decide whom you would like to have near you at this time, sharing your experience. Many fathers find it particularly difficult to contemplate being at a birth which is also a death. They may have felt uneasy at the prospect of being present for the birth anyway, and feel very unsure about how they will cope with supporting you through this birth. You will need to discuss this between you, and it may be that the mother's need to have her partner present will vastly outweigh any misgivings on his part. In the long run, it will probably help you in your grieving if you have been together for the birth and can share as many memories as possible.

IF YOUR BABY DIES DURING LABOUR

Should something go wrong during the actual labour, or if your baby is found to have died once you are in labour, the shock may make it more difficult for you to think or say what it is that you want. It may be that, in the immediate shock, you think you will not want to see, hold, name, or photograph your baby. Later, you might change your mind, and it is important to know that you can ask to see your baby when you feel ready — days later if you wish. Hospital staff should make it possible for parents to see and hold their baby whenever they wish, for as long as they wish, until the time of the funeral.

If your baby is stillborn and nobody has realized, the shock and surprise of hearing no sound, feeling no warmth or life, may seem intolerable — everyone is most acutely aware of the silence after a stillbirth. If your baby is born but lives only a very brief while, the wait will seem endless as you wonder what is happening, fearful for your baby's life. This is especially traumatic if there is no one available to be with you. If possible, a midwife who can stay with you and explain everything can be a great comfort, and can help you to feel less isolated and rejected at such a frightening and distressing time.

KNOWING YOUR BABY

SEEING YOUR BABY When your baby is first delivered, you may be fearful of seeing or holding her, but mothers and fathers whose babies died in the days when they were not permitted to see or hold them felt grief and regret for many years, often for the rest of their lives, because they did not have the opportunity to know for whom they were mourning. It is easier, and more natural, to mourn somebody you know and can visualize. After all, you, the mother, will have known this baby to a large extent already; the baby who has died today is the same baby who has been kicking and squirming inside you all these months; the one to whom you may have been speaking and for whom you have made so many plans.

You may want to hold your baby immediately after delivery or prefer to wait a little. Your midwife could wrap your baby in a little nest on your bed, or she could sit beside you, holding the baby so that you can look at her until you are ready to hold her.

If you feel afraid of what your baby will look like, explain this to your midwife, who can wrap the baby up and show you the perfect parts at first, gradually unfolding the rest of her. Most stillborn babies look very beautiful and quite perfect, and it can be very reassuring to parents to see how perfectly formed the baby is. Even a profoundly handicapped baby will not look as awful in reality as in your imagination. To have seen your child, and taken pleasure in those parts which are perfect, is comforting both for this experience and for any future pregnancy.

Your baby's presenting part may be rather bruised as a result of the pressure of birth; this will be more obvious on your baby's head and face than if it has been a breech presentation. If you want to take photographs of your baby, it is a good idea to take them fairly soon, while the condition of the baby's skin is still good.

Memories **HOLDING YOUR BABY** Many parents do not realize that they can see and hold their baby again if they want to. You will have such a short time with her anyway that you can make the most of whatever opportunities are available before the funeral. It may be a good idea for other members of the family to see and hold your baby too; if close family members share the experience, the more likely they are to understand what you, the parents have lost. You will also be creating a greater wealth of memories of your baby.

You could use any time you have with your child to unwrap her clothes and examine her, counting fingers and toes, admiring eyelashes and fingernails, just as you would with any baby.

PHOTOGRAPHS Take as many photos as you want. If you can remember and be sufficiently organized to do it, it is a good idea to take two separate films in case of loss or damage. Hospitals will usually take photographs too, and will keep them even if you think you will not want any. Hospital photographs may not be exactly to your taste, however, and taking your own may be a more certain means of ensuring you have the sort of memory you want. However sad the occasion is, you may later be aware of how important it was to have made this record for yourselves. You may wish to bath her and dress her in special clothes you had bought 'for best'.

SERVICE OF BLESSING Most hospital chaplains will be happy to conduct a service of blessing for your baby — with your baby present if you would like that.

REGISTERING THE BIRTH You will have to register your baby's birth *and* death — a painful and poignant reminder of what has happened. The certificates can become a valuable part of your store of memories.

FUNERALS A funeral is also a part of the memory-creation, as well as part of your grieving process. You will not have to make any decision immediately about whether or not you want a funeral, and if so, what form it should take. Thinking about the kind of service you would like and arranging the details often help people to cope with their grief in the early days. Others feel too overwhelmed by the events to be able to concentrate on planning anything. If you are recovering from a difficult delivery as well, it may be several days before you feel ready to think about funeral arrangements. There is a great value in both parents working out a funeral procedure for themselves with a clergyman or with a trusted friend.

The service can be as informal as you wish — at the hospital, your local church, or in your own home. You may decide to have the baby buried or cremated, but most parents find it useful to have somewhere which reminds them of their baby — a grave, a place in the crematorium, a tree in the garden, any special place where you can go to be with your child on important anniversaries.

Most parents also feel happier with a funeral service which involves a small intimate group of people rather than a crowd of mourners.

NAMING YOUR BABY Choosing a name for your baby is important, as it gives your child an identity; a means for you and your other children to be able to identify and remember the missing member of the family.

Memories are important — make the most of whatever you have.

AFTER THE BIRTH

Nature does not differentiate between a live birth and a stillbirth, and many women find it particularly hard that they should have to go through all the usual postnatal stages as if their baby were alive.

You will lose the lochia and experience all the other aspects of the postnatal period: sweating, constipation, and tiredness; but possibly the most distressing is the production of breast milk.

BREAST MILK If you have lost one twin, you will have a baby to feed, but for a mother with no baby and plenty of breast milk, this is a miserable time. Doctors can prescribe drugs to dry your milk up, but these are strong drugs and you may decide to let it happen naturally. Without the baby's suckling to stimulate milk production, lactation will eventually cease. If your breasts become uncomfortably engorged or full of milk, you might try any of the methods for relieving this, as described in Chapter 24, Feeding your Baby. You may need pain-killers to ease the pain. You might also need to express a little milk sometimes to relieve the discomfort and fullness. You may wish to offer your expressed colostrum to save the life of another very ill baby.

ACHING ARMS It is normal for women who have lost a baby to feel a physical ache in their arms from the need to hold a baby. You may need lots of cuddling with family, your partner, and your other children at this time. They will need it too. If you have a friend from your antenatal class, and you would like to hold a tiny baby, perhaps you could ask your friend to let you hold hers occasionally, to relieve the ache.

Grieving for your baby

The grieving process is complex, but is similar for the loss of any child, and the variety and intensity of feelings associated with a bereavement should not be underestimated. Neither can they be dictated by others who are not in your particular situation. Allow yourselves plenty of time to grieve for your baby in your own ways, and try not to expect too much of yourself or each other too soon.

Fathers

Fathers often feel forgotten or pushed to one side when something as momentous as a stillbirth has occurred, because everyone seems to be concentrating on the mother who has given birth.

They may feel angry that others have forgotten that this was their child too, and they need to be cared for and cuddled as well. It may be tempting to try to be 'strong' and not become too involved or express emotions, but it is as essential for fathers to live through their grief and express their feelings as it is for mothers and other children. Crying, and expressing anger and sorrow, are not signs of weakness, but an integral and vital means of coming to terms with your bereavement.

Other children

Children are very deeply affected by the loss of a baby brother or sister, whom they will have looked forward to meeting and for whom they too will have made plans. They will need plenty of encouragement to express their feelings of grief. Children appreciate honesty, but may ask all sorts of difficult, even unanswerable, questions about why the baby died, whose fault it was, or where she is now. They may feel angry with you, the parents, for somehow failing them — for not bringing the baby home as promised.

It is as important to let your children express their feelings as it is for you, though there may be occasions when you find them hurtful, or find the raw nakedness of their emotions too painful for you to watch.

Children may feel especially vulnerable themselves after a stillbirth, wondering if it will be their turn next, or if their other siblings will also die. Encouraging your children to speak openly about their worries and fears, however distressing, will enable you to reassure them and explain to them as appropriate. Children can also be immensely kind and supportive at such times — the sympathy and understanding a small child can offer, the freshness of his or her perspectives on life and death, can be incredibly touching.

It does sometimes happen that parents attempt to use their other children to compensate for the baby who has died, putting all their plans and dreams on to another child. This is particularly common where one twin has died, when all the parental hopes and expectations are passed on to the remaining twin. The more you have been able to express your grief and loss, the more memories you have been able to create, the easier it will be to see that baby as a separate person who cannot be replaced, leaving your other children the space to be themselves.

If you decide at some point to have another baby, it will also be easier to see your new baby as a separate person if you have allowed yourselves sufficient time to grieve for the baby who has died. Then you will be able to approach this new pregnancy full of positive feelings about the future rather than guilt at having betrayed your dead baby by trying to replace her.

SUPPORT FOR BEREAVED PARENTS

Support groups

As well as the support of friends and family, there are ways in which you can find support from others who have had similar experiences and are ready to contact bereaved parents. The Stillbirth and Neonatal Death Society (SANDS) has many branches nation-wide. SANDS befrienders (contacts who have lost a baby themselves) will sometimes visit bereaved parents in hospital, or there may be self-help groups where you can meet other parents in the same situation. Some NCT branches also have Baby-Loss groups and hold Experiences Registers both nationally and at branch level, so parents can be put in touch with others in similar circumstances who have suffered a stillbirth or neonatal death, but now feel ready to support and listen to any newly bereaved parents. (You will find addresses of relevant organizations at the back of this book.)

Helping the bereaved

If a friend or member of your family loses a baby or child, and you would like to help, but are not sure how to, here are some suggestions that others have found useful:

○ BE AVAILABLE — YOU DO NOT HAVE TO WAIT FOR A PHONE CALL, BUT VISIT THE HOME OR MAKE THE FIRST CALL YOURSELF.

○ DO NOT BE JUDGEMENTAL.

○ LET YOUR FRIEND TELL HER STORY IN HER OWN TIME AND IN HER OWN WAY.

○ TRY TO LISTEN TO THE STORY SHE IS TELLING, AND BE AWARE OF THE FEELINGS BEHIND THE WORDS.

○ TRY TO THINK OF THINGS FROM YOUR FRIEND'S VIEWPOINT.

○ WHEN SHE IS READY, HELP HER TO ASSESS THE GOOD THINGS SHE STILL HAS — OTHER CHILDREN, PARTNER, WORK, FRIENDS, FAMILY.

○ TRY TO BE OF PRACTICAL HELP: OFFERING TRANSPORT, A COOKED MEAL, WHATEVER YOU FEEL YOU CAN OFFER.

○ TRY TO FOCUS ON HER (OR HIM), NOT ON THE PROBLEM, SHOWING HER THAT YOU CARE ABOUT HER AND HER FEELINGS.

• *On 9 May 1989 I went to the hospital to have my 40 week check. After an examination by a student doctor, the registrar also had "a feel and a listen". I told him the baby had been quiet for a few days, but expected this, due to the extent of the pregnancy. At this stage he asked me to have a go on the small scanning unit they had in the clinic. However, after what seemed hours on this machine, and a lot of very quiet midwives trying to work it, he asked me to go to the main scanning unit and have a proper Ultrasound scan — and he then told me they were having a problem finding a heartbeat. A midwife accompanied me to the unit, and a very brusque lady gave me a scan — I could see her looking at the midwife and shaking her head, and at this point I knew there was no hope for the baby. The woman then asked if I knew why I was there, to which I replied, "To see if the baby has a heartbeat," and she then said she was sorry, there wasn't one.*

I was taken to a small room, where the nurses came in and offered me tea, and my consultant came to see me very quickly. I was asked if I wanted to phone my husband — but as he was miles away and not contactable, I rang my mother and blurted down the phone that the baby was dead, could she please come to the hospital, which she did. We then had to go through what I was to do. All I wanted was a Caesarean, then and there, but the consultant was insistent that I go through a normal labour, with as much pain relief as I needed, as I could then go back home as soon as I wanted.

My husband arrived later in the day, with our older daughter Danielle, and my mother left, taking Danielle with her. We agreed to go ahead with an induction early the next day. I was allowed to go home during the evening, but this was even worse, and I wanted to get back to the hospital — we didn't know what to say to each other, and all I could do was cry.

At 6.00 a.m. a pessary was inserted to soften the cervix, and from then on everything went quite well. I was fitted up with an epidural, and the midwives, who stayed with me all the way through, were totally fantastic. They actually helped me enjoy the labour and see it in a positive way. My consultant was very much in evidence all day, and after a lot of pushing, trying to move the baby down, he decided to do a forceps delivery as we were getting nowhere except tired and frustrated. Roger went out at this stage and at 6.00 p.m. I gave birth to a little girl — Eleanor. I was allowed to hold her almost immediately, for which I am very glad; she was lovely, with gingery hair, and a peaceful, beautiful face.

The staff then took her off, cleaned her up, took photos and dressed her in our own baby clothes. Another midwife came and explained about the procedures we should follow, with the registrar, etc., and also telephoned various people for us — our doctor, vicar. Eleanor was brought back to us in a beautiful Moses basket, and I was able to hold her and just cuddle her. There were so many things I wanted to say to her, how sorry I was and how I loved her. Roger put her back into the basket and the midwife took her to the Chapel. We were able to go and see her if we wanted.

I was allowed home the next day, once I had feeling back in my legs. Once I got home, feeling absolutely awful by this time, I just went to bed and my daughter came with me, and we hugged and hugged and cried our eyes out.

We held the funeral at our local church on 18 May. It was a lovely sunny day, very hot and peaceful. Our vicar had been coming to see us about this, and he held a very simple, caring service. It was a shock to see the small coffin there, even though Roger and I had been to the funeral directors' and sat with Eleanor there. But once the service was over, we all felt better, and I'm ashamed to say I got extremely drunk.

That summer passed in a blur and I don't remember too much of it now. We go up to the church whenever we feel like it, and sit with Eleanor, looking at the view, and

I think about it all. This week I took my daughter with me; we tidied up the grave and sat down and "introduced" my new daughter, Alexandra, to her sister. **9**

Part 3
PARENTHOOD

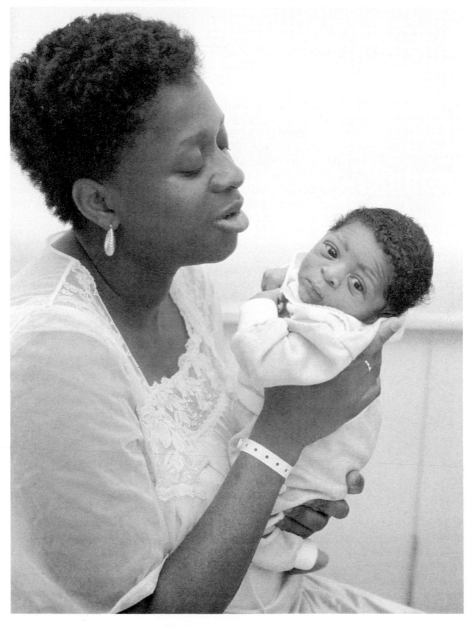

22　EARLY DAYS

(Opposite) The early days after the birth, when you are getting plenty of rest, allow you time to get to know and enjoy your new baby

The first days as a new mother come as a revelation to most women, as a whole new world is opened up for them. Even women who have had a baby before may have forgotten just what it feels like to be newly delivered. The complex variety of emotions, coupled with the need to care for the baby, whilst coping with your own physical recovery, can all add up to make everything seem extraordinarily strange — at times, almost overwhelming. You may be experiencing a mixture of emotions, which change from one moment to the next: pride, wonder, responsibility, awe, anxiety, excitement, and fear are all common feelings. You may be on an absolute 'high', or you may swing between wild euphoria and utter lack of confidence and misery. Your physical well-being and the baby's health and progress will often have much to do with how you feel from day to day.

THE NEWLY DELIVERED MOTHER

Babies often have long periods of sleep in the first two or three days after birth. This is a natural reaction as they sleep off the after-effects of labour, and you can use this as an opportunity to recuperate from the pregnancy and labour yourself. It is not possible in these early days to attempt to do anything other than look after yourself and your baby, be entertained by the occasional visitor, and maybe read or talk a little with other mothers. Enjoy as much as you can of these first few days as you regain your strength and come to terms with what it means to be a new mother.

Physical discomforts

Although it may be a relief not to be pregnant any longer, the discomforts of late pregnancy will have been exchanged for some postnatal discomforts.

FLUID LOSS You may feel as though you are leaking everywhere.

You will need to empty your bladder very frequently for the first forty-eight hours or so, as your body gets rid of the excess fluid gained during pregnancy, and you may also be sweating rather profusely, especially at night. Sweating sometimes continues for several weeks, being particularly noticeable when you wake at night

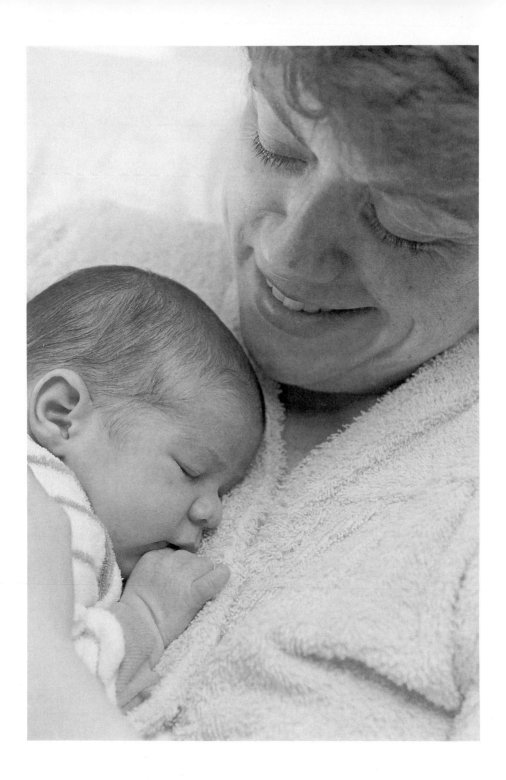

to feed your baby. The sweating is usually hormonal in origin, but do contact your doctor if you are feeling at all unwell.

You will be bleeding from the vagina, and from about the third or fourth day, will be producing quantities of milk as well. If you are in hospital, it may be harder to keep yourself cool and comfortable, because hospitals are such very warm places and the muggy atmosphere there can contribute to your stickiness. Baths and showers are therefore very welcome, though it is not always easy fitting these into the hospital routines, your baby's feed-times, and the bath-times of the rest of the ward! Unless you feel fit enough to clean the bath, you may prefer to take showers.

LOCHIA Lochia is the name given to the vaginal bleeding which is coming from the wound in your uterus at the placental site. For the first twenty-four or forty-eight hours the bleeding can be quite heavy; if you have only ever had light periods, you may feel a bit frightened by losing so much blood. Medical staff will soon tell you if it is enough to cause concern.

You will probably need the large maternity pads to cope with the loss in the first day or two. After this, the bleeding will gradually lessen, and will soon change colour from the bright red of the early days to reddish-brown, then from brown to a pinkish-yellow. Bleeding may last for as long as six or more weeks, but it may cease after only a couple of weeks.

You may experience sudden bursts of red blood in the first few weeks, especially as your uterus contracts when you are feeding your baby.

If your bleeding continues to be bright red for several weeks or starts being very red again once you have been discharged from your midwife's care, do ask your doctor to check that everything is all right. Sometimes bleeding is caused by retained placenta, which will need to be removed before causing infection or haemorrhage.

CLOTS You may pass clots of blood after the birth. These feel rather soft and bulky as they slip down the vagina, usually when you are on the lavatory. Tell a midwife if you have passed a clot and show it to her, so that she can examine it to check that it is not retained placenta. If the clot has landed down the lavatory and you would prefer not to fish it out yourself, call for someone to come and deal with it.

AFTERPAINS Occasionally with a first baby, then increasingly with subsequent babies, you may notice afterpains or strong contractions as the baby begins to feed. This is the uterus returning to its normal size, and can be quite painful. Try to remember to relax and breathe as you did during labour to ease the discomfort. If necessary, ask your midwife for a pain-killing paracetamol tablet about half an hour before feeding, so that feeding does not become discouragingly uncomfortable. Smiling can help to relax your muscles too!

BRUISING AND SORENESS You may well feel extremely bruised and tender for a day or two and will probably be well aware of the fact that your vagina has been stretched and the muscles worked hard. You may feel some discomfort in the pelvic regions, as everything starts to return to its non-pregnant place. Your coccyx might also feel sore from having moved back out of the way during delivery. Putting an ice-pack into your pad if you are very bruised and have a lot of swelling will help to ease the discomfort. Hospitals should provide these; if not, you can make your own, or use a small packet of frozen peas which can be endlessly frozen and refrozen. You just have to remember not to eat that particular pack afterwards! If you choose to refreeze and re-use your ice-pack or packet of peas, it must be covered in a disposable fabric at each use so that it cannot cause an infection. If you have stitches, it is best not to let the scar become too cold as a drop in temperature can delay the healing process, but even tepid water sponged on to the tissues feels marvellously soothing.

PILES Many women have piles as a result of the delivery and this could be an added discomfort. If you have no ointment available, rubbing ice on to your anus can be temporarily soothing.

EMPTYING YOUR BLADDER You may find it difficult to pass urine at first, as everything feels so numb and bruised. Try doing your pelvic-floor exercises to improve muscle tone generally and to encourage your bladder to empty itself and remember what it is supposed to do. If you have a tear, or slight graze in the vulva, it may sting as you empty your bladder. Sluicing a jug filled with warm water over the vulva as you empty your bladder will reduce the stinging. If a jug is not available, use a well-washed squeezy washing-up-liquid container instead.

YOUR BOWELS You will almost certainly be asked during the first twenty-four hours after delivery if you have opened your bowels, and will be asked regularly from then on. It is quite usual for a woman not to need to open her bowels for a day or two, bearing in mind that she may have gone for a day or so with very little to eat, and have emptied her bowels thoroughly in preparation for labour.

Constipation is nevertheless a problem for newly delivered women, as much fluid will have been lost in the days after birth and your breasts will also be preparing to make milk which requires fluid. Drinking plenty to quench your thirst may help to counteract this, but you will need to make sure your diet is full of fibre as well. A bran-rich breakfast cereal plus plenty of wholemeal bread, fruit, and vegetables should help. Laxatives are best avoided if you are breastfeeding, as they can affect milk production and are passed through the milk to your baby as well, where the effects can be extremely messy! Your midwife could leave you some suppositories if you become desperate, but prevention is better than cure.

Another problem with postnatal constipation arises if you have had stitches and are worried that straining to open your bowels could burst your stitches. Holding a clean pad over the stitches when you are on the lavatory will help you feel less anxious that they might not hold out and will be less painful too. You will need to make sure the lavatory seat is clean, so take a tub of antiseptic wipes and a pack of disposable paper lavatory seat covers into hospital with you. You may well feel a good deal happier once you are at home and can use your own lavatory in privacy and comfort.

Care of stitches

If you have had a tear or episiotomy repaired, you may be feeling exceptionally sore and uncomfortable for several days. It tends to feel worse with a first baby, and, generally speaking, episiotomy stitches are more painful and take longer to heal than tears, depending on your individual circumstance of course.

It is quite usual to see women shuffling round the postnatal ward, unable to walk upright or speedily because of their painful perineums. The scar itself may feel horrendous and you may wonder if you will be permanently deformed! It may help to have a look at your perineum with a hand-mirror to see just how big the actual scar is. Scars almost always feel much worse than they are. If you have had a look at your perineum before birth, too, you will know what it looked like before the stitches, which can also be reassuring. The scar should begin to settle down in a few days, and any bruising will soon fade.

Not everyone finds their stitches unpleasantly sore, but, if yours are painful, here are a few suggestions for helping yourself.

COMFORTABLE POSITIONS Sitting may be difficult; try half-lying or resting on one side instead. Some hospitals supply rubber rings to sit on. It is not a good idea to use these for any length of time, because the pressure they put on the pelvic floor can have a detrimental effect, but using them while you feed may be helpful.

More effective than a rubber ring is a Valley Cushion. This is an inflatable cushion, which shapes itself more to your contours, and can be adapted to avoid any sore areas. You can sit without pressure on your perineum or your piles without hindering the healing processes. A few hospitals do keep Valley Cushions, but if yours is not one of these, or if you have had your baby at home, you can hire one through your local NCT branch.

MOBILITY Walking around aids the healing process; try to avoid sitting or standing still for long periods.

PELVIC-FLOOR EXERCISES Doing your pelvic-floor exercises as soon as you can feel what you are doing, will help (see Chapter 6, Looking After Yourself). You can be doing as many as four tightenings every ten or fifteen minutes during the first few days. Exercising your pelvic floor increases blood flow to your pelvis, lessening pain and speeding healing. You may initially feel as if you have not actually got any muscles to tighten; the whole area may feel numb and useless, but the more you practise, the sooner you will notice an improvement. If your muscles are numb, simply being as mobile as possible during the early days will be useful. You can test how quickly things are improving by practising stopping your flow of urine mid-stream. Remember to finish emptying your bladder if you do this.

BATHING Frequent baths can ease any discomfort and may feel very relaxing. Adding salt to your bath will not aid healing, but might feel pleasant. You will not be allowed to use salt in some hospitals, as it can corrode the bath enamel.

It is unwise to sit for too long in the water, as water eventually breaks down scar tissue; it is better simply to dunk yourself up and down in the water a few times to avoid soaking your tissues. Never use a bidet with a vertical spray — lochia drips from one woman can be sprayed on to the next user.

USING THE LAVATORY If it hurts to pass urine, take a jug of water or squeezy bottle with you as described earlier.

Sit well back on the lavatory so that your urine is less likely to sting your stitches.

You can support your stitches with a clean pad when opening your bowels.

DRYING YOUR STITCHES It is sensible to make sure you keep your stitches dry. Some people may suggest you use a hair-dryer to help, but this may have too drying an effect which will slow healing. In any case, hair-dryers may harbour all sorts of germs better not puffed over a wound. An electric light bulb shone on to your perineum several times a day is effective in helping keep the tissues dry but not overdry.

When you are drying yourself after a wash, it may be easier to pat the area dry with a pad of tissues rather than rubbing it with a towel. In any case, make sure you keep a separate towel for your genital area.

SOOTHING REMEDIES Spreading honey on to your pad has antiseptic and healing properties, though it does feel a bit sticky. It can also soothe.

The homoeopathic remedy Arnica 30 or 200 is available to aid healing and reduce bruising. It can be taken during labour as well as afterwards. Tincture of Hyper-cal on the pad aids healing, reduces soreness and bruising, and feels cooling even at room temperature. Put a few drops of the tincture on a clean saucer, add a few drops of water, and dab the pad on to it; make it up freshly for each use.

RELIEVING PAIN If you are in a lot of pain, ask for paracetamol to ease it. The hospital physiotherapy department can help by suggesting other ways of easing the pain and may give you ultrasound treatment to speed up healing. You may have an infection, so your stitches need to be checked carefully.

PROLONGED PAIN OR DISCOMFORT Any discomfort from stitches should be feeling much easier after about a week. If you are still experiencing any pain or discomfort after this time tell your doctor, who can look to see what the reason for the pain is. You need not wait until your six-week postnatal check to sort out any problems. It is totally unacceptable for any woman to have to put up with a sore perineum several weeks or even months after delivery. If you are not satisfied, keep on asking and, if necessary, make an appointment to see a consultant to discuss the problem. It is miserable and de-bilitating to go on week after week feeling tender and uncomfort-able, afraid to make love because it hurts, when this can be rectified. It may mean that your perineum has to be restitched, but this will ultimately be better than living with a badly-stitched wound.

Breastfeeding This is an important factor in how you are feeling in the days after the birth, and is discussed fully in Chapter 24, Feeding your Baby. It is a good idea to ask a midwife who seems supportive to sit with you for the first few feeds until you feel confident to try it out on your own. If you are experiencing any difficulty at all, do contact your local breastfeeding counsellor, who can come into hospital, if you would like that, to help you over any initial hurdles. Experienced mothers on the ward can be an excellent source of help and support as well. There should be no need for any mother with a problem, however small, to struggle on unaided. Use whatever help is available and which appeals to your way of doing things.

SURVIVING IN HOSPITAL

If you have had your baby in hospital and are staying for longer than six or twelve hours, you may have ambivalent feelings about your stay on the hospital ward. Some women enjoy life in hospital, away from the worry of coping with domestic arrangements, pleased to have experts constantly at hand to help them grow in confidence in handling a new baby. You may like the idea of being with other new mothers, enjoying the camaraderie that is often built up as you all learn to cope with your bodies and your babies. For others, the period of time spent in hospital is less satisfactory, marred by constant interruptions day and night, from staff and from other women. You may feel you have little time to get to know your baby on your own at your own pace, little constructive help from your medical carers, poor food, lack of sleep, and an enforced absence from your family. You may find any or all of these feelings surfacing at different times. If the routine of life in an institution does not appeal to you and you do feel confident about going home, you can leave when you feel ready, provided there is no medical problem for either of you, and as long as there will be a community midwife available to care for you once you are home. Whether you have booked in for two, five, or seven days is largely irrelevant; it is an administrative guideline.

What your stay in hospital should be is an opportunity for you to rest and recuperate, plus the first stage in learning to handle and feed your baby confidently and with pleasure.

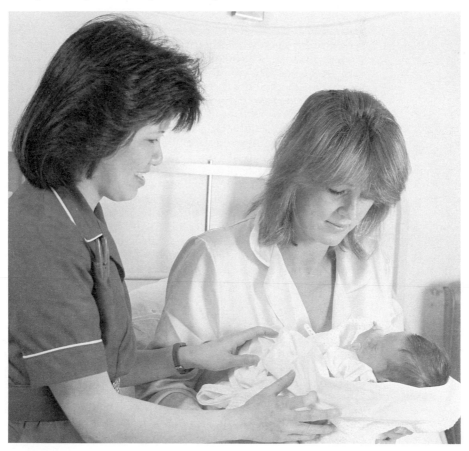

DEALING WITH ADVICE Conflicting advice is frequently mentioned as the biggest single problem for the majority of women during their hospital stay, particularly over the breastfeeding issue. As in pregnancy, new mothers are showered with advice from every quarter, often conflicting, so that they are left feeling more confused than ever. The baby will have the same problem. If you are constantly being advised to try out different things, it is difficult for the baby to grasp a sensible idea of what is expected of her. Most women feel it best to find one person — a midwife, an NCT breastfeeding counsellor, or another, more experienced mother — whose ideas seem logical, appropriate, and sympathetic, and then follow through her suggestions. If something does not feel right for you, or if it is not working, you do not have to go against your own instincts because someone else has told you to do it one way; you will know what feels best and most sensible to you, so trust your own judgement and stay with that.

SLEEP The usual advice to new mothers — to rest as much as possible and sleep when their baby sleeps — does not always work in hospital. The sleep times you might normally choose may not coincide with theirs. There is always a light on somewhere in a ward, which causes problems for many women. Some hospitals have entirely flexible visiting periods, so that it becomes hard to rest during the day while listening to other people's visitors laughing and talking. Others have rest times which are strictly adhered to, but you have no guarantee that your baby will not wake up during this hour. Hospitals are inevitably busy, noisy places and this may make sleep elusive. If you have been up with your baby during the night, you may not appreciate the usual hospital routine of waking everyone bright and early to ensure the wards are ready for doctors' rounds later on. You may decide to rest while your baby is sleeping, only to find someone comes in to empty the waste bins or to take a blood sample. It can be difficult having so little control over your own sleeping and resting conditions; once at home, you will still have an unpredictable baby to look after, but otherwise you will be able to make your own routines.

ROOMING-IN Many hospitals allow babies to remain with their mothers at all times of day or night. A few positively encourage mothers and babies to sleep in the same bed for warmth, security, and easy feeding. Others, often those with large wards, prefer babies to be taken to a nursery for the night. If you are breastfeeding, this means that you will have to be woken by the night staff when your baby wakes for a feed, and either have to walk to the nursery or have your baby brought to you. The reason for a hospital choosing nurseries rather than rooming-in is usually the possible effect of babies' crying on other mothers' sleep. Many women wake easily to all sounds in a strange place, including a baby crying, and have very disturbed nights in hospital, rooming-in or not. Other women remain oblivious, waking only to their own babies. Mothers who have experienced rooming-in often say that the babies hardly cried when next to their mothers all night, for, as soon as they murmured, the mothers would pick them up. Other women have lain awake hearing the sounds of a baby crying in the nursery, wondering if it is theirs and if they will have to get up.

AMENITY ROOMS If you feel very strongly that you would like your baby to remain with you at all times and you do not yet feel ready to go home, you might consider asking for a side room. Most hospitals have these available, though you will normally have to pay for them. Some mothers say that they were ignored in the side room and missed out on some of the help and companionship they would have liked, whereas others welcome the extra privacy gained.

NIGHT FEEDS Getting up to feed at night also has its advantages and disadvantages. If feeding is taking a while to become established, it can be helpful to sit in a nursery where there is often company and a member of staff who can help you to get the baby well latched on. On the other hand, it is possible that it will be far more tiring, and wake you more fully, to have to get up and trail down the corridor to sit on a chair, rather than snuggle up in bed with your baby. Some hospitals have adopted a system whereby babies are brought in to the mothers for feeding. This works reasonably well, given an enthusiastic staff.

One of the problems with the night-time is that staff on duty may be agency staff, without the same degree of commitment and experience that the regular ward staff have. You may find the attitudes of some staff during the night less than helpful and may feel upset if there is a lack of positive encouragement, help, and reassurance just when you are at your lowest ebb.

If you are worried that night staff may fail to wake you, or may give your baby a bottle of cow's milk or dextrose water while you sleep, it is worth making a notice to stick on your baby's cot to prevent this; 'Mother breastfeeding; please wake' or 'Breastfed baby; no bottles, thank you' should do the trick. If you are particularly concerned that your baby should not receive artificial milk, it may be worth writing a letter to the Director of Midwifery Services, expressing your wish that at no time should your baby be given a bottle of artificial milk without your consent.

FOOD It is rare for hospital catering to meet the needs of healthy, hungry, newly delivered, breastfeeding mothers. Neither the quality nor the quantity may be what one would normally choose. Added to this is the fact that for your first twenty-four hours or more you will have to have what your bed's previous occupant ordered. The main benefit is that it appears without any effort whatsoever on your part.

It is tempting, faced with the unappetizing, meagre fare so often served up to postnatal women, to fill up on cakes, sweets, and the like. This may fill the odd corners but will not do much for you nutritionally, or for your weight. You will probably want to order large portions on your menu sheet, though in practice this may make little difference to what arrives. If you can, always order sandwiches or biscuits and cheese in addition to your meal.

If you are desperate, your partner could bring in a take-away meal, or a ready-cooked meal to heat up in the microwave oven which many hospital wards now have.

Going home to food, cooked as and when you want it, can be a powerful influence on your decision about returning home.

VISITORS Not everyone wants to be surrounded by visitors in hospital. Your partner can do some judicious negotiating behind the scenes here, letting others know whether or not you want visitors, and if so, who and when.

Postnatal infection

It is an unfortunate fact that far too many mothers suffer from infections caught in hospital as a result of unhygienic conditions. You are less likely to catch anything unpleasant at home, since there are only your own germs, to which you are accustomed.

There are three main potential sites of infection:

○ **THE PERINEUM IF THERE ARE STITCHES**
○ **THE UTERUS, WITH ITS OPEN WOUND**
○ **A CAESAREAN SCAR**

AVOIDING POSTNATAL INFECTION There are ways and means of avoiding infection as far as possible, which do entail a little forethought and a bit more effort but are worth it for the problems they avoid.

○ **DO NOT USE A TOWEL FOR DRYING YOUR GENITAL AREA BUT PAT IT DRY WITH SOFT TISSUE. AVOID ACTUALLY TOUCHING ANY STITCHES.**
○ **DRY YOUR HANDS ON DISPOSABLE TOWELS IN HOSPITAL RATHER THAN USING ROLLER TOWELS.**
○ **CLEAN OUT THE BATHS AND BIDETS IF THEY HAVE NOT ALREADY BEEN CLEANED BY THE PREVIOUS OCCUPANT OR THE CLEANING STAFF. IF NO EQUIPMENT IS PROVIDED,**

AND THIS IS OFTEN THE CASE, TAKE IN YOUR OWN CLOTH
AND CLEANING MATERIALS.

○ STICK TO SHOWERS IF YOU ARE REALLY UNHAPPY ABOUT THE
STATE OF HYGIENE IN THE BATHROOMS.

○ WASH YOUR HANDS BOTH BEFORE AND AFTER CHANGING
YOUR SANITARY TOWEL.

○ CHANGE YOUR SANITARY TOWEL FREQUENTLY AND DISPOSE OF
IT CLEANLY, IN A BAG.

○ RE-WRAP ICE-PACKS OR PACKETS OF FROZEN PEAS AT EACH
USE.

○ WASH YOUR HANDS BOTH BEFORE AND AFTER VISITING THE
LAVATORY.

○ TAKE IN ANTISEPTIC OR ALCOHOL WIPES TO CLEAN THE
LAVATORY SEAT; TAKE IN A PACK OF PAPER LAVATORY-SEAT
COVERS AS WELL, IF YOU WISH.

○ SIT RIGHT BACK ON THE LAVATORY SO THAT YOUR VULVA IS
NOT IN CONTACT WITH THE SEAT AT ALL.

○ DO NOT USE LAVATORY PAPER WHICH HAS BEEN STANDING ON
THE FLOOR; TELL THE STAFF AND GET A NEW ROLL.

○ SPRAY WARM WATER ON TO YOUR VULVA WHILE ON THE
LAVATORY TO CLEAN THE AREA AS WELL AS TO SOOTHE.

○ AVOID SHARING SUCH POTENTIALLY BACTERIA-SWAPPING
ITEMS AS HAIR-DRYERS.

BABY BLUES

Many women find that they have a day or two when they feel really low. They may even be happy but be unable to stop crying all day. Baby blues often seem to coincide with the milk coming in and seem to be more commonly experienced by first-time mothers. Babies are usually becoming much more wakeful and demanding by about the third or fourth day, having recovered from the labour. You may be feeling physically stronger but find that the demands of being a mother and coping with everything at once seem just too much, particularly when your body is not yet back to normal, and you may be short of sleep. If you can relax and accept that this is a phase that will pass, that you will not always find looking after your baby quite so bewildering and exhausting, that you will soon feel more confident in mothering her, you can then enjoy a good cry.

Some women do feel very lonely in hospital without their partners, which can exacerbate miserable feelings around now. If feeding is taking a while to become established, this too may come to a head about now. Making sure you have the encouragement and support of a midwife or breastfeeding counsellor will help you over any initial hurdles. If you are tempted to think that it is breastfeeding which is causing your baby to be more demanding or yourself to feel so tired, it is worth remembering that bottlefeeding mothers are by no means immune from exhaustion and crises of confidence. You have the wherewithal to feed and comfort your baby whenever she cries; bottlefeeding mothers can only offer a specified amount of feeding and any other comfort needs will have to be met in other ways.

GOING HOME

If you have been in hospital for several days, going home again may feel rather strange, especially when someone has been living there without you. It may feel unreal that you are actually in your home with a new member of the family. You may be concerned about how you will cope, how your other children will react, even how you will know what to do. Babies also respond to changes in their environment and it is not at all unusual for a baby to behave quite differently at home from how she did in hospital. You may have been able to settle her to sleep quite nicely there, yet she seems impossible to settle now. Homes are quieter than hospitals and she may be reacting to this as much as to your understandable nervousness. Research has shown that babies who happily go three hours between feeds in hospital may need feeding every 1 hour 55 minutes when first at home!

Many new parents decide to arrange for the father to take some time off work, so that they can concentrate on finding out what life is like with an extra person and so that they can enjoy the new baby together, gradually working out ways of managing life with this new baby.

Some women choose to have their mothers or mothers-in-law to stay and help them look after the baby in the early days or weeks. Parents who choose this option find it works best when both parents are happy with the arrangement and when everybody has a clear idea about the precise role the new parents would like the mother to play.

Visitors   Women have said that the worst aspect of having a new baby was that too many visitors came too soon and stayed for too long, which felt like an intrusion into their day rather than being a welcome relief. There are ways to avoid this problem:

○ **ASK EVERYONE TO RING BEFORE COMING.**
○ **DO NOT FEEL AFRAID TO TELL UNEXPECTED OR UNTIMELY CALLERS TO RETURN AT A MORE SUITABLE TIME.**
○ **UNPLUG THE PHONE WHENEVER YOU FEED OR HAVE A BATH.**
○ **HANG A NOTE ON YOUR FRONT DOOR OR GATE EXPLAINING THAT YOU AND YOUR BABY ARE RESTING AND DO NOT WANT TO BE DISTURBED.**

○   **REMOVE THE BATTERY FROM THE DOORBELL.**

○   **MAKE A DETERMINED EFFORT TO REMAIN SEATED WHILE VISITORS ARE THERE AND INVITE *THEM* TO MAKE THE TEA, COFFEE, ETC.**

○   **MAKE A POINT OF SAYING YOU ARE GOING FOR A REST, IF VISITORS ARE OUTSTAYING THEIR WELCOME; THIS IS RATHER DIFFICULT TO MANAGE POLITELY, BUT IT MAY BE THE ONLY WAY.**

○   **ACCEPT ANY OFFERS OF HELP, HOWEVER TENTATIVELY OR UNCONVINCINGLY PROFFERED; SHOW VISITORS THE PILE OF IRONING OR THE BREAKFAST WASHING-UP AND THANK THEM FOR THE HELP. BEWARE OF LETTING VISITORS CUDDLE THE BABY WHILE YOU DO EVERYTHING ELSE. IF NECESSARY, HANG ON TO HER.**

THE NEW-BORN BABY

New-born babies do not always look round and placid like the babies in the advertisements, any more than you feel like the slim, serene mothers pictured there. New-born babies have all sorts of physical peculiarities which are quite normal, but not necessarily what you may have been expecting. Some of these have been described in Chapter 20, The First Few Hours, but there are others which can surprise new parents.

Appearance

HAEMATOMA Some babies are born with haematomas or swellings on their heads from the delivery; these usually disappear in a few days.

SWOLLEN SCROTUM Baby boys may appear to be very well endowed, with enlarged testicles. This is caused by fluid, takes a while to subside, and does not seem to cause the baby any discomfort.

MILK IN THE BREASTS Some babies have swollen breasts and may even pass 'witches' milk'. This is caused by hormones passed from you to your baby at birth.

VAGINAL BLEEDING Some girl babies have vaginal bleeding or 'mini-periods'; again this is a result of your hormones crossing to the baby.

DRY, FLAKY SKIN Lots of new babies have rather dry skin. A little moisturizing oil in the bath can help, though it will make for a slippery baby. You may feel more confident massaging your baby with oil after the bath.

SPOTS New babies tend to come up in all sorts of rashes. These do not normally mean anything, but ask if you are not sure. See Chapter

26, Looking After your Baby, for further information on caring for your baby's skin.

COLOUR Babies' hands and feet often remain rather grey or blue-ish for a few days. Whatever her skin colour, your baby's tongue and lips should be pink.

Mothers do sometimes feel alarmed by their baby's appearance — new babies seem so vulnerable and can change so quickly. If you are at all worried, ask your midwife, GP, or the paediatrician.

Medical care

Some of the procedures which are carried out on babies in these early days will be carried out by a paediatrician, others by a midwife.

THE CORD The cord will soon shrivel up, eventually falling off after about ten days or a fortnight. You may be given some powder to shake on to keep the area free of infection and will be shown how to keep the cord clean. If you are given the little bottle of powder, you will probably have plenty left once the cord has gone; this comes in very useful for sprinkling on to sore spots, minor blisters, or grazes etc. in other members of the family.

GUTHRIE TEST The Guthrie test involves taking blood from your baby's heel. It is performed routinely to find out if a baby is suffering from phenylketonuria, a metabolic disorder which causes mental retardation unless controlled by a special diet. The test can be as distressing for the mothers as for the babies, and some women prefer to stay out of the way while it is being done. Breastfeeding your baby immediately afterwards is comforting for both of you. Some midwives suggest putting an extra pair of bootees on your baby for a while before the test so the baby's foot is warm and the test easier to do.

TESTING FOR HYPOGLYCAEMIA Your hospital may test for hypoglycaemia, or low blood sugar, in babies considered to be at risk. A baby who has not the normal necessary nutritional reserves may have problems maintaining a good blood-sugar level. A prolonged period with a low blood-sugar level can lead to fits and, in some cases, brain damage. The test involves heel-prick blood tests taken several times during the first forty-eight hours of life.

Babies who may need to be tested for low blood sugar include small-for-dates babies, those who are particularly large, and those who have suffered a traumatic or prolonged birth. Small-for-dates babies are those who are fully mature but weigh less than is usual for their gestational age. Though these babies will be able to benefit from your colostrum, they may need to be given complementary feeds of artificial milk until your breast milk comes in if their blood sugar is found to be low. Once lactation is established, they can be fully breastfed.

If you and the medical staff decide there is a good reason to have

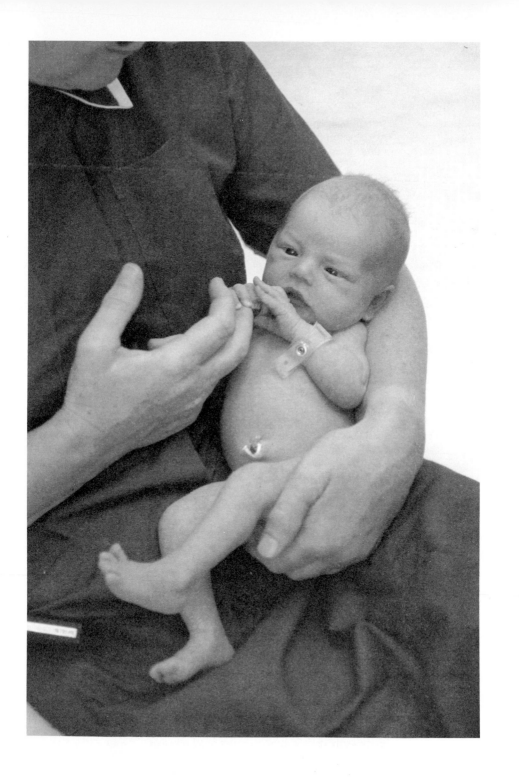

your baby's blood sugar tested and the level is found to be low, it will be well worth giving your baby another breastfeed, as this may be sufficient to raise her blood-sugar levels without further action. If breastfeeding does not have enough of an impact on her blood sugar immediately, then you will normally be advised that she will have to have a feed of artificial milk. If you intend to breastfeed, and your baby does have to have a formula feed, you may prefer it to be given through a naso-gastric tube rather than a bottle. New-born babies find it confusing to learn to suckle on a bottle as well as on a breast, and, unfortunately, it is often the breast which loses out. Using a naso-gastric tube avoids this possible confusion.

Healthy, full-term babies will have plenty of reserves to keep their blood-sugar level sufficiently high and will rarely have any problems with low blood sugar. Indeed, if there are allergies in the family and if you are concerned to establish breastfeeding as soon as possible, it may be disadvantageous for your baby to receive a bottle of formula milk (see Chapter 24, Feeding your Baby).

STOOLS The first stool a baby passes is meconium, which has collected in the rectum while the baby was in the uterus. Meconium is a peculiarly sticky, tarry substance and you may need lashings of soap, water, and patience to clean it all off your baby, and perhaps her clothing, her bedding, and even you.

Once the meconium is passed, your baby's stools will change to a greenish-brown, then after a few days will settle to being bright yellow, curdy, and usually rather loose if you are breastfeeding. The stools of a bottlefed baby will be a darker yellow, more solid, and will smell more strongly.

VOMITING Some babies are prone to bringing back some milk after a feed. This is known as 'posseting'. Vomit from a breastfed baby does not smell very much, just a bit milky; but artificial milk will smell sour, of stale milk. Keeping a good supply of tissues or muslin nappies about you can be useful if you have a sicky baby. It may seem as though she is wasting a good deal of her feed, but, like any spilt liquid, a little goes a long way, particularly once it is mixed with saliva.

A common cause of posseting is 'winding' a baby — if you pat her back, holding her against your shoulder or sitting on your lap, you can actually give her wind. Instead, hold her sitting on your hip, facing you but leaning away from you, her spine and head supported on your hand and forearm. The heavy milk will stay in her stomach and the air will move up or down.

If your baby vomits up what seems to be a complete feed once or twice, ask your doctor to check her for possible infection (most unlikely in a breastfed baby), or pyloric stenosis, a condition where vomit is regularly shot literally across the room. The occasional vomiting of large amounts in the early days is, however, not at all unusual.

JAUNDICE Many babies develop jaundice at about three days, because the immature liver cannot excrete bilirubin — the blood pigment responsible for yellow staining of the skin. Keep an eye open for any yellow discoloration of the skin — staff will take a blood test if they are concerned. Jaundice rarely does any harm, but could have serious repercussions if left untreated. You may be asked to make sure you feed your baby more frequently if she has mild jaundice — at least every two or three hours, because frequent feeding helps flush the jaundice through her system. There is no evidence that giving extra water to jaundiced babies is of any use at all in clearing the jaundice and it is a positive hindrance to breastfeeding.

Jaundice makes babies sleepy, so you may have to wake her for feeds, and it may be difficult to keep her awake for very long. If the jaundice is at a higher level, she may have to be fed more often and also put under phototherapy. This involves the baby lying naked under a bright light, with an extra heater for warmth and some protection for her eyes. The light helps to break down the yellow pigment in the skin, speeding up the natural course of the jaundice. Babies under phototherapy usually pass a lot of very liquid stools. They often protest loudly and unhappily when first placed under the light without their clothes, but eventually settle down to quite liking it. You may feel rather helpless and sad at not being able to cuddle your baby as much as you would like, and your baby may have to be away from you in the nursery, but this is a problem normally resolved in a couple of days. You can, of course, remove the baby's eye covering during feed-times.

Part of the fun of being a parent is in discovering all the little things a baby can do, and watching her develop. A new-born baby is capable of a wide range of activities, many of which you can help her with, thus enjoying a closer relationship and exploring the world with her.

What your baby can do

SEEING Your baby can see, though she cannot focus beyond about 9 inches. This distance is just right for her when she is at the breast looking up at you. She will be able to distinguish light from dark, and will be able to watch and follow an object held in front of her. (By about six months her sight will have matured to a level similar to an adult's.)

Many new-born babies appear cross-eyed; this is normal, but if your baby seems to be squinting beyond about three months, you should discuss it with your GP or clinic doctor.

HEARING Your baby will be able to hear perfectly well and has been listening to the sounds of your body as well as to external noises since the fourteenth week of pregnancy. Some babies are easily startled and may jump or cry at sudden loud noises.

GRASPING Your baby will be able to hold on to any object, or a finger placed in her palm; she will hold on surprisingly tightly too. Her hands will be clenched for much of the time and her grasping of objects is purely a reflex response now, but over the months her hands will open more and more, and soon after three months she will be able to reach out for an object and take hold of it.

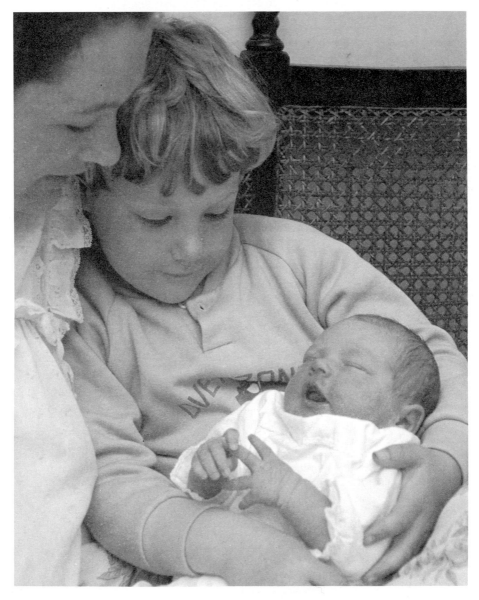

COMMUNICATING Babies can communicate; the problem, as often as not, is whether other people can understand what they are trying to say. Some cries are obvious in meaning — the sudden piercing cry which indicates fear or pain, for example. Other cries are less easy to interpret, and it may take you a while to work out what means what.

Babies can also express pleasure and contentment; although most books will tell you to expect the first smile at about six weeks, mothers and fathers know that babies as young as four or five days old are capable of trying out their first smiles. Some people will say this is wind, but you will soon know if your baby has wind or is attempting to respond to your face, your smiles, and your voice.

Babies quieten when they are picked up, and you can watch their fingers and toes curl and uncurl as they feed or play. A breastfed baby will spend much of her feed-time kneading, stroking, and pushing at the breast, partly to encourage the milk flow, but also as an expression of contentment.

Babies are able to copy you in ways other than smiling too. Try putting out your tongue and moving it from side to side. She will soon try putting out her own tongue in imitation, which is, after all, the key to all her initial development and learning.

The first days and weeks with your new baby may not be easy and may feel very strange and disorientating; but it will not always be quite so new, and gradually you will become accustomed to each other; you will feel more like your old self and you will begin to imagine that she has always been a part of your family, that there never was a time before she came. There are no short cuts to learning about your baby and finding ways of mothering which suit you. The more you can manage to rest and relax and enjoy your new role and your new baby, the better you will feel able to cope.

* *Looking back it was funny, all of us hobbling round the ward with painful perineums, edging ourselves into chairs and on to beds with the greatest care.* *

* *The hardest thing was trying to sort out for myself what I should do. Everyone around me — and there was no shortage of new faces! — seemed to have a different piece of advice to offer.* *

* *No one warned me how difficult the first bowel movement after the birth would be. Actually it was probably worse than having the baby.* *

* *My body didn't feel its usual self at all. I was very busy coping with this new body I was inhabiting, and on top of that I had a baby to care for.* *

* *It took me all my time to look after the baby and, if I was lucky, tidy myself up. Everything else went to pot.* *

23   THE NEW BABY IN THE FAMILY

You will have spent the last few months thinking about and, as far as possible, preparing for the arrival of your new baby, and now she is here; you have become parents for the first, second, third, or whatever time; your parents have become grandparents; your other children have a new brother or sister. Life is not quite the same any more. Most of the changes we encounter in our lives have at least two sides, and with a new baby also the rejoicing may well be coupled with some uncertainty about what the future holds in store. It can feel rather strange when everyone around you is pleased for you, expecting you to be delighted in your new roles, but you may be feeling rather unsure as to quite what you have let yourselves in for.

THE NEW FAMILY

Finding a balance

When the new baby arrives, the focus of attention inevitably shifts to her, and rightly so. But how long should life be like this? What about her siblings, her father and mother? Every member of the family has his or her own needs and this new baby will eventually have to fit into the existing structure as far as possible, although her very presence will alter the family dynamics to some extent. Too much of a change to the family's life-style is stressful and can cause resentment of this new baby who has brought about so much change. Trying to find a way round looking after your tiny baby's needs whilst ensuring that your partner does not start to feel left out, or your other children jealous, can be difficult but not insurmountable. It can help to discuss this with the rest of the family beforehand; talk about what a new baby needs, how much time she will take, and explain that it will not always be quite so disorganized as in the first few weeks. The more your partner and children can feel involved in the care of this new baby — the interesting bits as well as the nappy changes — the easier it will be for everyone to feel a valued part of the family.

Some tact may be needed here too. If others are helping to do things with the baby, they will need their confidence to be built up as well. If your partner offers to bath her, it may be kinder not to 'supervise' him, so that he can find his own way of doing things, just

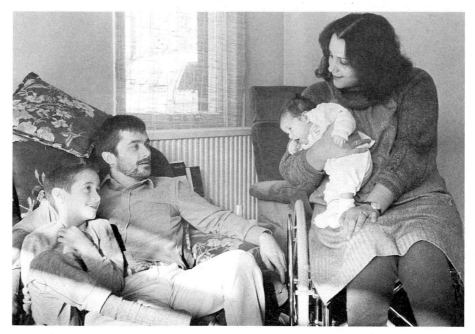

as you have been doing. If an older child wishes to cuddle the baby, try to let him or her do so — but with a reminder to hold the baby's head carefully. Equally, however, if others are sharing the care of the baby, it is only fair that things are done properly; there is nothing worse than someone else changing a nappy, then leaving the dirty nappy plus changing equipment strewn around the room.

As you all become more accustomed to life with this new member of the family, so you will be able to start doing the things you enjoy as a family again.

Out and about

Most babies are pretty adaptable people and there are comparatively few places you can visit with children that will not accommodate a baby. If your children are used to going to the swings in the park, to swimming lessons, to friends' houses to play, it is usually manageable while your baby is small and easily transportable.

If this is your first child and you are looking forward to socializing again, it may be more difficult. In this country, there are many places where babies are barely tolerated, and it can be difficult to get out and about. Pubs, restaurants, and cinemas often have a no-babies policy and you may not feel brave enough to confront intolerant adults just yet.

Loss of spontaneity in social activities is something new parents often find quite hard to adjust to. Whether it takes you three weeks or three months to feel confident enough to begin socializing again, as soon as you feel ready, have a go. As well as your new roles as mothers and fathers, you are also friends and lovers, and your other children have needs too which have to be met if they are not to feel pushed aside by this baby.

'STUCK AT HOME'? It is reasonably common to hear women talk about being 'stuck at home' with a baby, and it is worth considering how this might affect you. Will you possibly feel trapped, or are there plenty of ways for you to get out once you feel ready? If you are going to be short of adult company during the day, will you expect your partner to be a stimulating, entertaining conversationalist when he comes home from work? It can be rather difficult to maintain any sort of sensible conversation when the baby is crying, your toddler is fractious and over-tired, and you are both wondering how you are ever going to get a meal this evening. Finding some time when you can talk to each other is important; it just may be a bit hard to find many occasions for a few weeks or months.

Your new roles

It is worth discussing in advance what sort of role you each expect the other to have in your relationship once the baby arrives, and to try to make this fairly realistic, knowing your own characters and your family backgrounds. It is not easy to do this, because it is difficult to know precisely how you will react to becoming a mother, let alone how your partner will react, however well you feel you know him. Will either or both of you expect the child care to be undertaken by the woman, believing that it is 'women's work'? Women feel as vulnerable and uncertain as men when faced with a tiny baby for whom they are responsible. It may be hard for a woman to come to terms with the fact that being a woman does not necessarily mean she can automatically interpret and deal with every cry and scream. Sharing both the difficult and the enjoyable parts of parenthood is what makes it so rewarding for both of you. As with most things in life, the more you put into it, the more you get out.

You will find it valuable to think about your own mental images of mother- and fatherhood, seeing if they are realistic once the baby has arrived, and preparing to be flexible.

It will also help to know what you expect of each other. Does your partner expect to carry on playing football every Saturday and Sunday when you have a new baby? Do you expect him to give up his football because you have a new baby?

You will need to be prepared for things to be slightly different once the baby comes, and the best-laid plans can go straight out of the window once the reality of life with a baby hits you. You may, for example, have discussed both of you being awake to cope with the night feeds, yet, when it comes to it, your partner may find he cannot keep up with the broken nights and his day-time job. You may have agreed that night-time feeds will be the sole responsibility of the mother. What will happen when the mother has returned to work but the baby is still waking two or three times a night? New circumstances will alter your original plans, and you will have to renegotiate your position and roles in the family, sorting out what suits you best, being flexible enough to adapt to changing circumstances and attitudes. Above all, you need to work your lives round being able to get the maximum enjoyment from your baby and from all members of the family.

YOUR BABY'S DEVELOPMENT

Babies are a lot of fun as well as hard work, and watching yours grow and develop, delighting in her individuality, as she finds

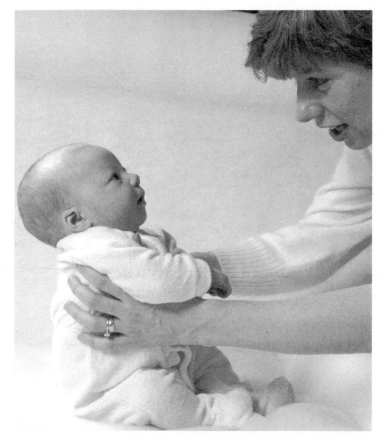

out about herself and the world around her, develops new skills, and gradually makes her own personality apparent, is one of the best aspects of parenthood. One of the best aspects of having a second or subsequent baby is that this development can be shared not only between the two of you as a couple, but also with your other children. The capabilities of a new-born baby have been mentioned in Chapter 22, Early Days. It is a source of immense fascination and interest to watch as she grows and progresses over the months. The lists that follow give you some idea of what your baby might be able to do at certain stages in her first year. Do bear in mind that these lists are only guidelines to a baby's development. Your baby will do things at a pace that is right for her, not necessarily according to the baby books. However, if you feel at all concerned that your baby is not progressing at the rate you would expect, do not feel afraid to consult your GP or health visitor and keep asking questions until you feel satisfied with the answers or help you are receiving.

THE FIRST MONTH

- ○ LIFTS AND TURNS HER HEAD IF PLACED FLAT ON HER TUMMY.
- ○ BEGINS TO BE ABLE TO SUPPORT HER HEAD.
- ○ STARTS TO TURN HER HEAD WHEN SHE HEARS YOUR VOICE.
- ○ LIKES LOOKING AT PATTERNS OR CONTRASTS BETWEEN DARK AND LIGHT; YOUR FACE IS A WONDERFUL PATTERN.
- ○ STARTS TO STARE AT YOUR FACE WHEN YOU ARE TALKING TO HER; MEETS YOUR EYES.

THE SECOND MONTH

- ○ STARTS TO HOLD HER HEAD UP FOR A WHILE WHEN ON HER TUMMY.
- ○ STILL CANNOT HOLD HER HEAD UP WHEN SHE IS SITTING, BUT THE SUPPORT IS STRONGER.
- ○ HOLDS AN OBJECT PLACED IN HER HAND, BUT WITHOUT ANY IDEA THAT SHE HAS IT!
- ○ BEGINS TO TALK BY 'COOING'.
- ○ FOLLOWS OBJECTS WITH HER EYES.
- ○ SEES LARGE OBJECTS SEVERAL FEET AWAY.
- ○ DISCOVERS HER HANDS — A FIRST TOY!
- ○ DEFINITELY AND UNMISTAKABLY SMILES AT YOU.
- ○ BANGS HER HEAD ON YOUR SHOULDER — A GREAT GAME, WHICH STRENGTHENS NECK MUSCLES AS WELL.

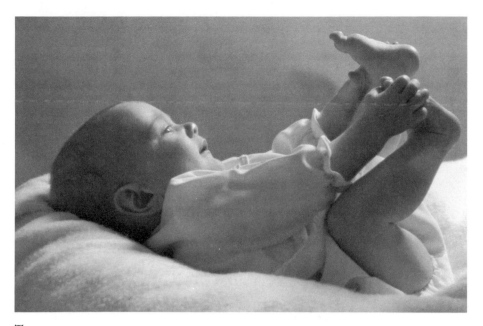

THE THIRD MONTH

- ○ PUSHES HERSELF UP WITH HER ARMS AND LIFTS HER HEAD AND CHEST WHEN ON HER TUMMY.
- ○ PUTS HER HANDS TOGETHER.
- ○ SUPPORTS HER OWN WEIGHT WHEN PULLED UP TO HER FEET.
- ○ MAKES NOISES FOR HER OWN BENEFIT.
- ○ MAKES NOISES BACK AT YOU WHEN YOU TALK TO HER.
- ○ SHOWS SIGNS OF MEMORY — E.G. BECOMES EXCITED ON SEEING HER BATH.
- ○ STARTS TO MAKE A GRAB AT OBJECTS — HAIR, GLASSES, AND EARRINGS ARE NO LONGER SAFE.
- ○ REALLY ENJOYS PHYSICAL GAMES ON THE FLOOR OR IN THE MIDDLE OF THE BED.
- ○ ENJOYS HER BATH; BATHTIME BECOMES MUCH MORE FUN, AND MUCH WETTER!

THE SIXTH MONTH

- ○ JUST ABOUT SITS UNAIDED IF LEANT FORWARD.
- ○ MOVES HER FEET WHEN SHE IS PULLED TO STANDING.
- ○ ROLLS FROM HER BACK ON TO HER TUMMY AND VICE VERSA.

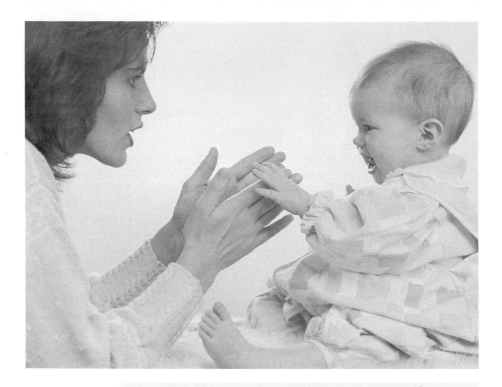

- ROTATES HER HANDS SO THAT EVERYTHING IS EXAMINED FROM ALL ANGLES.
- MAKES A VARIETY OF DIFFERENT SOUNDS IN HER BABBLING; YOU MAY RECOGNIZE THE EARLY BEGINNINGS OF WORDS.
- REACTS TO YOUR TONE OF VOICE.
- REACHES, GRABS, AND INSPECTS CAREFULLY WITH SMOOTH, ACCURATE MOVEMENTS.
- TURNS WHEN YOU CALL HER NAME.
- IS LESS HAPPY TO BE HELD BY STRANGERS.
- SEES EVERYTHING AS A POTENTIAL TOY.
- ENJOYS PEEK-A-BOO WITH YOU.
- ENJOYS A FEW ACTION RHYMES, E.G. 'ROUND AND ROUND THE GARDEN'.
- FINDS THAT FEET ARE AS NICE TO SUCK AS HANDS.
- IS JUST ABOUT READY TO BE ON THE MOVE; YOU WILL NEED A BABYPROOF HOME NOW — PREFERABLY BEFORE THE FIRST ACCIDENT!
- IS ALMOST READY FOR SOLID FOOD — PREPARE FOR THE MESS.

Teeth.

THE EIGHTH MONTH

- ○ GETS TO MOST PLACES BY WHATEVER METHOD SHE USES AS 'CRAWLING'.
- ○ STARTS TO BE INTERESTED IN PULLING HERSELF TO STANDING ON THE FURNITURE OR YOUR ARMS.
- ○ LEANS FORWARD WHILE SITTING WITHOUT TOPPLING OVER.
- ○ SHOUTS MOST EFFECTIVELY.
- ○ IMITATES AND SAYS TWO-SYLLABLE WORDS — USUALLY 'DADA'.
- ○ SEARCHES FOR SOMETHING IF YOU HIDE IT.
- ○ PUTS OBJECTS INSIDE OTHER THINGS.
- ○ HOLDS TWO THINGS SIMULTANEOUSLY.
- ○ MAY BE FRIGHTENED OF OTHER PEOPLE OUTSIDE HER IMMEDIATE FAMILY.
- ○ LIKES ROLLING THINGS.
- ○ ENJOYS PLAYING WITH YOUR SAUCEPANS AND WOODEN SPOONS.
- ○ ENJOYS WATCHING HERSELF IN A MIRROR.

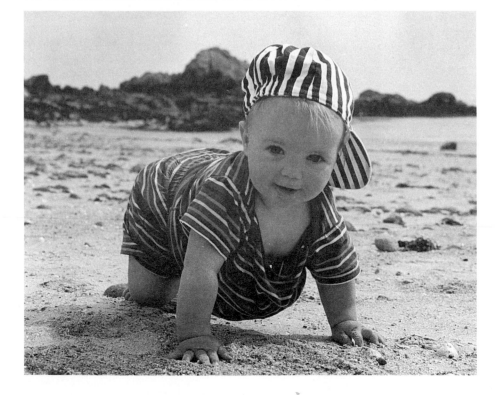

THE TENTH MONTH

○ CAN POSSIBLY STAND UP WITHOUT PULLING HERSELF UP.
○ BEGINS TO CRUISE AROUND FURNITURE.
○ BEGINS TO CLIMB.
○ RECOGNIZES SEVERAL WORDS.
○ SPEAKS ONE OR TWO WORDS OF HER OWN.
○ STARTS TO BE FEARFUL — OF BATH, VACUUM CLEANER, DRILL.
○ TRIES TO HELP YOU DRESS HER.
○ DISCOVERS THAT SHE CAN SAY 'NO' — AND YOU DISCOVER SHE MEANS IT!
○ ENJOYS SITTING IN A HIGH CHAIR OR PUSH-CHAIR AND DROPPING THINGS OVER THE SIDE FOR YOU TO PICK UP SO THAT THE GAME CAN START AGAIN, AD INFINITUM.

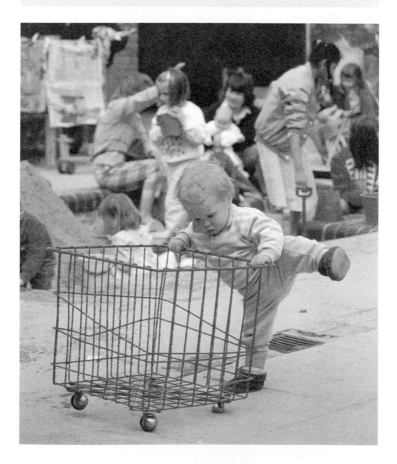

THE TWELFTH MONTH

- ○ FINDS STAIRS FASCINATING AND GOES UP AND DOWN THEM.
- ○ POINTS.
- ○ REMOVES LIDS.
- ○ STARTS TO SAY A FEW CLEAR WORDS.
- ○ STARTS TO IMITATE OTHER THINGS, E.G. A CAT, NOISE OF CAR.
- ○ RESPONDS TO REQUESTS.
- ○ MAY START WALKING.
- ○ RECOGNIZES PARTS OF HER BODY.
- ○ ENJOYS LOOKING AT BOOKS.
- ○ HAS HER FIRST BIRTHDAY PARTY!

When you all look back over the year, it will be difficult to imagine that this laughing, cheeky toddler was a helpless little baby only twelve months ago. There will never again be a year of such rapid and incredible development.

Comparisons

What your friend's baby does at what stage will be different from what yours does. Because we are all different, it is pointless making comparisons, though it does seem to be the favourite pastime of many mothers — usually those with rather forward children! Remember too, that when you are 25 no one cares how old you were when you first stood up unaided, or when you spoke your first intelligible word. Just enjoy your baby for who she is and what she can do — whenever she decides to do it.

OTHER CHILDREN

Each time a new baby comes along, the balance within the family is altered; everyone has to 'move up one'. This can be a source of problems for your other children and you may find a certain amount of sibling rivalry creeping in. Children prefer to be the centre of attention themselves, so, when someone else turns up, who is new and hogs all the attention for a while, it is understandable if children feel put out. They may behave in all sorts of different ways in order to regain the limelight.

Unusual behaviour

- ○ SOME ARE NAUGHTY, BECAUSE, EVEN IF A PARENT IS ANNOYED WITH THEM, THAT IS STILL ATTENTION.
- ○ SOME ARE RATHER OSTENTATIOUSLY AND SELF-RIGHTEOUSLY 'GOOD'. (THIS IS RARELY A PROBLEM, JUST IRRITATING.)
- ○ SOME TRY VERY HARD TO MAKE SO MUCH COMMOTION

THAT THEY DISTRACT THE BABY FROM FEEDING, OR MAKE
SURE THEY ASK FOR A DRINK OR THE POTTY IMMEDIATELY
YOU BEGIN TO FEED. IT MAKES SENSE TO TRY TO FORE-
STALL POTENTIAL DISRUPTIONS BY HAVING THE BOOK,
POTTY, DRINK, ETC. READY BEFORE FEEDING.

○ OTHERS WORK OUT, QUITE LOGICALLY, THAT IF BABYISH
BEHAVIOUR GETS SO MUCH ATTENTION, OBVIOUSLY THE
WAY TO ACT IS LIKE A BABY! IT IS QUITE USUAL FOR
CHILDREN TO REVERT TO WEARING NAPPIES OR TAKING UP
A BOTTLE INSTEAD OF A CUP.

○ MANY CHILDREN EXHIBIT CLEAR INDICATIONS OF ILL-WILL
TOWARDS THE NEW BABY — POKING, HITTING, KICKING,
ASKING YOU TO TAKE HER AWAY.

○ OTHERS HIT OUT AT THEIR PARENTS, BLAMING THEM FOR
CAUSING THIS UPSET.

○ SOME CHILDREN DO NOT HIT THE BABY, BUT TAKE THEIR
FEELINGS OUT ON THEIR TOYS OR OTHER CHILDREN AT A
TODDLER GROUP OR PLAYSCHOOL. BOTH OF THESE LAST
TWO SUGGEST REPRESSED JEALOUSY, AND WITH SUCH
BEHAVIOUR YOU WILL NEED TO TALK GENTLY AND
LOVINGLY WITH YOUR CHILDREN, AND, MOST IMPOR-
TANTLY, GET THEM TO TALK TO YOU ABOUT THEIR
FEELINGS. THEY MAY BE FEELING VERY GUILTY AND
HORRID THEMSELVES AND NEED A CHANCE TO KNOW
THEY ARE LOVED AND UNDERSTOOD, AND TO EXPRESS
THEMSELVES OPENLY.

Whatever your child does or does not do, try to give as much attention as you possibly can, showing the older children that, although a new baby has arrived, it does not mean they are loved any the less. This may be a little difficult if your previously angelic toddler has just turned into a shrieking monster, but understanding the reasons for this transformation and continuing to treat him or her with sensitivity and love will eventually work wonders.

Preparing your children

Preparing your child or children for the impact a new baby will have on family life will help to lessen the surprise when the baby actually arrives. A very young child, still a baby herself, may be able to understand very little, but will have had less time as the only child so may feel less threatened by a new baby. Talk about the baby, look at books, get the baby clothes and equipment ready together, so the excitement is shared. Talk about how much bigger your toddler is than this new baby will be, and how nice it is that he or she is old enough to paint pictures, ride a sit-on car, play on the swings, go to playschool, etc.

It is not a good idea to suggest that your child will be getting a brother or sister to play with. This is asking for trouble, as there is no way a baby is interesting enough for a toddler to play with safely. Even a much older child may be quite disappointed when he or she realizes how little a very new baby can do, and how little he or she can do with her. Sharing the baby's development over the weeks and months, pointing out little changes of behaviour and new skills as she learns them, will help any older children to feel more involved; once the baby is a toddler and into the Lego and playdough herself, they may well wish she were a good deal less interesting!

You may think it is a good idea not to be holding your new baby when she and your other child first meet, though this may be difficult if you come home on an early discharge and carry your baby in, but, whatever you do, try to concentrate on making it obvious that you are really pleased to see your other child. You do have two arms — one to hold the baby, the other to hug the toddler. Making time for your child alone is a useful start. *Introducing the baby*

You may like to give the child a present; some parents say it is from the baby, but it is truthful to say it is from you. You could have this ready in or beside the cot (unless it is too large, of course), but presents are substitutes for what your child really needs, which is love and attention.

Try not to make too many changes all at once, as this may be too much for a small child to cope with. If the baby is born just as a child is due to start playschool or nursery, it may be better to delay this for a term until life at home is more settled. Older children who are about to start primary school will not have this option, but should be able to cope better because they are older, can understand more, and can explain better how they are feeling. It is sensible to extend this sensitivity to any baby equipment too. Now is not the time to move your child out of his or her cot 'because the baby needs it'; your older child needs time to adapt to this new situation, just as you do. *Minimizing disturbances*

GRANDPARENTS

New grandparents usually want to visit you and your new baby fairly soon, and it is worth discovering precisely what you are all expecting from visits, especially in these very early days. Your parents may be looking forward to admiring the baby, holding and cuddling her, while 'you have a chance to get on with some cooking and cleaning'; whereas you may feel you are more in need of some practical help around the house — while *you* do the holding and cuddling. It is a good idea to make it clear from the beginning what help you do need and would like, so that you avoid becoming a worn-out and tearful new mother, attempting to cope with demanding guests as well as a new baby.

If you suspect things may not run smoothly for you, it is better to discuss this with your partner beforehand, so you can have a plan of campaign. It may be that you would like to have a week or two alone together as a new family, before inviting guests round. It may work better for you if your mother or mother-in-law comes to stay once your partner returns to work, helping you over those first uncertain days on your own with your baby. You might feel better and more capable of handling potentially tricky situations if you have several weeks to build up your confidence before having relations to stay. You know your families and their strengths and limitations best, and it is far easier to have worked out in advance what you think you will feel able to ask for, and what you can cope with, than be lumbered with all sorts of family difficulties when you have a baby to care for.

Some grandparents have very definite ideas about the right ways to treat a new baby. These may or may not be appropriate for your situation. If your ideas do not coincide, you may have to make it extremely clear about what is or is not acceptable as far as your baby is concerned. The sooner you speak up and explain what it is that you want to do with your baby, the better it will be for your self-confidence.

Some grandparents are quite wonderful, managing to offer the right sort of help just when it is needed: being interested but not suffocatingly so, supporting you both in your new roles, and knowing how long to stay. This is not a problem. Accept all offers of help, and enjoy yourselves.

JEALOUS ADULTS

It is not only children who suffer from jealousy when a new member of the family arrives. If you are used to being a couple, having time only for each other, it can be quite disconcerting to find that someone else has appeared on the scene who demands, and gets, rather a lot of attention. Traditionally, fathers are almost expected to feel jealous and may be prepared to feel slightly left out of the inevitably close bond between mother and baby. It can come as a surprise, therefore, if a mother also finds she is jealous of the close relationship between a father and baby. This may happen immediately or as the relationship develops over the months. Sometimes, if there is a child already, the father may take over much of the care of this child for a while and the older child may begin to want his or her father's attention and company more than the mother's, particularly as he or she may be feeling a bit annoyed at her having brought home this new baby. This can be irritating to the mother, knowing she is 'second-best' at the moment, especially if she is still

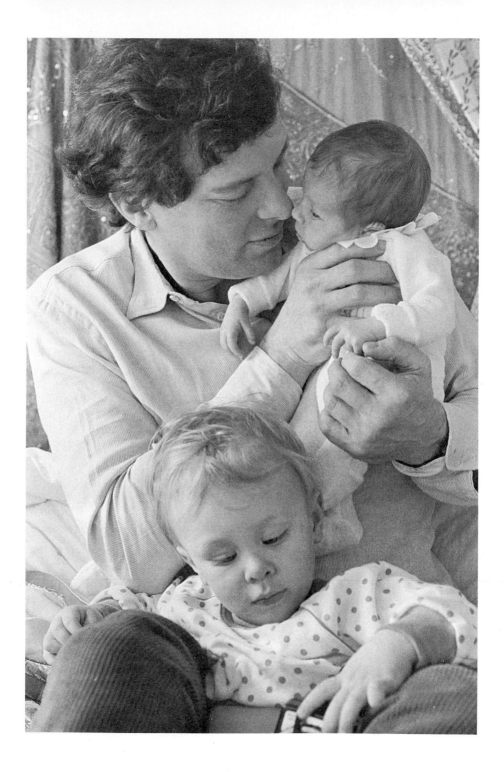

the primary child-carer during the day. As with everything else, it is important that you talk about your feelings too. Unless you each know what the other is worried or upset about, there is no way you can begin to help each other come to terms with the changes this baby has brought to your lives together as a family.

* *From the time I arrived home with Kate until she was about five months old, there was no let-up in Tom's awful behaviour. Given a chance, he would prod, poke, punch, bite, and scratch her. He was forever wanting us to take her back to the hospital. I could never leave them alone together. I tried not to be too cross with him, because, in my heart, I felt sorry for him — he'd gained an unwanted sister and had lost the kind, patient mother he'd once known.*

* *One of the nicest things that's happened since becoming a mother is the feeling of empathy and closeness with my own mother and father. Suddenly I appreciate all they've done for me.*

* *Martin was aware he might feel left out once the baby was born, so he was expecting it and didn't actually feel resentful, but there were more changes to our daily lives than we'd imagined.*

* *Having a new baby when the other children are a little older is fantastic — they love her dearly, and are fascinated by all she does. Each time she does something new, there are four other children as well as her parents watching her and sharing in her progress.*

FEEDING YOUR BABY: BREASTFEEDING AND BOTTLEFEEDING

24

Talk to anyone starting something new — a change of job, meeting someone important, learning to drive — and they usually say that what they really need is a 'spoonful of confidence'. So it is with a new mother starting to breastfeed her baby; she needs confidence in herself and her ability to do it, and confidence in her baby, knowing that the baby can let her know when she would like to be fed, when she has had enough, and whether or not she wants the other side.

Relying on your own instincts can be extremely difficult, however, when there are so many different people, so many books and magazine articles, all offering you different advice, until it becomes impossible to know which way to turn. So, how can you work out what is best for you and your baby? You may find that the best way for you is to make an effort during pregnancy to get as much information as you can, not only about birth, but also about breastfeeding. As with your preparations for the birth, you can read widely, and talk to other mothers who are breastfeeding. Your local breastfeeding counsellor may hold regular 'open house', where pregnant women can meet and talk with mothers with tiny babies. Reading and discovering other people's experiences will give you a good starting-point. Most importantly, though, remember that you and your baby are special, an entirely different partnership from any other mother and baby. What is right for you may not be right for anyone else.

THE BENEFITS OF BREASTFEEDING

AVAILABILITY The benefits of breastfeeding for a baby are numerous, but possibly one of the most important advantages for both mother and baby is that it is always there. Unlike a bottle of artificial milk, there is always some milk in a breast — it can never be completely emptied. There may be times in the day when your milk supply will seem more plentiful than others, but there will always be milk there for your baby. This could be a benefit for the father too, of course — no bottles to make in the middle of the night.

For the baby

COLOSTRUM As soon as the baby is born, your breasts will feed your baby colostrum, which is full of antibodies to help protect your baby against the many diseases you have either had or been immunized

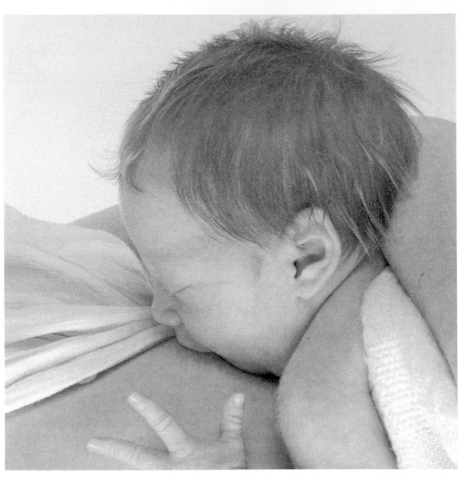

against. It is a high-protein fluid, and helps to protect babies against the bacteria which cause gastro-enteritis. Bottlefed babies are very much more likely to get gastro-enteritis than breastfed babies, especially if their bottles or teats are not properly sterilized.

These are sound reasons for giving your baby a few days of breast milk, even if you have already decided that you would prefer not to breastfeed.

'THE PERFECT FOOD' Breast milk itself is quite amazing. Unlike cow's milk, which needs to be modified before it is suitable for feeding to a human baby, breast milk is perfect. It is made by your breasts as your baby feeds. First of all your breasts will produce and store foremilk in 15–24 reservoirs behind the areola (the darker area behind the nipple). As the feed progresses, your breasts will start to produce hindmilk. Foremilk will quench the baby's thirst, while the rich hindmilk will act as her main meal. Just as your body produces all your baby's food requirements as she grows inside you, so your body will produce all that she needs from your breasts.

PROTECTION AGAINST ALLERGIES There is some evidence to suggest that breastfed babies are less likely to develop allergies such as eczema or asthma while they are totally breastfed. If you know that either you or your partner or anyone in your respective families suffers from allergies, you will be encouraged to breastfeed totally for at least six months before introducing any solid foods to give your baby maximum protection. Many experts advise that, where there is a family history of allergy, the introduction of cow's milk should be left until the baby is at least a year old. Just one bottle can initiate an allergic reaction in a sensitive baby.

You will also need to avoid any foods to which you are allergic whilst you are breastfeeding, even if you do not normally do so.

PROTECTION AGAINST INFECTION Breast milk also serves to line your baby's stomach and gut flora, providing a means by which the baby is not alone when fighting any infection. All your own antibodies, past and present, will be there ready to fend off any unwanted bacteria throughout the breastfeeding period, and setting up protection over longer periods too. As well as offering protection against infection, breastfeeding also ensures that your baby can recover more quickly after an illness. Even older babies who have had stomach upsets can often manage to drink breast milk, which prevents them becoming dehydrated.

PROTECTION AGAINST OBESITY The fat stores of a breastfed baby seem to be different from the fat stores of a bottlefed baby. The breastfed baby is less likely to become a fat adult, and fat adults are more prone to heart disease, arterial disease, and diabetes. Fat babies and children also seem to be more liable to catch colds and chest infections.

DEVELOPING INTELLIGENCE Recent research has shown that children who were breastfed are more intelligent than those who were bottlefed, because the constituents of breastmilk are exactly right for developing the brain fully.

PLEASANT NAPPIES The different fats in breast milk will make your baby's motions smell less strongly than those of a baby being fed artificial milk. Breastfed babies' stools do not smell unpleasant at all — rather like yoghurt, in fact.

NATURAL LAXATIVE Nearly all mothers find that a baby who is totally breastfed does not become constipated, but can go for several days without passing a motion, though very young babies seem to produce dirty nappies at every feed. Breast milk is easily absorbed by the baby and consequently she will not produce hard, dry motions.

For the mother

GETTING BACK TO NORMAL Breastfeeding helps the mother's uterus to contract back to its non-pregnant position and size. You may find that, for a few feeds, you experience some 'afterpains', but these soon disappear.

After mothers have breastfed for some time, they usually discover that they are gradually losing the fat stores they put on during pregnancy. Some mothers, however, do find that they do not regain their pre-pregnancy figures until they stop breastfeeding.

TIME Some mothers say they feel they actually have more time available to play and talk with their baby (as well as looking after the rest of the family!) without feeds to make up and bottles and teats to sterilize.

EXPENSE Breastfeeding can work out cheaper, in that there is no need to buy all the bottlefeeding equipment, in particular the artificial milk. You may find you have to eat a bit extra yourself at the beginning, but this is unlikely to be a major expense.

REST AND RELAXATION One good reason for breastfeeding is that it is easier to sit down to do it, thereby guaranteeing yourself several occasions during the day when you will be resting and not trying to

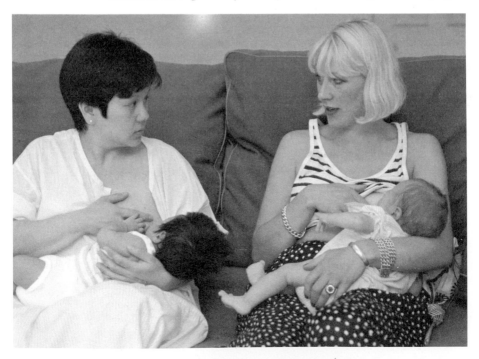

rush round catching up on the chores. If you have an older child, this is an ideal opportunity to enjoy a book and a cuddle together. If not, you can sit down with a drink and some time for yourself and your baby.

SENSE OF ACHIEVEMENT In the same way as most mothers feel a sense of satisfaction at having grown their babies inside them for so many months, breastfeeding mothers feel this same pleasure at knowing that they are providing everything their babies need to thrive and grow.

PROTECTION AGAINST BREAST CANCER It has also been shown that mothers who have breastfed are less at risk of developing breast cancer. Studies so far suggest that the longer a mother breastfeeds, and the more babies she feeds, the greater the protection against this disease.

CLOSENESS Probably the very best reason to opt for breastfeeding for both mother and baby is the closeness that breastfeeding will bring. For your baby, it will provide warmth, comfort, security, love, food, and drink all rolled into one. For you, the mother, there is a special closeness with your baby and the knowledge that you are doing something for her which no one else can do.

Many fathers say that they feel a special pride when they see their partners breastfeed their baby. Some do feel rather left out, on the periphery of this close relationship. Others would like to be able to feed their baby themselves. It is a good idea to talk about this; providing food is not the only way of showing you love your baby, and there may be lots of other things you can do to help your partner enjoy closeness with your baby.

For the father

PREPARING FOR BREASTFEEDING

So, talk about it, and if you decide you are going to breastfeed, then go ahead and enjoy it. When friends ask what you intend to do, tell them you *are* going to breastfeed. Try not to say, 'I'll try.' You can if you want to. When you decide, for instance, to learn to drive, you do not say you are trying, you tell your friends and yourself you *are* going to learn. The same is true for breastfeeding. Like driving, or any other skill, it takes a while to master the art, but with patience and practice you can and will pass your driving test. So, with the same patience and practice, you will be able to breastfeed.

Try thinking about tasks you have mastered — learning to use a word-processor perhaps, or a food-mixer — then apply the same techniques to breastfeeding. Everyone will rally round to help if you have any problems to overcome — your midwife, your health visitor, or your NCT breastfeeding counsellor. NCT breastfeeding counsellors are mothers who have breastfed themselves and have been trained to give information and support. You do not have to be a member of the NCT to ask for help; just phone and they will do their best to help you. Breastfeeding counsellors are available not only during the day, but in the evenings and at weekends as well. So, while you are pregnant, find out who your nearest counsellor is. If you have any concerns or questions while you are still pregnant, your breastfeeding counsellor will be happy for you to ring her whenever you like. Try to meet her once your baby has arrived, or phone her with any worry you would like to talk about; nothing will be too small.

Thinking about how you want to feed your baby is about the only preparation you need make for feeding, although clearly, if you are going to bottlefeed, you will need to buy all the necessary equipment. If you decide to breastfeed, there is nothing you need do to prepare your breasts in any way for feeding. You may like to choose a well-fitting and comfortable bra to wear, but this is a very personal choice. There is no need either to express colostrum during pregnancy, nor to rub your nipples to try to 'toughen them up', as some people may have suggested to you.

BREASTFEEDING: GETTING IT RIGHT

Once you have made the decision to breastfeed, there are ways and means of making it work for you and your baby. It will help you approach breastfeeding with confidence if you understand how breastfeeding works, and how you can get it right.

Positioning

Many experts say that successful breastfeeding is almost totally dependent on 'a good latch', that is, the baby getting into a really good position on the breast. What does this mean?

If a baby is incorrectly positioned and not feeding from the breast properly, then the following may happen:

> ○ **YOUR BABY MAY NOT STIMULATE YOU SUFFICIENTLY, AND MAY NOT DRAIN YOUR BREASTS WELL ENOUGH FOR THEM TO MAKE MORE MILK, SO GRADUALLY YOUR MILK SUPPLY WILL DECREASE.**

(Opposite) A good starting-point for offering the baby your breast is to bring her chest close to your body with her nose in line with your nipple

A baby who is not in a good breastfeeding position may only get the foremilk, thus missing out on the calories. She may put on less weight and be unsettled, even colicky if her tummy is full of lower-calorie foremilk. She may also be missing the fat-soluble vitamins, such as Vitamin K. If your breasts are not being well drained by your baby, your milk production will be inhibited, and uneven drainage may lead to problems with engorgement, blocked ducts, or mastitis (you will find further information about these conditions later in this chapter).

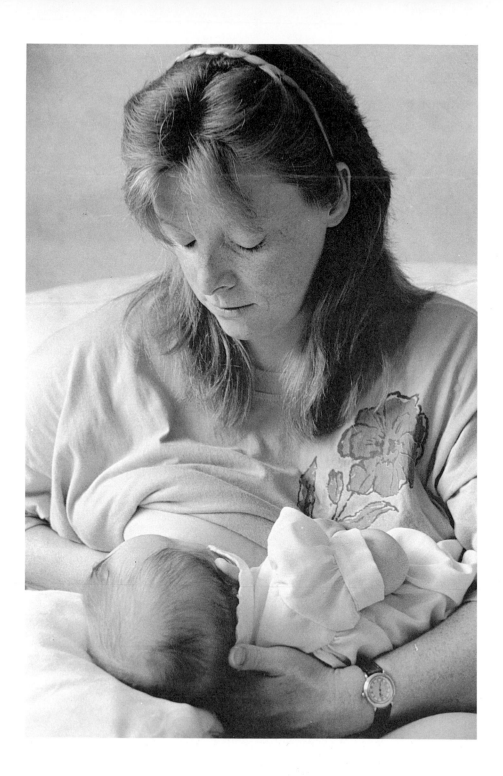

Looking at this mother you can see that both she and the baby are relaxed, and the baby's head is in a straight line with his body. Breastfeeding should not be uncomfortable for either mother or baby

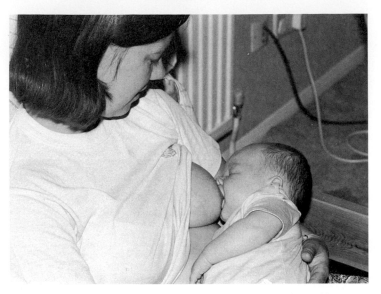

It is worth spending time and care in these early days of learning to breastfeed to make sure you and your baby are getting things absolutely right.

How can you make sure your baby is feeding properly?

GETTING COMFORTABLE First of all, make yourself comfortable. If you have had stitches, then you might find it helps to use a Valley Cushion (see Chapter 22, Early Days), or a pillow when sitting down, or maybe you would prefer to feed lying down. Some mothers find it helps to change positions, sometimes breastfeeding sitting up and at other times lying down. If you are sitting up to feed your baby, it is best to sit upright, leaning neither forwards nor backwards.

If you feed sitting up, you will probably find it more comfortable to lift your baby up to your breast by using a pillow or cushions. If your arm becomes tired during the feed, you can rest it on the pillow. This will also stop the baby 'dragging' on your nipple and making it sore, because she is at the right height already. Some mothers find it hard to get the hang of feeding lying down to begin with, but for some it can be a life-saver. You need to lie on your side rather than on your back so that your baby can get a good mouthful of breast.

HOLDING YOUR BABY Hold your baby with her whole body facing towards you — it might help to say to yourself 'chest to chest, and chin to breast'. To begin with you might find it easier to hold her head. Some babies dislike having their heads held, particularly if they have had a difficult birth. It works equally well if you hold her at the top of her shoulders, with a couple of fingers up to stop her head falling back. This position gives you plenty of control whilst allowing her head to be free of any pressure. Her head should be just underneath your breast rather than in the crook of your arm. If she is too far over, she will find it hard to get both your nipple and the areola in her mouth. By the time she is ready to take your breast in her mouth, her nose should be actually touching your nipple; this encourages her to reach up so that her chin is well off her chest and your nipple will go right into the top of her mouth.

'Teasing' your baby Now tease her with the smell of your skin and breast, perhaps expressing a little milk to get her excited by the taste, so that she will open her mouth nice and wide, searching for the breast. As soon as this happens, draw her close to you and offer her the breast. Remember to bring your baby to the breast, not your breast to the baby. Her tongue should be down underneath your nipple and areola, not over it. It is not easy to see this yourself, but perhaps your partner could check as you begin to feed. More of the areola should be taken in underneath than on top.

Watching your baby feed As soon as your baby starts sucking, you should be able to see the muscles at her temple working, possibly

If you are worried about your breastfeeding position ask someone to see if it's like this:
1. lower lip beautifully curled back allowing baby's tongue to press the milk out of the breast
2. baby's chin in the right place — against the breast — so that he has no difficulty breathing

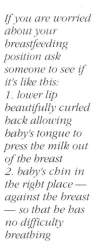

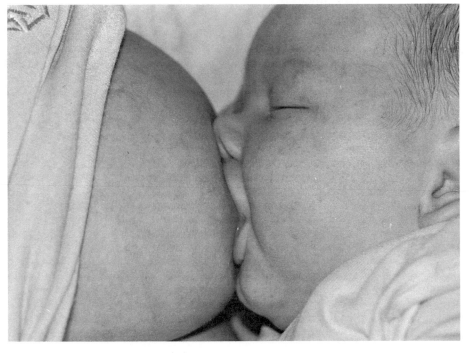

even an ear wiggling. If you have ever chewed gum for a long time, then you might have felt a dull ache at your temple, and it is these same muscles your baby will be using as she suckles at the breast.

You will notice that your baby does not suckle all the time; she will probably suck a few times and then have a rest. Do not worry about this; remember that we do not eat all the time, that we have rest periods between mouthfuls! She will probably suckle strongly at the beginning of the feed to get the let-down reflex working, and then gradually suck more slowly and strongly as the rich hindmilk lets down.

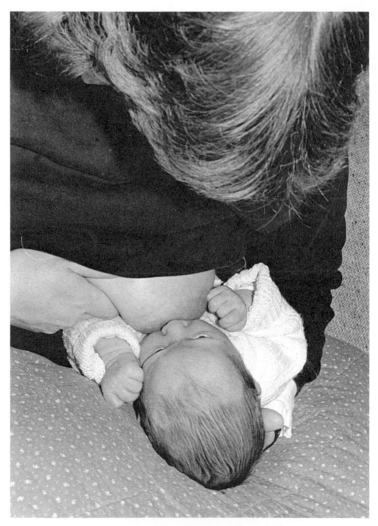

Mothers with blocked ducts or mastitis may find this a helpful alternative position

MAKING AN AIRWAY You need not worry about trying to clear a breathing space for your baby. Although it may seem, when you look down, that she cannot breathe and her nose is buried in your breast, if she could not breathe, she would come off the breast and find another feeding position. It is impossible for her to suckle if she cannot breathe properly. Using a finger to make an 'airway', as you may have seen some women do, often means that the nipple becomes tilted and can then rub against your baby's hard palate.

WHEN TO FINISH A FEED Allow your baby to decide when the feed is finished before offering her your other breast. Most mothers find that their baby decides when the feed is over, either by falling asleep at the breast, or by 'spitting' the nipple out. Not all babies will want to feed from both breasts at each feed. Whether your baby has one breast per feed or both breasts at each feed, just remember always to start from alternate breasts so that they both receive the same amount of stimulation.

IF IT HURTS If your nipple hurts, your baby is badly positioned, so start again. A little bit of soreness at the beginning of a feed with a very new baby is normal, as she suckles hard to encourage your let-down reflex; anything more than this suggests you need to reposition her.

TAKING YOUR BABY OFF Wait until your baby has stopped to take a breath, or put your little finger in the corner of her mouth, break the suction, and take your breast away. Do not try to drag your baby off the breast: it will hurt and possibly make you feel even more sore.

So, have confidence in yourself and your baby, relax, spend plenty of time getting the position right, and enjoy breastfeeding.

CARING FOR YOURSELF

Breastfeeding mothers need care and attention in the early days. You should not feel pressurized to do anything except look after yourself and your baby in these early days and weeks while you are getting to know your baby and establishing a plentiful milk supply for her. You may need to eat some extra snacks between meals as well if you are particularly hungry. Some of the hormones involved in breastfeeding often make a mother feel drowsy towards the end of a breastfeed, just as the baby often goes to sleep finishing the hindmilk. This is nature's way of encouraging mothers to make up for any sleep lost during the night. This is possibly what some mothers mean when they say they found breastfeeding exhausting. If you can let nature take its course and enjoy a short nap or rest while you are feeding, you will probably find you wake up refreshed for the rest of the day. If you have other children, you can usually find a time when you can rest while they are watching television or a video, just as you may have managed during pregnancy. Making the most of opportunities to rest and relax when they come along also means that you will have more energy for the days when you do need to be alert and busy. Many new mothers find that learning to pace themselves, although difficult at first, is a remarkably useful skill, which means they can adapt themselves easily to all sorts of changing circumstances. You may find it helps to sit down with a drink when you breastfeed, as most mothers feel incredibly thirsty when feeding. Try to make sure you are eating well right through the day too, not just managing on little snacks, then having one meal in the evening. Eating regularly may help you feel less tired so that you can cope better with the nights as well. If you are sensible about taking care of yourself, there is no reason why breastfeeding should be especially tiring or prevent you from leading as normal a life as having a small baby will permit. Many women have several children yet manage to breastfeed a new baby successfully, pacing themselves so that they adapt to the needs of breastfeeding whilst maintaining their usual activities with the rest of the family.

It does take several weeks to establish breastfeeding fully, so keep going and get as much help as you can at the beginning.

HOW BREASTFEEDING WORKS

Some mothers find it helps them to know how the breast actually works. The production of breast milk is controlled by hormones, the principal ones involved being prolactin and oxytocin.

PROLACTIN Prolactin is responsible for the amount of milk being made. It is released into your bloodstream while your baby is feeding, so, the more often she feeds, the more prolactin is produced, ensuring a good supply of milk for the next feed. This is the principle of demand and supply which is the basis of breastfeeding.

OXYTOCIN Oxytocin is also released as your baby feeds, but, whereas prolactin makes milk, oxytocin makes it available to the baby by causing the milk-producing cells to contract, squeezing the milk down the ducts and out of the nipple. This is called the let-down reflex, and you may feel it working as you feed your baby. Some mothers never feel it, but that does not mean it is not working all the same. Other mothers find it works so strongly that the pleasant, rather tingly feeling of the milk letting down becomes more like a 'full-to-bursting' feeling, so that they welcome the baby's eager feeding to relieve this initial tension.

THE LET-DOWN REFLEX Your let-down reflex sometimes makes milk drip from one side while your baby is busy feeding from the other.

You can stop these drips by pressing on your nipple with your arm or heel of your hand, or you can mop it up with a breast pad of some sort. Some mothers catch this milk in a sterilized shell, freeze it for use later on, or donate it to the local Special Care Baby Unit. Occasionally mothers worry that their let-down reflex is not working. If you think this may be the case, it may be worth talking to a breastfeeding counsellor. Normally any problems with a let-down reflex are sorted out once the baby is in a good position at the breast.

Sometimes, if your let-down is very strong, it can overwhelm your new baby and she will come off spluttering, unable to keep up with the flow. You can try letting this first gush of milk subside before putting the baby on to your breast, so that she can cope without feeling afraid of being overwhelmed.

Composition of breast milk

COLOSTRUM Your baby's first food will be the colostrum which your breasts have been making during pregnancy, and gently starts your baby's digestive system working. Although there is not much of it, colostrum is high in quality, containing all the protein, minerals, fats, and vitamins your baby needs. It is rich in antibodies, offering protection for many months beyond the breastfeeding period. If she is given adequate feeds of colostrum, she may sleep as much as six, eight, or more hours between feeds. This will give your nipples a chance to recuperate, whereas limiting suckling time will not allow your baby an adequate feed, so she will either not settle or will soon wake to be fed again. Babies have been around far longer than any clocks, and timing of feeds is associated with cow's milk and is totally inappropriate for breastfed babies.

After the first couple of days, the colostrum is gradually replaced by milk. Transition milk, which, though not as rich-looking as colostrum, still looks yellowish and creamy, follows on for several weeks. By about 6 weeks you will be producing mature milk, watery-looking and bluish. Towards the end of lactation (whenever that happens to be), smaller quantities of milk are supplied, and this is known as regression milk. Both colostrum and regression milk are proportionally higher in antibodies than mature milk.

FOREMILK The composition of breast milk actually changes as a feed progresses. At the start of each feed, your baby will be getting foremilk, which is low in fat and calories, so satisfying her thirst.

HINDMILK As the let-down works, the richer hindmilk becomes available, which provides your baby with a high-calorie, satisfying meal. Once the fat content of the milk becomes too high for her (it will be rather like drinking butter), she will come off the breast, either to sleep or ready to move to the other breast, where she will get another thirst-quenching drink followed by the richer food. If feed-times are restricted, the richer hindmilk will not be taken, and your baby will not settle after feeds or gain much weight, despite having frequent, short feeds.

COMMON BREASTFEEDING PROBLEMS

Getting help

Many mothers find that, if they can get the positioning right, then breastfeeding is relatively plain sailing, though they may occasionally experience one or two difficulties. Knowing how to get help is often the first step to overcoming any problems, so do not let a small problem become insurmountable; contact your midwife, health visitor, or NCT breastfeeding counsellor as soon as you can. If you do not happen to know the phone number of your nearest breastfeeding counsellor, ring NCT Headquarters; you should be put in touch with a breastfeeding counsellor who will be able to talk through your problem with you.

Primary engorgement

Some mothers find that, as their colostrum changes over to milk, their breasts can become swollen and engorged, so that, if they are not careful, the baby finds it difficult to feed from the breast, grabs at the nipple, and makes it sore. Primary engorgement is caused by increased blood pressure in the breasts to open up the ducts, and oedema. Using cold compresses in between feeds, and warm ones at the start of a feed, can help. You may also find it helps to express a little milk at the start of a feed to make your breast softer and easier for your baby to feed from. Your breasts may feel almost too tender to touch, and it can help to try expressing, with your breast in a basin of warm water to encourage the milk flow. See p. 329 for how to express breast milk.

This can be the time when you wonder if it is all worth while and perhaps it would not hurt if you just let your baby have one bottle of artificial milk while you carry on sleeping. Your breasts hurt, you are tired, and you may be wondering whose idea it was to have a baby in the first place! It may seem a good idea to let your baby sleep in the nursery for the night while you sleep, so that you can face tomorrow. This is the time when it helps to grit your teeth and hang on. Your new baby might get confused by the different way of getting milk through a teat and could possibly reject the breast, having discovered how much easier it is to get formula milk. The milk flows out easily and immediately. Giving your baby even the odd bottle means she will have to learn a different way of sucking. Some babies quickly learn to suck on a teat, using little mouths, and they rapidly abandon the gaping mouth they need to breastfeed. An older baby for whom breastfeeding is well established may be able to cope with using two different methods of sucking, but most tiny babies seem to find it confusing, and may well refuse to breastfeed after just one bottle.

Do not forget about the nutritional value of your milk — the way it changes from feed to feed; the vital antibodies it contains; how breastfeeding helps teeth and jaw formation — and speak to someone who you know will be supportive and will encourage you to keep going.

You may experience a blocked duct; this is often caused by the milk from one segment of the breast not being drained sufficiently.

Blocked ducts

SIGNS The signs you might experience are:

- ○ **A TENDER, LUMPY AREA IN PART OF YOUR BREAST**
- ○ **REDDISH SKIN, WITH PERHAPS A RED STRIPE TOWARDS THE NIPPLE**
- ○ **PAIN IN THE AFFECTED BREAST AS YOUR MILK LETS DOWN**
- ○ **A FEELING AS THOUGH THE BREAST IS BRUISED**
- ○ **A SLIGHT TEMPERATURE**

CAUSES There are several reasons why a segment of the breast might not be adequately drained.

- ○ **YOU MIGHT HAVE HURRIED A FEED, PERHAPS NOT ALLOW-ING YOUR BABY TO FEED FOR AS LONG AS SHE WANTS.**
- ○ **YOU MIGHT HAVE CLEARED A PASSAGEWAY FOR YOUR BABY TO BREATHE BY PRESSING A FINGER AGAINST YOUR BREAST.**

Lots of mothers find that this can be a very relaxing way of feeding their baby — a good feeding position after a Caesarean, or if you are tired or ill

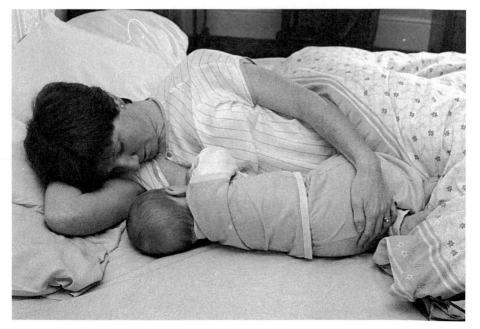

- ○ YOU MIGHT HAVE WORN A BRA WHICH IS TOO TIGHT, OR PERHAPS A SWIMMING COSTUME THAT IS NOT BIG ENOUGH.
- ○ YOU MIGHT HAVE GONE TO SLEEP ON YOUR FRONT, 'SQUASHING' YOUR BREAST, OR PERHAPS CATCHING YOUR BREAST BETWEEN YOUR BODY AND ARM.
- ○ YOU MIGHT HAVE DROPPED A FEED, PERHAPS IF YOU WERE OUT SHOPPING AND IT WAS NOT CONVENIENT.
- ○ YOU MIGHT HAVE A WHITE SPOT ON YOUR NIPPLE, WHICH MIGHT BE BLOCKING ONE OF THE OUTLETS.

CLEARING A BLOCKED DUCT If you have problems with blocked ducts, you may find it helps to examine your breasts every morning to see if you have a red patch anywhere. If you find one, then it is best to clear the blockage as soon as possible, so that it does not develop into non-infective mastitis, which can be really painful. The following steps may be helpful:

- ○ FEED THE BABY OFTEN, AND FROM THE AFFECTED SIDE FIRST, PERHAPS USING A GRAVITY FEEDING POSITION (ALLOWING THE BREAST TO HANG INTO THE BABY'S MOUTH). FEEDING FREQUENTLY WILL FEEL MORE COMFORTABLE TOO — PERHAPS EXPRESSING IF THE BABY IS NOT KEEN TO WAKE UP.
- ○ APPLY A WARM COMPRESS AT THE START OF A FEED TO GET THE MILK FLOWING.
- ○ SOAP THE BREAST AND USE A WIDE-TOOTHED COMB TO COMB THE AFFECTED AREA, WHICH CAN HELP TO BREAK UP THE BLOCKAGE; TRY NOT TO GET SOAP ON YOUR NIPPLE.
- ○ DO SOME ARM-SWINGING EXERCISES, OR PERHAPS SCRUB THE FLOOR OR WASH WINDOWS TO ENCOURAGE GOOD CIRCULATION.
- ○ IF YOU FIND A WHITE SPOT ON THE NIPPLE, THEN YOU MAY BE ABLE TO REMOVE IT CAREFULLY, OR OTHERWISE CARRY ON FEEDING FROM THAT BREAST FIRST.
- ○ LAST, BUT NOT LEAST, TRY TO DISCOVER WHAT CAUSED THE BLOCKAGE.
- ○ WHAT CLOTHES HAVE YOU BEEN WEARING IN THE LAST FORTY-EIGHT HOURS? HAVE THEY CAUSED IT?
- ○ HAS THE FEEDING POSITION BEEN THE CULPRIT?
- ○ DID YOU NOTICE A WHITE SPOT?

You might find it helpful to talk this through with a breastfeeding counsellor, who can do some further detective work to try and find out the cause, so that you can minimize the likelihood of having another blockage in future.

Mastitis

There are two types of mastitis which a breastfeeding mother can get.

INFECTIVE MASTITIS Infective mastitis is not very common and normally occurs during the hospital stay, or fairly soon afterwards. It may be extremely difficult, if not impossible, for either a midwife, a doctor, or you to distinguish between infective and non-infective mastitis. It usually occurs when the nipples have been cracked or sore, allowing bacteria to enter the crack (possibly via the baby's nose), causing an infection. If infective mastitis is diagnosed, it is generally recommended that you stop feeding and express your milk until the infection has cleared up. You can then resume breastfeeding your baby. Some doctors will treat infective mastitis in precisely the same way as non-infective mastitis (see below).

NON-INFECTIVE MASTITIS Non-infective mastitis often follows on from a blocked duct which has not been treated swiftly. The symptoms are very similar to blocked ducts except that you will probably feel as though you are getting flu. The hot, shivery feeling is most likely due to milk leaking into the breast tissue. The treatment for mastitis is the same as for blocked ducts, except that, if it does not clear up after a little while, you should visit your GP, who will probably prescribe antibiotics. Do remind your doctor that you are breastfeeding, so that he makes certain that whatever is prescribed is suitable for your baby as well.

You can help prevent the after-effects of antibiotics (thrush or a further spate of infections, for example) by taking the complete Vitamin B formula and/or natural, live yoghurt to replace the correct flora balance in the gut. Some doctors prescribe homoeopathic remedies to avoid these problems with antibiotics.

Abscess

This is a comparatively rare problem, but it can follow from untreated mastitis. Usually the breast no longer feels tender and the only visible sign is perhaps where the skin looks pitted, a bit like orange peel. Sometimes breast milk will have some pus or blood in it. Neither will harm the baby, but the blood might make her vomit. Treatment is usually to incise and drain the abscess, but more recently abscesses have been treated by aspiration — the insertion of a hypodermic syringe to draw off the pus, which will allow you to continue breastfeeding. This may have to be done several times before all the pus has gone.

Having read through this list of potential disaster situations, you may be wondering whether to bother about breastfeeding at all. Do not worry. It is most unlikely that any one woman would experience all these problems, but it is better to be prepared for any eventuality so that you can recognize if things seem to be going wrong.

UNUSUAL SITUATIONS

BLOOD IN BREAST MILK Very occasionally a mother may notice some traces of blood in her breast milk. The blood might come from a cracked and bleeding nipple or sometimes from a duct which bleeds

— rather like blowing your nose so hard it bleeds a little. This usually disappears within a few days, but, if it does not, talk to your midwife or GP.

MEDICAL CONDITION Occasionally, a mother's or baby's health might be affected if you have to take drugs while you are breastfeeding. This is fairly rare; sometimes it is possible for the drugs to be changed so that they are compatible. Do check with your doctor during pregnancy and, if you are not happy with his advice, ask for a second opinion. You may find it helpful to discuss the situation with a breastfeeding counsellor as well, particularly if you are feeling distressed at the possibility of being unable to start, or having to abandon, breastfeeding.

HIV AND AIDS Mothers who are HIV positive or who have full-blown AIDS are advised not to breastfeed, in case the baby becomes infected via the breast milk.

MULTIPLE BIRTHS Some mothers wonder if it is possible to breastfeed more than one baby, and mothers who are expecting twins may have been told that they will be unable to produce sufficient milk for two (or more) babies. Getting in touch with other mothers who have had twins and breastfed successfully will help you to realize that you can indeed breastfeed both your babies, though it might take a little longer to get feeding established. You can find more information in Chapter 30, Twins and Supertwins: Life after Birth.

THE ILL OR PRE-TERM BABY The benefits of breast milk are widely accepted and most Special Care Baby Units will encourage you to express your milk for your new baby. See Chapter 29, Babies in Special Care, and p. 329 for information on expressing and storing breast milk.

JAUNDICE If your baby is jaundiced, it is important that you encourage her to breastfeed as often as she wants and that you make sure your position is right. Feeding a jaundiced baby extra fluids is unnecessary. If your baby is sleepy because of the jaundice and is having a problem breastfeeding, you could try expressing some milk and offering it with a cup or spoon instead. (See also Chapter 22, Early Days.)

ADOPTING A BABY

If you are considering adopting a baby, you might wonder if you can breastfeed. Some mothers find it is possible to stimulate their milk supply by hand-expressing or by using an electric or hand breast pump.

NURSING SUPPLEMENTER A nursing supplementer can also help. This enables you to feed your baby with either expressed breast milk or formula milk through a tube fixed to your nipple. This means that, as your baby sucks at your breast, she will not only be fed but will also stimulate your milk supply. The nursing supplementer cannot ensure you make enough milk for your baby unless you combine using it with increased breastfeeding and checking your feeding position. If you would like more information, you can contact Anne Buckley (her address is listed at the back of this book).

A nursing supplementer can be useful in:

    O   **GETTING A BABY BACK ON TO THE BREAST AFTER**
        O   **AN ILLNESS**
        O   **TUBE-FEEDING**
        O   **BOTTLEFEEDING**

    O   **INTRODUCING BABIES TO AN ADOPTIVE BREAST TO**
        O   **BREASTFEED FULLY**
        O   **BREASTFEED PARTIALLY**
        O   **PROVIDE BOTH COMFORT AND SPECIAL 'CUDDLES'**
           FOR MOTHER AND BABY
        O   **SUPPLEMENTING MILK SUPPLY**

See also Chapter 31, Parenting in Special Circumstances.

EXPRESSING AND STORING BREAST MILK

There are many reasons why you might want to express some breast milk. Some of them are:

    O   **IF YOUR BABY IS ILL**
    O   **IF YOUR BABY IS IN SPECIAL CARE**
    O   **IF YOU ARE RETURNING TO WORK**
    O   **IF YOU ARE GOING OUT FOR THE EVENING**
    O   **IF YOU WANT A WHOLE NIGHT'S SLEEP!**

BREAST PUMPS Looking in any chemist shop, you might imagine that you need to buy lots of gadgets to help with breastfeeding, and one essential item would appear to be a breast pump. There are several different pumps on the market, but many mothers find they do not need a pump at all, and can hand-express lots of milk very quickly. So, before rushing off with your hard-earned money, it is worth trying hand-expressing. You might find it takes several attempts before you become proficient and happy with the amount you can express.

When you first start to express milk, whether by hand or by pump, try to choose a time when you do not feel hurried and there is no urgency for you to express a certain quantity ready for a feed. Many

Expressing breast milk

mothers find that at the beginning they can only squeeze a few drops out, but this will increase with practice. You may find that expressing milk first thing in the morning means you can get more milk.

Before you start to express, it is important that you wash your hands thoroughly and dry them on a clean towel. Any container you use to catch your milk should be properly sterilized before you use it. If you decide to buy a hand pump, do make sure it is the type that can be properly cleaned and sterilized.

How to hand-express

Begin by encouraging the milk to flow down the milk ducts: you can do this either by breastfeeding your baby first, and expressing the second breast immediately afterwards; or by applying some warmth to your breast with a warm flannel or a warm hot-water bottle.

To encourage the milk to make its way to the ducts, you may find it helpful to massage your breasts both before and during expression. You can use the flat of your hand, or your fist if that feels more effective. It is better to start massaging from your shoulders or rib-cage, moving your hands towards the areola.

TO EXPRESS THE MILK Gently place your fingers on the underneath part of the areola, along the line where the areola and the breast meet. At the same time, place your thumb as flat as possible along the top of the areola, on the line where it joins the breast.

Very gently move your fingers and thumb together in a backwards direction towards the ribs, so pressing on the wider milk ducts behind the areola.

Storing breast milk

As soon as you have expressed your milk, you should cool it as quickly as possible, then store it in a refrigerator. Breast milk will keep for a couple of days on the top shelf at the back of the fridge or three months if deep frozen. You can buy sterile plastic bags to store your milk, or you might find a plastic ice-cube tray works well. A plastic tray can be sterilized and then small amounts of breast milk frozen, as long as the tray is covered. When defrosting milk, stand the container in the fridge for several hours or, if necessary, defrost it more quickly by standing it in a container full of warm water. Defrosting milk using a microwave oven is not recommended.

Hygiene

You will need to avoid introducing bacteria into your milk, and it is therefore important to make sure your hands are always scrupulously clean before expressing, and that you dry them on a fresh, clean towel. All containers, bottles, teats, etc., should be washed and sterilized exactly as for bottlefeeding artificial milk.

Drip-catching

Some mothers collect drip milk for their babies by using a drip catcher on one breast while feeding from the other. If you do this, you will also need to express some hindmilk, because drip milk is only foremilk. Drip catchers should not be used between feeds as germs may multiply over a long period. The drip-catching shells may also put pressure on your milk ducts and cause your nipples to become sore.

Some babies are reluctant to feed from a bottle if it is being offered by the mother — after all, they know the real thing is just there! A breastfed baby may well feel unkindly disposed to a hard teat when she is used to a soft, warm breast. She may find it all very confusing! Often a father, or other person, will be able to persuade the baby to feed from a bottle. It may take a little while, but some mothers find that their baby will readily feed from a cup or spoon, and once a baby is older, she will probably be happy drinking from a cup.

Encouraging the reluctant bottlefeeder

LOOKING FOR SUPPORT

It is really important to try to find someone you can trust, who is able to offer you plenty of sensible information, and will help you work out for yourself which is the right way for you and your baby. It sometimes helps to remember that there is no one correct way of looking after a baby, and it is up to you to sift through all the information available to you, then to have confidence in yourself to do whatever you want. It is a bit like trying out a new recipe — after you have used it a few times, you try out slight variations until you discover what you prefer.

Older babies become adept at feeding in a variety of positions and situations

You can get your support from lots of sources: your partner;

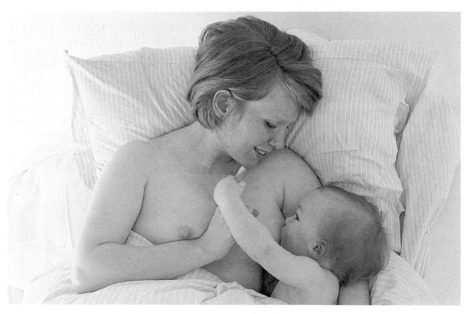

friends; midwives; your health visitor; breastfeeding counsellors; the chemist's shop; your next-door neighbour; the greengrocer's; another mother . . . accept it, sift through it, then do your own thing!

The father's role

Some women are concerned that breastfeeding means that their partner may feel left out. It is possible to equate love with giving food; if someone is upset, for instance, people often rush for the teapot, whereas it might be more valuable to sit and listen.

It is important that both you and your partner understand that breast milk is the best nutrition a baby can have, that breastfeeding is very much more than just food, and that it is something men cannot do. Only women can breastfeed. But that does not mean that the father cannot be involved in all sorts of other ways. A new mother may come to rely very heavily on the encouragement and support of her partner to help her whilst she is breastfeeding. Many women say they could not have managed to breastfeed successfully if they had not had so much help from their partners. Your partner can give you confidence when other people are not being particularly supportive, can reassure you by telling you that you can do it, and can always be there, encouraging you to carry on.

Men can cuddle their babies, change nappies, rock them to sleep — everything in fact that a woman can do, except breastfeed. Your partner may offer you practical support in various ways as well: leaving a packed lunch in the fridge while he is out at work; cooking the evening meal; doing the shopping; caring for your other children whenever possible so that you can rest. Understanding that your new job is important and is extremely time-consuming is a valuable part of his support for you as well. Perhaps the most important thing to remember is to talk to each other, to say how you are both feeling, and to share with each other not only the awful things that have happened, but the delightful ones as well.

OLD WIVES' TALES

Some of the advice you might be given will come into the category of old wives' tales, containing no truth whatsoever. These myths can be difficult to ignore, as so many people may believe in them, but you will know better!

'Timed feeds stop sore nipples'

You might be advised to time the minutes your baby feeds from the breast, perhaps starting with one minute each side every four hours on Day 1, gradually building up to ten minutes each side every four hours by Day 10. This will not stop you getting sore nipples and can be truly disastrous for breastfeeding. The effect is liable to be a hungry baby who cries a lot because she is never really allowed to enjoy a good feed from the breast. Sore nipples are nearly always caused by incorrect positioning at the breast, and timing the feeds simply means that the breast will be inadequately stimulated to make enough milk for your baby. The same applies to those hospitals who suggest feeding 'on demand' — between three and five hours! Your baby will know what she needs and will not understand about time.

In fact, quite the reverse will happen. The breast will not know how much milk your baby needs, and will start to slow down milk production. It is important to allow your baby to feed whenever she wants and for as long as she needs.

'Skipping a feed means there will be more milk for the next one'

Many mothers do not realize that their prolactin levels are higher at night-time, and breastfeeding during the night will help the breasts produce enough milk for the baby. There is no reason why you should not breastfeed in bed, providing neither you nor your partner has been taking sleeping-pills, drugs, or alcohol — or, indeed, anything else which might alter your normal responses!

'A bottle at night will not hurt'

Colostrum tends to be really thick and creamy, so it is possible to feel confused once your milk supply starts to come in. Foremilk is quite watery-looking, and you may not actually see the hindmilk as the breasts are making it while you are feeding.

'Your milk looks too thin'

It used to be believed that rubbing the nipples with a flannel or rough towel or perhaps using methylated spirits would harden the nipples ready for breastfeeding, as though they were off on a cross-country run! The opposite is the truth. The skin of your nipples needs to be supple, as they get longer while your baby is suckling. Mothers find that rubbing some hindmilk into their nipples at the end of a feed can help keep their skin soft and supple, as the hindmilk is rich in fats.

'Unprepared breasts lead to sore nipples'

Several studies have shown that neither the colour of a woman's hair nor the colour of her skin has any effect on her ability to breastfeed or her propensity for getting sore nipples.

'Red-haired or fair-skinned women will get sore nipples'

Although some babies are happy to feed immediately after birth, some are not ready. If you can find a quiet time together when your baby can nuzzle at the breast and just lick your nipple for a while it can help. You will probably then find that, a little while after your placenta has been delivered,

'Babies must be breastfed immediately after birth for breastfeeding to succeed'

she will be quite keen to feed. A baby who is allowed to have a good feed at the breast within an hour of birth does, however, triple her chances of establishing breastfeeding.

Remember that not all babies are able to breastfeed straightaway — perhaps having to go into Special Care or having had a Caesarean birth — but it is still possible to breastfeed once your baby is well enough or you are ready. Using an electric breast pump can help to stimulate your milk supply and any colostrum or milk you express can be tube-fed to your baby.

See the section on Expressing and Storing Breast Milk on p. 329 and also Chapter 29, Babies in Special Care.

'Babies must feed from both breasts at each feed'

In the early days in particular, many babies do not want to feed from both breasts at every feed. Sometimes they will feed from only one breast, in which case it is important to remember to start the next feed with the other breast. Listen to your baby; she will clearly show you whether or not she is still hungry and wants to feed from both breasts.

'Breastfed babies need extra fluids'

Even in the height of the hottest summer, your breasts will make exactly the right food and drink for your baby. Foremilk, the first milk to be given during the feed, is high in volume and will quench your baby's thirst. There is no need to worry, as long as you allow her to decide when she has had enough and wants the 'second side'. If it is hot, you may simply need to drink more yourself.

'There are some foods you must not eat while breastfeeding'

Although some mothers do find their babies are affected by some foods which might give them a tummy-ache, there are no rules about what to eat while breastfeeding. The best solution is to continue with your normal diet, but think carefully about what you might have been eating if your baby seems particularly distressed or has unusually loose stools. Certain fruits and spicy foods are often cited as culprits, but most mothers find that they have absolutely no problems maintaining what is for them a normal diet. Occasionally mothers report reactions when they have overdosed on some seasonal fruits, but this is not normally a problem.

'Cow's milk is as good as breast milk'

Now that you have read this far you know that this is not so. Your breast milk is made exclusively for your baby, and brings benefits to both you and your baby. Cow's milk has to be modified to make it suitable for babies, and, as more and more is discovered about the properties of living breast milk,

> the clearer it becomes that cow's milk simply cannot match up to all the natural advantages breast milk has to offer.

POSSIBLE REASONS FOR CHANGING FROM BREAST TO BOTTLEFEEDING

Many mothers cite many reasons for giving up breastfeeding. The suggestions offered here may help you keep going. Taking one day at a time will help, as will not being over-ambitious with the goals you set yourself. It is also worth remembering that changing over to bottlefeeding is no guarantee that your problems will cease.

During the early weeks, when a baby might be asking to feed very frequently, it is easy to imagine that you do not have enough milk. Talking to other mothers who have found that it does take a few weeks to establish breastfeeding fully can help. Talking through the situation with a breastfeeding counsellor, midwife, or health visitor may be useful as well; they may be able to suggest all sorts of ways of building up your milk supply.

Fear of not enough milk

This is a reason often given by mothers. You may be so tired that you do not know which way to turn and become increasingly confused. Ask your partner if he can have some time off to be at home and help. Accept all offers of help. Having some confidence in yourself will help, which is easy to say but less easily achieved, especially when you are exhausted by your new role as a mother.

Misinformation or conflicting advice

Contact your midwife or health visitor, if you find them supportive — they may be able to suggest ways of getting help. Get in touch with your local NCT group too. Maybe the postnatal supporter for your area could help by taking your toddler for a walk or helping with the evening meal while you go to bed. Find some way to cheer yourself up too, even if it is only a visit to the hairdresser.

Lack of positive help and support

Some mothers are not prepared for the length of time it can take for a baby to breastfeed. You may have imagined a feed would last only about five or ten minutes; you may not have realized how many feeds per day your new baby would want; maybe you had not been able to talk with other mothers before the birth. Every baby is different. Like adults, some will rush through a meal, while others will take their time. Perhaps you could look at your timetable and work out why you are wanting to gallop through this important time in your life.

Feeds take too long

This can be a real nuisance. If you are always looking down only to see yet another wet dress, it can become quite depressing.

Leaking breasts

Foremilk stored in the reservoirs behind the areola can start spurting out if you hear a baby cry, if you simply think about feeding, or even if you drink a cup of tea! Sphincter muscles which control the reservoirs might be lax, and away goes the milk. Helpful people can remind you how lucky you are to produce so much milk, but that does not help if you are into your third T-shirt of the morning. Splashing your areola with cold water can tone up muscles, and wearing thick breast pads will help, but there is little you can do except try to disguise the wet patches by wearing dark or patterned clothes. You might also try holding the heel of your hand against your breast to stop the milk flowing once it has started.

Baby is sick after feeds

A few mothers find that their let-down reflex works so swiftly that the poor baby can hardly cope with the way the milk gushes out. The baby coughs and splutters and then manages to feed well once the flow settles down. Unfortunately, though, the baby may have gulped down pockets of air, which means that she is sick after the feed is over.

If this seems to be happening to you and your baby, you might find it helps to express a little milk at the start of a feed, or to feed your baby so she is sitting up a little more. If you have ever tried drinking on your back, you will know how easy it is to cough and splutter.

If yours is a sicky baby, the problem might not be any different if you were bottlefeeding — and the smell would be a lot worse!

Baby cries a lot

Some babies do cry a lot and it is not always easy to work out why. Perhaps your baby has just been fed, changed, and winded and should be ready for a sleep, but carries on crying. If you have eliminated all the other problems to do with comfort, boredom, etc., it may be that she is crying because you have taken her off the breast too soon and she is still hungry, in which case let her feed a little longer, until she indicates that she has finished. Some babies do, however, seem to manage to extend some feeds for an inordinate length of time, possibly because they need the extra comfort the breast offers; this can be wearing, but may be preferable to the crying.

Perhaps your baby associates breastfeeding with discomfort. Some mothers say that, while they were learning to breastfeed, they perhaps held the baby's head too tightly and pushed her on to the breast. If you think this happened with you, you might find it will help to comfort her by holding her close, with skin-to-skin contact but without offering the breast. Then, when she has calmed down, carefully offer her the breast. With gentleness and time, she will learn to associate breastfeeding with love and be eager to feed.

Food intolerance

Some mothers find that their baby appears to cry a lot after they have eaten a particular food themselves. If you are wondering whether the food you eat is affecting your baby, you could try keeping a chart of the times when your baby cries a lot and what you have eaten.

You may find some connection between the two. Some mothers recognize that dairy products affect their babies, and, after cutting them out, the babies have stopped crying quite so much. Your baby may be a bit more upset for a day or two after eliminating the food, but it can take up to two weeks to notice a big improvement. You can check if your suspicions were correct by eating a test dose of the food, then noticing if the baby is very upset again. If you do not do this, you might be avoiding a useful food which has no bearing on your baby's behaviour. It is important not to eliminate a lot of things at once, or you will never find the real culprit! While you are breastfeeding, it is important that you have an adequate diet and that you do not starve yourself, and you should be able to get help from your local dietician. Your hospital or GP's surgery will have a contact number. There is also some evidence that smoking or drinking a lot of coffee, tea, and some soft drinks can cause a baby a lot of discomfort and make her cry. Smoking also reduces breastmilk, because it discourages the production of the hormone oxytocin.

Embarrassment at feeding in front of people

With practice, it is possible to feed very discreetly from underneath a large T-shirt or shawl, so why not practise at home in front of a mirror? You may not have realized how little of your body you need show while breastfeeding. You can also keep an eye open for the Babycare symbol when you are out — this sign indicates that a shop, café, etc., offers somewhere private for a mother to feed in comfort and change her baby's nappy.

Returning to work

No matter when you return to work, and whether full- or part-time, it is still perfectly possible for you either to express milk and bring it home for the baby for the next day, or combine breast and bottlefeeding. It is up to you. However, do remember that, if at any time you do decide to change to total bottlefeeding, your baby will have a good start in life even if you breastfeed for only a few days or weeks.

Relationship with partner

Some couples find that making love during the months that a woman is breastfeeding can be rather a messy business. Milk may suddenly start spurting which can be off-putting for both partners. You could resolve this by dashing off to bed together immediately after the baby has been fed, but this is not always practical.

On the other hand, you may find that you are not at all interested in making love during the early months of breastfeeding and, indeed, do not really want your partner to touch your breasts as you feel they are for the baby.

Whichever way you feel, it is important that you talk it through together and share your emotions. Many couples feel that being shut out from a partner's thoughts and feelings is more damaging to a relationship than being told that the baby is uppermost in the woman's mind at the moment. There are, of course, other ways of enjoying your long-term relationship which do not revolve around making love, and giving priority to breastfeeding your tiny baby for these first few months of her life may not seem such a terrible sacrifice for a man if he can look at it in the context of their family life and relationships as a whole.

BREASTFEEDING WITH PLEASURE

A lot of the information about breastfeeding so far relates very much to the early days, and many mothers find that, if they can keep going, breastfeeding quickly becomes established and feeding becomes a real pleasure. As your baby gets older, so the feeds gradually become more spaced out and take less time. If you talk to mothers who have breastfed, many say that there are no real words to describe the joy they have felt feeding this living creature, knowing that they grew the baby inside their body, and this body can still produce all that the baby needs to continue growing into a strong healthy baby. As your baby grows older, she will stop breastfeeding to give you a wonderful smile, and, as she goes back to feeding, she may well stroke your breast, showing the pleasure she feels feeding from your breast.

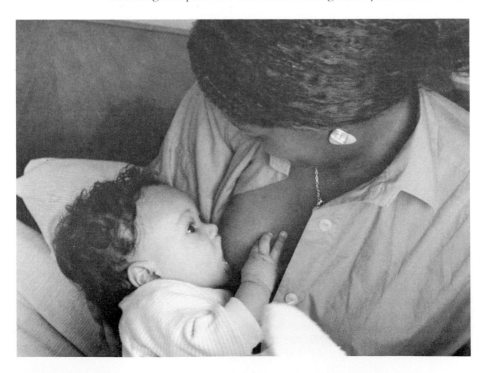

WEANING YOUR BABY

Your body is capable of producing enough milk for your baby until she is around six months old, when you might start thinking about weaning or giving your baby tastes of new foods. Once again, be guided by your baby. She will let you know when she is ready — perhaps she will be sitting on your lap while you are eating or drinking, and a small hand will stretch out to grab at the glass or your sandwich! There is no need to rush into weaning or giving solid foods and there is no competition to be the first one eating a roast dinner. You need not be in too much of a hurry to make her grow up!

As the amount of solid foods she eats increases, so she will probably demand fewer breastfeeds, and many babies stop breastfeeding by the time they are about one year old. Not all babies are the same though, and many mothers find they are still breastfeeding an older baby.

Toddlers can find breastfeeding a great support in this new large world which they have discovered. Breastfeeding is of nutritional value, and you are still passing across many vital antibodies to your baby, even if you are breastfeeding only once or twice a day. There is no need to stop unless you want to. | *Breast-feeding a toddler*

COMMON REASONS FOR MOTHERS GIVING UP BREASTFEEDING, AND WAYS OF OVERCOMING THEM

SIGNS | *Not enough milk*

- BABY CRYING AT END OF FEED
- POOR WEIGHT GAIN
- ONE FEED MERGES INTO ANOTHER
- SORE NIPPLES
- FEW WET NAPPIES
- SCANT DARK-GREEN, HARD MOTIONS

POSSIBLE CAUSES

- FAULTY BREASTFEEDING POSITION
- INADEQUATE STIMULATION OF BREASTS
- GROWTH SPURT BY BABY REQUIRING EXTRA MILK PRODUCTION
- RIGID TIMING OF BREASTFEEDS
- RIGID TIMING OF INTERVALS BETWEEN FEEDS
- SLEEPY BABY NOT FEEDING OFTEN ENOUGH

(Opposite)
Successful
breastfeeding
can be enjoyed
for as long as
you and your
child want it to
continue

- O   MOTHER NOT EATING OR RESTING SUFFICIENTLY
- O   TENSION INHIBITING LET-DOWN REFLEX, SO BABY ONLY
      GETS FOREMILK
- O   FEEDING PAINFUL, SO LET-DOWN REFLEX NOT WORKING
      PROPERLY
- O   MEDICATION AFFECTING MILK SUPPLY

STRATEGIES

- O   CHECK FEEDING POSITION (SEE P. 316 FOR MORE INFORMA-
      TION).
- O   REMEMBER LAW OF DEMAND AND SUPPLY; FEED MORE OFTEN
      — WHENEVER THE BABY WISHES, EVEN IF THIS MEANS VERY
      FREQUENT FEEDS.
- O   CHECK THAT BABY IS FEEDING FROM BOTH BREASTS 6–8 TIMES
      IN TWENTY-FOUR HOURS. WAKE AND FEED BABY MORE
      FREQUENTLY. (SOME BABIES DO ONLY FEED FROM ONE
      BREAST AT A FEED.)
- O   ALLOW BABY TO COME OFF BREAST NATURALLY RATHER THAN
      TIMING FEEDS.
- O   CONSIDER WHETHER BABY IS HAVING A GROWTH SPURT.
      THESE TEND TO OCCUR AT ABOUT 3 AND 6 WEEKS AND 3
      AND 6 MONTHS.
- O   STIMULATE BREASTS IN BETWEEN FEEDS USING A HAND OR
      ELECTRIC BREAST PUMP OR BY HAND-EXPRESSING.
- O   EAT ENOUGH — LET YOUR APPETITE BE YOUR GUIDE.
- O   DRINK ENOUGH — BUT MAKE SURE YOUR FLUID INTAKE IS
      NOT ALL IN HIGH-CAFFEINE DRINKS.
- O   REST ENOUGH.
- O   CONSIDER ANY MEDICATION — CONTRACEPTIVE PILLS,
      DIURETICS, LAXATIVES, ANTIHISTAMINES CAN ALL AFFECT
      MILK SUPPLY.
- O   TAKE VITAMIN B AND E TABLETS, BUT CONSULT YOUR GP
      FIRST.
- O   CONSIDER ASKING YOUR GP TO PRESCRIBE FOR YOU —
      METOCLOPRAMIDE AND SULPIRIDE MAY POSSIBLY INCREASE
      MILK SUPPLY.

Sore or cracked nipples

SIGNS

- O   RED SORE NIPPLE
- O   STRIPE ACROSS NIPPLE
- O   WHITE END TO NIPPLE
- O   CRACK WITH BLOOD
- O   BLISTER ON END OF NIPPLE

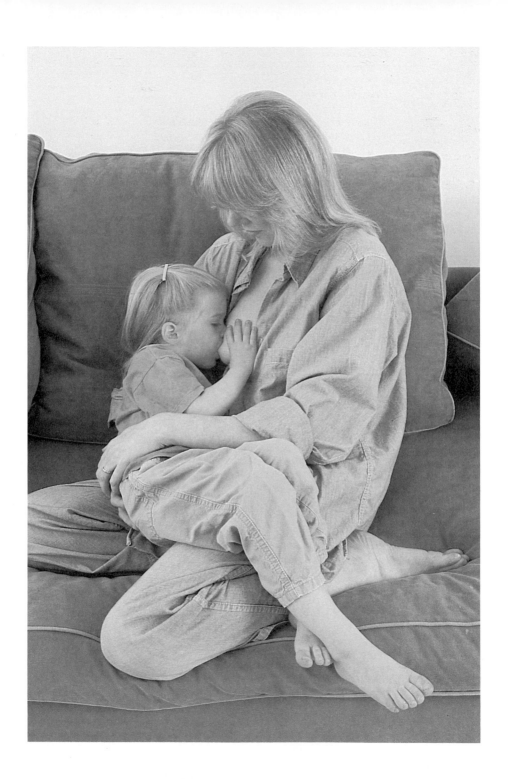

POSSIBLE CAUSES

- ○ INCORRECT POSITIONING AT BREAST
- ○ BABY NOT SUCKING PROPERLY
- ○ PULLING BABY OFF BREAST
- ○ LEAKING NIPPLES
- ○ PLASTIC-BACKED BREAST PADS
- ○ SOAP, ANTISEPTIC SPRAY, OR OTHER IRRITANT
- ○ NIPPLES NOT DRY AFTER FEED
- ○ THRUSH IN BABY'S MOUTH OR ON BREASTS

STRATEGIES

- ○ CHECK FEEDING POSITION AND PERHAPS CHANGE IT FRE-QUENTLY TO ENSURE DIFFERENT PRESSURE POINTS.
- ○ LIFT BABY TO BREAST; SUPPORT BABY ON PILLOW.
- ○ SUPPORT BREAST BY PUTTING HAND AGAINST RIB-CAGE AND UNDERNEATH BREAST TO LIFT IT AWAY FROM BODY.
- ○ DO NOT LET BABY DRAG ON BREAST.
- ○ USE A COTTON BRA.
- ○ FEED ON LEAST SORE SIDE FIRST.
- ○ EXPRESS AND RUB IN BREAST MILK AFTER FEED.
- ○ DO NOT WASH BREASTS AT START OF FEED.
- ○ MORE FREQUENT FEEDS MAY HELP.
- ○ COOLED BOILED WATER SPRAYED ON NIPPLES CAN BE AS EFFECTIVE AS PROPRIETARY SPRAY.
- ○ SPLASH COLD WATER ON AREOLA TO HELP TONE UP SPHINC-TER MUSCLES IF LEAKING IS A PROBLEM.
- ○ IF THRUSH IS THE CAUSE, GET A PRESCRIPTION FROM GP BOTH FOR BREASTS AND FOR BABY'S MOUTH.
- ○ IF NIPPLES SEVERELY CRACKED, IT MIGHT HELP TO REST BREASTS FOR TWENTY-FOUR HOURS, BUT YOU MUST THEN EXPRESS AND FEED BABY EXPRESSED BREAST MILK WITH AN ORTHODONTIC TEAT.

‘ *Breastfeeding is natural, so I expected it to come naturally. It was a shock to discover we'd both have to work at it!* ’

‘ *I wasn't prepared for how much I'd enjoy it. I'd thought of it as a chore, like changing nappies or doing the washing. I loved every moment.* ’

‘ *I found breastfeeding my second child much easier, because I felt confident enough to relax and let it happen the way we both wanted.* ’

⁶ *It surprised me that it took three or four weeks before feeding settled down this time. She found it hard to latch on properly on one side, so we were forever starting then stopping to re-position. It's working very well now.* ⁹

BOTTLEFEEDING

Some mothers know straight away that they will not wish to breastfeed for whatever reason. Others begin by breastfeeding, but circumstances mean that they have to change to bottlefeeding at a later date. There are many reasons why women make the decision to bottlefeed, and the NCT is there for all mothers, to support them in whatever choice they have felt is the right one for themselves and their family. Whether you choose to bottlefeed from the beginning, combine breast and bottlefeeding, or change from breast to bottle, you may find it helpful to talk over your decision with a supportive breastfeeding counsellor. If you are moving from breast to bottle, there may well be useful tips she can pass on to help make any transition as straightforward as possible.

If you have decided to bottlefeed, either from the beginning, or at some later stage, you will need:

- ☑ **SIX BOTTLES**
- ☑ **SIX TEATS**
- ☑ **A SUPPLY OF FORMULA MILK**
- ☑ **STERILIZING EQUIPMENT**

STERILIZING Everything will need to be sterilized very thoroughly. You can either use sterilizing tablets in cold water, in which case you will need a large plastic container with a lid; or you can sterilize using boiling water, when you will need a large saucepan with a lid. You could also use a steam sterilizer. Whichever way you choose, everything will need to be washed very thoroughly first.

Wash the bottles and teats using hot soapy water and a bottle brush. If you have used salt on the teats, make sure it is well rinsed off. Rinse everything in cold water before sterilizing.

If you have decided to use the chemical means of sterilizing, you will find full instructions on the packet or bottle. If you are using the boiling water method, everything needs to be submerged in boiling water for ten minutes, then left in the saucepan until you are ready to use it.

Most authorities would recommend sterilizing until your baby is a year old.

CHOOSING A FORMULA MILK There are a bewildering variety of formula milks on the market, all claiming to be as close as possible to breast milk. So how do you know which to choose? You could

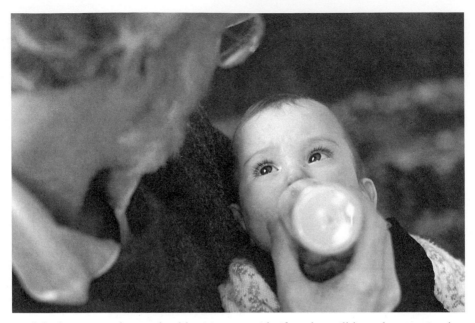

Bottlefeeding also provides opportunities for close and loving contact with your baby

ask your health visitor or midwife, who will have been trained to help. It is not a good idea to keep changing brands. Give your baby a reasonable chance to get used to one and stay with it unless either of you is particularly unhappy with it. Ask as many other mothers as you can what they have used and what they thought of the different brands.

FLEXIBILITY The routine of giving six bottles of 4 oz. a day to new babies will not necessarily be appropriate for your baby. As with everything else, different babies will have different requirements. As long as you are offering the correct amount a baby of her weight should be having, it does not matter whether you offer it in large amounts fewer times a day or smaller amounts more often. Wait, and work out what your baby seems to prefer. Bottlefed babies can have water between feeds, and may well become rather thirsty, especially in hot weather. Any water you give should be boiled and cooled first, of course.

You may find it easiest to make up all the feeds for a day at once and store them in the fridge. This may entail you having more than six bottles and teats. If you have no fridge, you will need to make the feeds as you need them, as milk left standing around at room temperature rapidly grows harmful bacteria.

FOLLOW-ON MILKS You may see so-called 'follow-on milks' on the supermarket shelves, or you may read about them in magazines and leaflets. These are milks aimed at babies who are over 6 months. The Department of Health has stated that these milks have absolutely no advantage over ordinary formula milks, and that the extra iron they contain is mostly not bio-available to the baby. Only 3–4 per cent of this iron can be absorbed by the baby. New regulations also mean that these milks are allowed to be 48 per cent glucose.

There is no reason at all why your baby should not continue receiving ordinary formula milk until she is old enough to drink unmodified cow's milk. Follow-on milks are usually more expensive than formula milks, and do not benefit your baby in any way.

ENJOYING FEEDS Just because you have chosen not to breastfeed for whatever reason does not mean that you and your baby cannot enjoy the same degree of closeness in a feed that a breastfeeding mother and baby would have. When you are feeding, hold your baby as close to you as possible, perhaps against your naked breast, talk to her and smile at her, enjoy the experience of feeding your baby. It is better, particularly in the early days, to make sure that only you or your partner feed your baby. It is tempting for other people to want to help feed the baby, but she will not be able to take in too many new people at once and needs the security of knowing those who are feeding her. Just as with a breastfed baby, a bottlefed baby will not want to wait for feeds either. She has not learnt to tell the time yet, so, if she is hungry, feed her. A cross baby who has been kept waiting for a feed will be too upset and angry to feed well, and will only need feeding again in a short while.

Bottlefeeding reminders

- ○ MAKE SURE YOU USE PRECISELY THE AMOUNT OF FORMULA SPECIFIED ON THE TIN, USING ONLY THE SCOOP PROVIDED AND NOT PACKING IT DOWN FIRMLY TO GET MORE IN.
- ○ BOTTLES ARE BETTER HEATED BY STANDING IN A JUG OF WARM WATER THAN IN A MICROWAVE WHEN THE MILK MAY BE UNEVENLY HEATED AND COULD SCALD A BABY; IN FACT, YOU ONLY NEED TO WARM THE MILK UP IF YOUR BABY PREFERS IT THAT WAY.
- ○ COVER ANY MILK AS SOON AS YOU HAVE MADE IT.
- ○ NEVER LEAVE A BABY PROPPED UP WITH A BOTTLE, AS SHE COULD EASILY CHOKE.
- ○ YOUR BABY WILL KNOW WHEN SHE HAS HAD ENOUGH. DO NOT FORCE THE REST OF THE BOTTLE DOWN HER IF SHE IS NOT KEEN.
- ○ THROW AWAY ANY UNUSED MILK AT THE END OF A FEED.
- ○ DO NOT LEAVE MILK STANDING AROUND AT ROOM TEMPERATURE FOR ANY LENGTH OF TIME.

‘ It may seem odd, but I decided to bottlefeed because my partner very much wanted to feed the baby. I wasn't honestly all that bothered about which I chose, so we did what suited him. ’

‘ Imogen was bottlefed after I became ill and had to go into hospital when she was 6 weeks old. I felt too ill to feel any sadness or sense of failure at the time, but I do feel a bit sorry now that she missed out on breastfeeding after those first few weeks. ’

‘ I put Mark onto a bottle when I went back to work at 3 months. Actually, I did manage to carry on with a couple of breastfeeds a day for a while, which helped me to feel more settled about all the changes. ’

‘ I tried breastfeeding my first baby and felt utterly miserable when it didn't go right. So this time I decided from the beginning not to start breastfeeding. Everything's fine now—no fretful baby, no sad, frustrated, guilty mother, no husband wanting to help and not knowing which way to turn. ’

‘ Getting bottles in the night sounds terrible, but it wasn't any problem at all —like everything else, you just get used to it. ’

FEEDING YOUR BABY: MOVING ON TO SOLIDS

25

Your baby has no need of any food other than breast milk for the first six months of her life, and this is what most experts would recommend; some advise leaving the introduction of mixed feeding even longer. What you decide to do is up to you and your baby. Many mothers feel they want to start earlier, or are advised to by other people, even health professionals. It is not, however, a good idea to introduce solids to a baby under four months, as the gut is still too immature to cope with different foods at this stage. If your baby of four months or less seems hungry all the time, what she needs is more milk, so you will need to work at building up your milk supply (see p. 340).

STARTING OFF

You may find the following suggestions helpful once you have decided to start. Remember, though, that if you have tried and your baby has not taken to mixed feeding, you can always leave it for a few more weeks until she seems more ready to try something new.

EQUIPMENT You will not need much equipment — a special bowl and spoon, of course, and a hand-held blender is useful for small amounts. Electric blenders work better with larger amounts, which is fine if you are freezing quantities at a time. An ordinary sieve will do very well too. Once your baby can manage slightly lumpier food, from about seven or eight months, you can mash most of it with a fork. You will, of course, need to be sure that everything is spotlessly clean.

FIRST FOODS You might start with puréed fruit or vegetables or a rice cereal mixed with milk (breast milk is fine). It is better to avoid cereals other than rice, in case your baby happens to be allergic to gluten, the protein in wheat. Puréed stewed apple, carrots, cauliflower, potato, mashed pear or banana are all suitable. Never add any sugar or salt to your baby's foods — the salt is bad for her kidneys and sugar is a taste better not acquired.

THE FIRST TASTE It is usually best to try mixed feeding at a feed around the middle of the day to start with. You can give her half

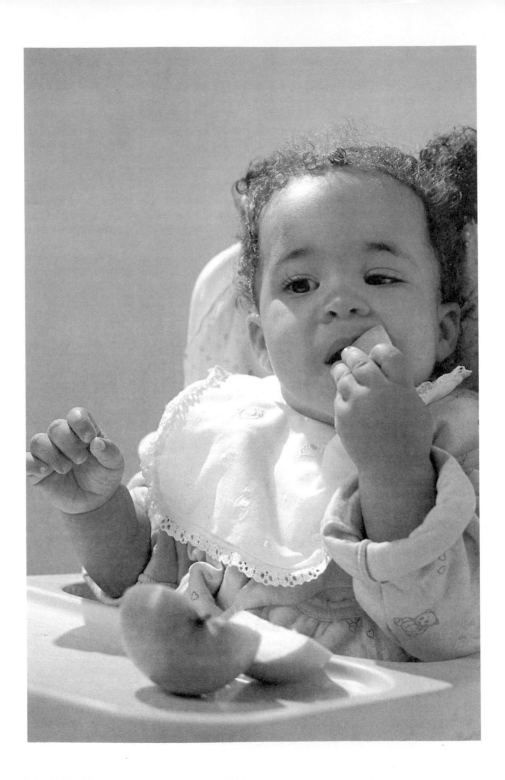

of her breastfeed, then offer her a tiny spoonful of whatever you have on offer. Once she has sucked at this or pushed it around with her tongue a few times, you can give her the rest of her breastfeed. Do not force anything, just let it happen gently and at your baby's pace. These are, after all, only tastes, not the real meal.

MOVING ON

Once your baby has tried a few tastes of foods, you can start offering her a little more, until after a few weeks she is eating a meal at lunch-time. You can offer her a drink from a cup after her meal, or her breastfeed, whichever you and she prefer. Gradually you can introduce some solid foods at breakfast and tea-time as well. Deciding on the amounts to give can be difficult, but most babies will decide for themselves when they have had enough. As soon as she begins to seem interested, let her have her own spoon. Either keep another spoon yourself, or let her do it all herself, with a spoon or fingers; feeding herself is an important part of discovering about the world — about texture, about manual dexterity, about dropping things, and about your reactions too! Make sure mealtimes are fun. Do not expect her to eat alone, as it is unsociable as well as dangerous in case she chokes, and try to let her eat with the rest of the family at least once every day, so that she comes to enjoy the social rituals associated with eating as well as the actual food.

Early foods

FRUITS Many fruits are excellent starters; try apple, banana, pear, or avocado pear, and, as your baby gets older, from about eight months, let her hold thin slices of fruits to eat herself. Make sure she does not choke though.

VEGETABLES Virtually any vegetable is suitable and they are wonderful because they are so easily puréed. Once your baby can chew well, you can give her well-washed and scrubbed vegetables to hold and eat raw — carrot, celery sticks, or cauliflower chunks are all ideal.

Use as little water as possible for cooking and cook for as little time as possible, though you will need to ensure the fruit or vegetables can be mashed well.

MEAT Meat is fibrous, does not mash easily, and so must be cooked very thoroughly. It is better to avoid minced meat from the butcher as it tends to be high in fats, and the surfaces will have been handled, but you can always mince your own meat. Some babies like chewing on a defatted and meaty cooked bone, but you will have to make sure there are no sharp edges or splinters first.

FISH You could cautiously introduce white fish from about six months, but oily fish are best left until your baby is over a year old, and babies

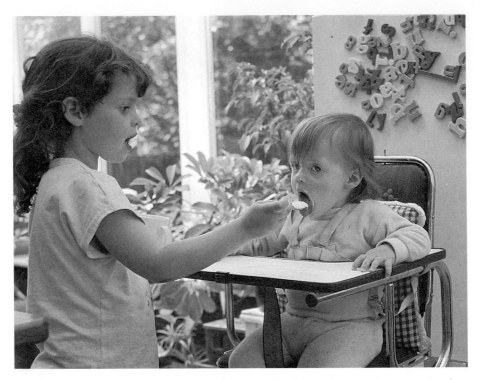

should not have smoked or salty fish such as smoked mackerel or haddock or shellfish. Make sure you have removed all the bones.

PEAS, BEANS, PULSES Pulses and beans are good sources of protein which mash up well, but they need careful cooking.

EGGS You can give egg yolk from six months onwards, but do not offer egg white until you are sure your baby can tolerate egg yolk. Do not give raw or lightly-boiled eggs to a young child, because of the risk of salmonella.

CHEESE Any mild, finely grated hard cheese is suitable, added to a cool sauce or mashed up with some cool vegetables. Cottage and curd cheeses are useful, too, perhaps sieved and added to food. Babies may like a mixture of mashed cottage cheese and banana, or curd cheese and avocado pear.

BREADS AND CEREALS Breads and cereals should not be the most important parts of a meal at this stage. Introduce rice first, leaving wheat, oats, and barley until later in case of gluten allergy. Once your baby can hold foods, she can have toasted bread-and-butter fingers, breadsticks, or rusks. You can make your own rusks by slowly drying out thick slices of bread in a warm oven — most of the commercial brands of rusk contain sugar, even low-sugar ones!

MILK AND YOGHURT You can introduce small amounts of cow's milk after the sixth month, but only in cooking, e.g. mixed with cereal, as custard, or as a sauce. Cow's milk is very low in iron and should not be given as a drink until your baby is on a good mixed diet. This will probably be at about a year old, or later for some babies. It is better to continue giving breast milk or formula milk, as these contain more iron. Whole cow's milk (full fat) should be given to children under 2, rather than skimmed or semi-skimmed. It does not need to be boiled as long as it is pasteurized.

Yoghurt can be introduced after the sixth month too. It is an excellent food and mixes well with all sorts of other foods, especially fruit, but also savoury foods. Natural yoghurt is best, as this will not contain sugar or additives.

Watching for reactions

If at any time you notice that your baby is having unusual bowel movements or seems unhappy after a meal, it may well be that something has disagreed with her. This food can then be left out of her diet for a few more weeks or months until she is older. Because of this, it makes sense to introduce any new foods very gradually, one at a time, so any problems can immediately be pinpointed and the offending food eliminated.

Convenience foods

Tinned and packet baby foods are very useful at times — they are easily made up and handy to carry around. Make sure you read the labels though: many contain sugar in one form or another (dextrose, sucrose, glucose, and fructose); most are predominantly water; some contain large quantities of cereals or wheat starch; many use vast amounts of thickener, which is a waste of your money. Many also contain milk, which you might be anxious to avoid. Although it may be fiddly, it might work out cheaper in the end to offer your baby foods that you have prepared most of the time, saving the expensive convenience foods for the odd occasion when you have run out of ideas, or for outings and holidays. The added advantage of this is that your baby will begin her experiences of mixed feeding with the taste of your cooking, and will probably adapt easily to the family's eating styles.

Cooking for and feeding your baby can become a very emotive subject. Since you have invested so much time, energy, and love in the preparation of her food, it can feel like a rejection of you if she rejects it. Try not to see it this way, as this may eventually cause mealtimes to turn into a battle of wills where the stakes are high. If she does not fancy something, however lovingly prepared, try to shrug your shoulders and leave it.

You can, of course, make your own convenience foods if you have a freezer. Freezing small quantities of puréed foods in ice-cube trays or other tiny containers means you will have a meal ready to hand whenever you need.

Foods to be avoided by babies

- [X] VERY SPICY FOODS
- [X] SUGAR
- [X] SALT
- [X] FRUIT SQUASHES
- [X] UNRIPE FRUIT
- [X] FRUIT WITH LOTS OF SEEDS
- [X] COFFEE AND TEA
- [X] CANNED FIZZY DRINKS
- [X] CREAM CAKES
- [X] SWEETS
- [X] PROCESSED CEREALS, LIKE CORNFLAKES
- [X] SMOKED FISH OR MEAT
- [X] CHUNKY PEANUT BUTTER
- [X] NUTS
- [X] CRISPS
- [X] PROCESSED MEAT PRODUCTS

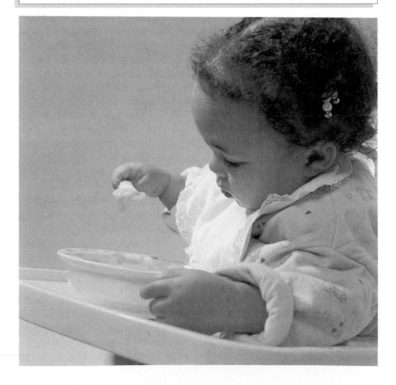

Looking After Your Baby

26

Looking after babies, like parenting as a whole, is essentially a mixture of commonsense and personal inclination. Whatever your experience, or lack of it, so far, you will soon establish a way of life which suits your family. This will not necessarily be your friend's way, or your mother's or great-aunt's, but if it feels right for you, that is what is important. You will almost certainly be inundated with advice from every quarter once your baby is born. Everyone you meet will appear to have some stake in the baby's upbringing and welfare, from your health visitor, mother, or sister-in-law, to assorted baby-goods manufacturers and the woman in the supermarket queue. If the advice offered happens to suit your preferred life-style, then you will welcome it; the rest you will quickly become adept at discarding. There are, in any case, no fixed rules about how to care for a baby. Babies need to be fed, played with, and cuddled; to be kept clean, warm, and comfortable; to be allowed to sleep when they wish, and to feel secure. How you choose to achieve this with your child is a matter for you and your partner. Your baby will not mind whether or not great-aunt approves of disposable nappies, as long as she is comfortable and can sense that you are happy and confident in what you have decided to do.

SLEEPING

Babies have very different sleep requirements, but an average amount is around 13–14 hours a day. At first this may or may not fall into patterns which are convenient to you. Your baby will not know the difference between night and day for some while, and it may be many months before she sleeps through the night. This is not a problem for the baby. It is a problem for adults because we expect our sleep to fall into a routine; we are used to a certain number of hours' sleep, at times decided by ourselves. Your baby will not understand this, and it will be several years before she is able to take into account the fact that lack of sleep makes people feel tired and irritable. Even then she may find it hard to do anything about it. However unlikely it may seem at first, parents do eventually get used to broken nights; you may grow so used to getting up several times a night that a whole night of unbroken sleep, when it comes, is a shock, leaving you feeling decidedly worse the following day. This is, unfortunately, of small consolation to new parents in the first throes of sleepless nights, who may find it hard to imagine that they could ever become used to it. In fact, many mothers come to welcome the night feeds, as a time of peace and quiet with their babies, away from any pressures of the day: a contented, unhurried time just to be together, enjoying a breastfeed.

What you will need

☑	**SOMEWHERE TO SLEEP**
☑	**A MATTRESS**
☑	**SHEETS**
☑	**BLANKETS**

SOMEWHERE TO SLEEP A new-born baby can sleep in her parents' bed, in a crib, Moses basket, carry-cot, or pram; even in a suitably lined drawer.

MATTRESS You may decide to use a fabric mattress, a plastic-covered mattress for easy cleaning, or the type with holes at one end. You may also prefer to use a new mattress rather than a second-hand one for reasons of hygiene. If you are using a second-hand mattress, do make sure that it is well cleaned and aired before use. You may have concerns about the safety of mattresses following certain reports into cot deaths. You will find further information about cot death and about your baby's safety while asleep in the section on cot death later in this chapter.

SHEETS You may need several sheets to keep up with the washing; try cutting up old sheets or using pillow cases.

BLANKETS You can use shawls instead of blankets, but watch out for holes where little fingers could get stuck. If you decide to use a duvet rather than blankets, tuck it carefully under the mattress so that the baby cannot pull it over her face.

Daytime sleeping

Your baby will need somewhere to sleep during the day. This could be the same place or receptacle she uses at night, but some mothers have a crib upstairs and a pram or whatever for daytime use, so that she can be near them. A carry-cot can double as crib and pram. Wherever she sleeps, the mattress needs to fit well, and babies should not have pillows.

If you have other children, you may find your baby spends so much time in her pram or car-seat going to and from playgroups, shops, and school that she rarely sleeps anywhere much at home during the day; all her sleeping is done on the move. Fortunately, most babies are agreeably adaptable and will willingly fit in with your routine most of the time, given a little forethought in terms of feeds and nappy-changes. If your baby does not like going off to sleep during the day and you have things you would like to do, or have run out of ideas for playing with her, try a sling. You can wander off for a walk or get on with the vacuum-cleaning this way. Perhaps surprisingly, most babies will sleep through noise; in fact your baby may be more liable to wake up if everyone is tiptoeing round the house than if your four-year-old and his friends decide to play football around her pram.

OUTDOORS When you put your baby outside in the garden to sleep during the day, watch out for cats (yours or other people's), stray insects, and any direct sun on your baby. A net with large mesh will keep cats off; a fine-mesh net will keep off most other things, including fallen leaves and the occasional bouncy ball thrown by an enthusiastic toddler.

IN YOUR ROOM Some parents prefer to have their babies near them for the first few weeks or months. This can work to the advantage of both parents and baby — mother and father will feel reassured by hearing the baby's breathing, knowing that she is nearby, and there is no trekking off to another room for a feed. The baby is similarly reassured by hearing her parents' breathing.

Night-time sleeping

IN YOUR BED Many parents have their babies sleeping in their bed with them. This is not dangerous, providing neither of you has been taking any drugs or alcohol, which might alter your normal responses. Because young babies are unable to regulate their own temperatures efficiently, you will also need to make sure that your baby cannot become overheated in your bed. You can lessen the chances of her becoming overheated by letting her sleep in just a vest and nappy and by keeping your bedroom relatively cool. Most importantly, you will need to take care that she is able to lose excess heat through her head. Babies lose most of their heat from their heads, so her head should not be buried under a duvet which traps the heat. There is no likelihood of either of you rolling on top of her, as you will be well aware of her presence even in sleep. If your baby does share your bed, night feeds are even easier, once you have got the hang of feeding lying down. Often a baby who is not happy to settle in her own cot at night will readily fall asleep, secure in her parents' bed, in her mother's arms, listening to their relaxed, calm breathing. It may take a few days to get used to having another person in your bed.

IN A DIFFERENT ROOM Not all parents like having their babies in the same room. Babies' breathing patterns are irregular and many parents find it nerve-racking waiting for the next breath to come, or find the sighs and snuffles disturbing. You may be concerned that letting your baby sleep with you now will make it difficult to move her into her own room later on. Parents who have had their babies with them have not usually found this a problem, but if you are not happy with the idea, then it will not feel right for you. Mothers do also worry that partners will not be getting enough sleep if they are disturbed by the baby's night feeds, so choose to feed in another room. In fact this can work either way: many partners are aware of a woman getting up and out of the bed to feed a baby who is crying for attention, whereas they might not even notice her turning over to pick up the baby next to her, who has just begun to make a few mutterings and is not left long enough to work up to full-scale yelling.

NIGHT FEEDS Babies will soon respond to the quieter atmosphere of the house during the night, and many mothers find they enjoy these rather special times together. There are ways to make night feeds easier:

○ **MAKE AS LITTLE NOISE AND FUSS AS POSSIBLE SO THAT YOUR BABY LEARNS THIS IS NOT A TIME FOR PLAYING.**

○ **USE A DIMMER SWITCH, LOW-WATTAGE BULB, OR GLOW PLUG INSTEAD OF HAVING TO TURN ON A BRIGHT LIGHT.**

○ **HAVE A FLASK OF A WARM DRINK READY FOR YOU AND MAYBE A COUPLE OF BISCUITS OR A SANDWICH.**

○ **MAKE SURE THE ROOM YOU ARE IN IS WARM AND YOU ARE ON A REALLY COMFORTABLE CHAIR OR WELL-PROPPED UP IN BED; IF YOUR BABY IS IN BED WITH YOU, YOU WILL BOTH BE WARM AND COMFORTABLE ALREADY.**

○ **DO NOT CHANGE HER NAPPY UNLESS IT IS DIRTY. IF YOU ARE WORRIED ABOUT LEAKS IN YOUR BED, YOU COULD USE A TOWELLING NAPPY AT NIGHT-TIME OR USE A WAD OF NAPPY-ROLL INSIDE A DISPOSABLE.**

○ **USE DIFFERENT BEDS FOR DAY- AND NIGHT-TIME SO THAT SHE LEARNS TO DIFFERENTIATE.**

The sleeping baby

SLEEPING POSITIONS Ideas on how a baby should lie to sleep change with every new generation of parents, and are different in the different cultures within a society. Even tiny babies are surprisingly mobile in sleep, determinedly working themselves up the cot until their heads are squashed in a corner, or wriggling around until they are in a favourite position. To lessen the risk of cot death, parents are now advised to lay their babies to sleep on their backs or sides. If your baby has a strong preference for sleeping on her side rather than on her back, you can bring her lower arm forward to prevent her rolling forward onto her tummy.

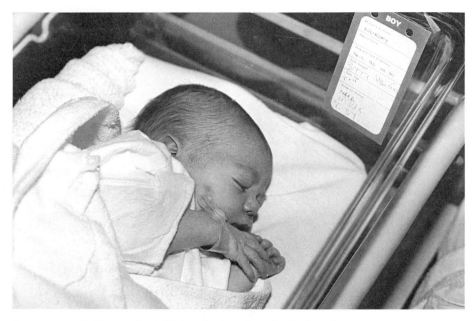

APPEARANCE Babies can look frighteningly pale and still when they are asleep. Virtually all parents have at some time prodded a sleeping baby because she appeared not to be breathing. Babies also make strange little noises in their sleep, but you will soon get to recognize what is a normal sleeping pattern for your baby and stop feeling quite so alarmed or disconcerted by every twitch and snuffle.

TEMPERATURE Babies need to be kept reasonably warm as they are unable to control their own body temperature very well as yet, but there is no need to live in semi-tropical conditions. A perfectly adequate temperature is 65 °F (19 °C) and, if it seems cold, you can always put an extra blanket on her. Layers of clothes and blankets will be warmer too, and a large blanket folded in four then placed over the top of the crib will trap the heat most effectively. Beware of overheating a tiny baby, especially if your home is centrally heated. Babies do not need layer upon layer of clothing and bed clothes if the room is already very well heated; they need to be able to cool off as well as to be kept warm. If your baby is sleeping in your room it is perfectly safe to have a window open at night; just wrap her up warm or, even better, snuggle her up with you on cold nights — better than a hot-water bottle!

You can test if your baby is warm enough by feeling her skin under her clothes at the back of her neck. The skin here is a more reliable indicator of her temperature than her hands and feet, which may often feel cold to the touch.

CLOTHING

☑ **VESTS**
☑ **STRETCH SUITS OR NIGHTGOWNS**
☑ **CARDIGANS**
☑ **OUTDOOR WEAR**

VESTS Choose vests with envelope necks or ties: babies do not like having clothes pulled over their heads.

CARDIGANS Cardigans are easier than jumpers, as they do not need to be taken over the baby's head.

FASTENINGS Avoid ribbons or strings on baby clothes, as these will be sucked or chewed and can be dangerous. Keep fastenings as simple as possible as babies hate being fussed. Poppers all down the front or back are preferable. Many babies absolutely loathe being undressed and will cling to their vests with pathetic determination.

OUTDOOR WEAR Choose this according to season: you may need a suit, mittens, socks or bootees, and a hat. Avoid mittens with holes where fingers could get stuck.

You will need as many clothes for your baby as will keep you ahead of the washing. (This also applies to bedclothes.) Babies do get through an amazing number of clothes, especially if they are sicky babies. You can save the occasional stretch suit by using muslin nappies to mop up small amounts of sick, but even so a baby can happily run through three or more complete changes of clothing in a day. Breastfed babies have soft bowel motions which tend to leak, however well-accomplished a nappy-changer you are. You can, unfortunately, expect to be doing a lot of washing and drying of linen and clothing — yours and hers.

It is not really worth buying vast quantities of clothes for the first size as babies grow so rapidly and clothes are expensive. If you are happy about using second-hand clothes, then many areas do have sales of second-hand babies' clothes, because people have bought too many and the babies have grown so fast. Try your local NCT branch, play-groups, or school jumble or good-as-new sales. You can then keep any special clothes you or someone else has bought for outings and visits.

NAPPIES

☑ **DISPOSABLE NAPPIES**

or

> ☑ **TOWELLING NAPPIES**
> ☑ **PINS**
> ☑ **LINERS**
> ☑ **PLASTIC PANTS**
> ☑ **BUCKETS WITH LIDS FOR SOILED NAPPIES**
> ☑ **STERILIZING SOLUTION, IF LIKED**
> ☑ **NON-BIOLOGICAL WASHING POWDER**

Nappies do seem to preoccupy everyone when discussing babycare, probably because nappy-changing is something that will happen so often — maybe seven or eight times a day at first. The general aim is to keep the baby clean and dry with a minimum of fuss. You may initially find the thought of nappy-changing mildly unpleasant and feel a bit squeamish, but you will soon find yourself coping with it very well, even when your baby wets the clean nappy before you have got it on, managing to soak everything else in sight at the same time, then repeats the performance with her next set of clean clothes.

DISPOSABLE NAPPIES Disposable nappies have improved vastly in terms of efficiency over the last few years. They are easier to put on, less work to change, and less trouble when it comes to cleaning. They do not work for everyone though. Some babies have legs and bottoms which will not fit comfortably into a disposable nappy. Other mothers find their babies are so wet that they are forever soaking right through disposables and their clothes. They are more expensive overall, even taking washing-powder into account. Also, anyone concerned about ecological arguments may feel they are an unnecessary extra drain on natural resources, as well as being impossible to dispose of properly. They are neither reusable nor biodegradable. You may object to the chemicals which go into manufacturing disposable nappies. You will also have to sluice off soiled ones in a lavatory and use sealed plastic bags for disposal because of the risk of infection, causing further long-term environmental problems. For all these drawbacks, they are very convenient and immensely time-saving.

TOWELLING NAPPIES Towelling nappies are more trouble to change, but you may not have to change them so often. Some babies are allergic to disposable nappies and have constant nappy rash when using them, so need to use towelling ones. Some mothers like to ring the changes, so they use towelling nappies most of the time and disposables occasionally, when going out or on holiday. An older baby cannot remove her towelling nappy as efficiently as she can a disposable one either!

If you are using towelling nappies, you will also need pins, liners, and plastic pants. One-way liners help to keep a baby's bottom reasonably dry. Plastic pants come in three sorts: the elasticated variety, which do not always fit very well and can be tight round the

Choosing nappies

legs; tie-pants, which work well on small babies if you tie them front and back rather than at the sides, but get too tight later on; and the sort with elastic plus poppers, which usually fit well and hold everything in place neatly, but are more expensive. They are all washable. Some babies cannot wear plastic pants at all because their skin is too delicate. One solution is to use two towelling nappies, or disposable nappy-roll inside the towelling nappy.

The better the nappy you buy, the longer it will last before being wet through or fraying at the edges or going into holes in the middle. It is well worth buying good-quality terry-towelling nappies as they last longer and retain their texture better. You will need about two dozen nappies — enough to allow for a day's dry supply, a load being washed or drying, and some soaking, or waiting to be washed.

You can now also buy varieties of towelling nappy which are shaped like disposable nappies, so are easier to put on and look less bulky, but are washable. Some come with a waterproof coating, others need plastic pants as well. Many mothers find these an excellent alternative to either disposable or straightforward towelling nappies. They are convenient, but more ecologically acceptable to many parents than disposables. Mothers have also said that they are effective in keeping babies dry and free of nappy rash. Although the initial outlay may work out rather expensive, as with ordinary towelling nappies, at least you have only the one packet to buy. You can get further information from other mothers, good local chemists, and most health food shops.

STERILIZING You do not have to go to the extra expense of soaking your nappies in sterilizing solution unless you want to; the hottest machine wash, nearly boiling, will sterilize effectively, and putting them out to dry in the sun will bleach them too. Some babies' bottoms react badly to the solution, as do some mothers' hands.

Folding nappies

KITE SHAPE

○ **FOLD SIDES INTO CENTRE AS SHOWN.**

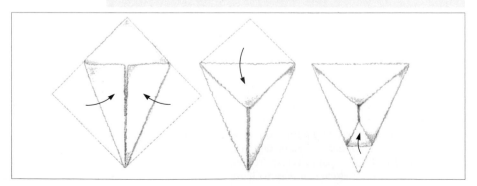

○ FOLD TOP AND BOTTOM CORNERS INWARDS, THUS PRODUC-
    ING EQUAL THICKNESS EVERYWHERE.

○ FOLD ROUND BABY'S LEGS AND PIN AT SIDES.

This shape works well with babies after the new-born stage, and can be adapted to suit the growing child by lessening the amount of nappy folded up from the bottom.

ORIENTAL SHAPE

○ FOLD NAPPY IN HALF UPWARDS.

○ FOLD IN HALF AGAIN, LEFT TO RIGHT.

○ DRAW TOP LAYER OF NAPPY FROM TOP RIGHT-HAND CORNER
    OVER TO THE LEFT, HOLDING OTHER LAYERS DOWN SO THAT
    THE BOTTOM RIGHT CORNER ARRIVES AT TOP LEFT CENTRE.

○ REVERSE WHOLE NAPPY, FACE DOWNWARDS.

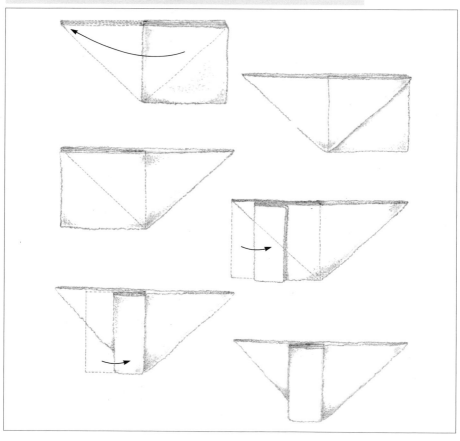

- ○ **FOLD STRAIGHT EDGE ON LEFT INTO THE CENTRE, LEAVING THE TRIANGULAR 'WING' BEHIND.**
- ○ **FOLD THICK STRIP BETWEEN BABY'S LEGS AND PIN TO 'WINGS'.**

This fold is excellent for new babies, who need a small nappy which will fit snugly.

AMERICAN SHAPE

- ○ **FOLD NAPPY SO THAT THERE ARE THREE THICKNESSES LENGTHWISE (FOR A TINY BABY FOLD INTO FOUR SO THAT THE RESULTING STRIP IS NARROWER).**
- ○ **FOLD LOWER THIRD UP TO MAKE A THICKER PART TO GO AT FRONT OR BACK, AS REQUIRED.**
- ○ **SIMPLY PLACE IT BETWEEN BABY'S LEGS AND PIN AT SIDES.**

KEEPING CLEAN

What you will need

- ☑ CHANGING MAT
- ☑ BABY BATH
- ☑ UNPERFUMED SOAP
- ☑ TOWELS
- ☑ NATURAL SPONGES OR COTTON WOOL
- ☑ CREAM FOR PROTECTION, IF LIKED

CHANGING MAT If you do not have a changing mat, you should have somewhere to change a nappy which is wipe-clean.

BABY BATH A baby bath is useful, but a large sink or washing-up bowl will do, provided it is kept scrupulously clean.

SOAP Make sure soap is unperfumed, and any liquid baby bath is not detergent-based — especially for little girls, as it can damage their vaginas.

SPONGE If you use a natural sponge or flannel to wash your baby's face, make sure you keep it just for her face; you can also use cotton wool.

CREAMS AND LOTIONS There is a bewildering range of creams and ointments for nappy changes. Try small pots, or share with friends, until you find one that suits your baby. Your baby may prefer you not to use mineral-based oils and creams on skin which is sore or broken, as they can sting. Creams can be prescribed if necessary.

A WORD OF WARNING

ALLERGIES Babies' skins are extremely sensitive. Try all products out carefully, and stop using them if there is any obvious reaction. If your baby has an especially sensitive skin, your health visitor or GP can help you find alternative products, which will not harm the skin and will prevent it from drying out. Most of these are available on prescription.

All the following products may contain strong chemicals to which your baby may have an adverse reaction:

○ **WET WIPES**
○ **PERFUMED SOAP**
○ **BABY SHAMPOO**
○ **LIQUID BABY BATH**
○ **FABRIC CONDITIONERS**
○ **BIOLOGICAL WASHING POWDERS, OR THOSE WITH ENZYMES**
○ **NAPPY STERILIZING SOLUTION**

ZINC-AND-CASTOR-OIL CREAM Avoid using zinc-and-castor-oil cream if your baby is taking antibiotics, or if you are taking them while breastfeeding; also if your baby has thrush.

BABY LOTION You may want to use baby lotion and cotton wool or wet wipes to clean a dirty bottom; however, baby lotion can feel very astringent and wet wipes particularly so. Using unperfumed soap and water works perfectly well, though it takes more time.

BABY POWDER Talcum powder is best left on the shelves. It may smell delicious, but babies can easily inhale the dust and it tends to dry out already dry skin and then settle in creases where it causes irritation.

COTTON BUDS Cotton buds may be useful for some things, but are best kept out of babies' ears and noses. They only pack earwax in harder anyway; wait for it to come right out, then wipe it off at bath-time.

HAIRBRUSHES Only babies with hair need hairbrushes, and even then, stroking the hair into place is usually enough.

NAIL SCISSORS The round-ended nail scissors are very useful for cutting babies' nails without risking catching tiny fingers. Many mothers nibble babies' nails short instead.

BATHING

Babies do not need bathing every day, as long as they are kept clean. If this is your first baby, you may well enjoy bathing her very much, and find the daily ritual extremely pleasant. If it is a second or subsequent baby, you may find yourself fitting in baths on days you can manage it!

There is not really any great mystery about bathing, though often much seems to be made of it. The main things to remember are:

> ○ **KEEP THE BABY WARM**
> ○ **HAVE EVERYTHING READY PREPARED**
> ○ **WASH HER FACE AND HEAD FIRST AND HER BOTTOM LAST**
> ○ **HOLD HER FIRMLY**

Getting ready

Whether you are using a baby bath or the kitchen sink, the technique is basically the same. If you are bathing your baby in a sink, it is a good idea to cover the taps with flannels as they stick out and will be sharp or hot.

Many babies have an intense dislike of baths in the first few weeks, often because they detest being undressed. The more you can prepare in advance, the easier it is to cope with — the last thing either of you wants is to have to keep dashing back and forth for something you have forgotten.

If you have the room nicely warm, you will be able to bath her in a leisurely way, staying to feed her afterwards if necessary. It does not really matter too much if you bath her before or after her feed. After a feed may make the baby sick — annoying if she does it after you have put clean clothes on. On the other hand, she may need a feed to settle her before her bath, and, if you feed her afterwards, there is a good chance she will mess up her clean nappy. You will soon work out which suits the two of you better.

Check that the water is the right temperature with your wrist or elbow — it should feel about blood temperature. You will not need very much water unless your baby already enjoys a good splash.

Bathing a baby

If you have a towel on your lap, you can lie the baby there while you gently wipe over her face. Use separate balls of cotton-wool to prevent cross-infection if her eyes are at all sticky.

It is safest to leave the nappy on till the last moment if you want to keep the towel clean and dry!

You can shampoo or gently soap the baby's scalp. You will need very little, as her hair will not have got dirty as an adult's would. Hold her firmly in one hand, with her head hanging over the edge of the bath, so that you can use your free hand to rinse off the soap. You may find it easiest if she is well wrapped in a towel to keep flailing arms and kicking legs out of the way. (Some babies are happier if still wrapped in a towel when they are lowered into the bath.)

Once her head is done, you can concentrate on her body. If you are using a liquid soap or emollient liquid which you squirt straight into the bath, you can simply lower her into the bath and gently smooth the soapy water over her body, into all the little creases. If you are using ordinary soap for your baby, soap her all over on your lap first, then lower her into the bath to rinse it off. Hold your baby with the back of her head resting against your wrist and your finger and thumb holding her farther arm just below the armpit. Your other hand can then hold her under her legs and bottom. Until you feel experienced, just swishing the water around her will be enough. If she seems frightened, try holding her arms firmly against her chest to see if this reassures her.

There is a knack to holding a slippery, wriggling little baby in the bath with one hand, and it may take time to acquire. Do not feel afraid of holding her firmly, as she would rather be safely held than be aware that you are afraid of dropping her.

Lift her out, then wrap her in a warm towel, letting her feel secure and comfortably enfolded before you begin patting her dry. Remember in particular the folds of skin

○ **UNDER THE ARMS**
○ **IN THE NECK**
○ **AT THE TOP OF THE LEGS**

Making sure you have actually patted the towel in all the creases should do the trick.

Some babies dislike bathing so much that it becomes a miserable chore for both of you. You could try simply wiping her down with a sponge of warm water, so she does not have to be in the water. Try varying the water temperature slightly too, as she may have a preference for cooler or warmer baths.

You can also take your baby into your bath with you. That way she will feel secure and cuddled still and you will have the extra benefit of the skin-to-skin contact. Do check the temperature carefully, as what feels fine for you may be too hot for her. Make sure you hold the baby firmly as you get in and out of the bath, or have your partner there to hand the baby to you. If you then lie in the bath, the baby can sit up or lie against you, supported and comforted by your body, yet still in the water. Most babies love bathing with either mother or father like this; the reassuring closeness of the parent and the lovely feel of skin against skin in the bath is good fun. If you are on your own, the drawback is having to get out at the same time as the baby. It is pleasanter if you have a large towel or a towelling robe waiting to wrap yourself in so that you can dry the baby first but keep warm yourself.

Topping and tailing

If you are not bathing your baby every day, she will at least need to be kept fairly clean. Topping and tailing her simply means washing her face and hands with cotton-wool or a clean flannel, then washing her bottom carefully with soap and water, making sure you wash and dry in all the creases as if you were bathing. Laying her on a towel or a nappy, so that neither any water nor her urine can seep up the change-mat soaking her clothes, saves time and energy.

CRYING

Life with a new baby is not all smiles and gurgles or a happily sleeping baby tucked up sweetly in her crib. Some babies cry and cry for hours on end. It can be hard to imagine how people actually enjoy parenthood when you have a baby who spends much of her waking time fretting, grumbling, or screaming the house down. Parents soon become practised at knowing which cries mean they really need something and which are whingeing. If you have worked out that your baby always cries a little before dropping off to sleep, or often wakes, cries a little, then goes back to sleep, you may become irritated by others who go to pick her up at such times. Let them know, tactfully, that you recognize what that particular cry means and you would rather the baby were left in future.

Why babies cry

Babies cry for all sorts of reasons, not all of them easy to detect. A baby may cry because she is:

- ○ **HUNGRY**
- ○ **BORED**
- ○ **UNCOMFORTABLE**
- ○ **ILL**
- ○ **IN PAIN**
- ○ **LONELY**
- ○ **TIRED**

She may also cry if you needed a lot of drugs during your labour (especially Pethidine or an epidural).

In the beginning, it will mostly be trial and error to discover what is making her cry. You may find that there are specific times of day when she is often fretful. Unfortunately, this all too often coincides with the late afternoon and evening, when you are tired after your day, you want to get a meal ready, your other children are tired and grumpy, and your partner was really looking forward to a quiet evening after working all day.

If you have tried feeding your baby, changing her (some babies mind about wet or dirty nappies more than others), checking there are no pins or bits sticking in to her, if she is not ready to sleep, and does not particularly want to be played with, there are various things you can try:

- ○ **FEED HER AGAIN. MANY BABIES JUST WANT TO BE CUDDLED AND SUCKLED. YOU CANNOT OVERFEED A BREASTFED**

are normal reactions and will disappear eventually.

Occasionally children develop a rash after having the MMR injection, and a few get a mild form of mumps about three weeks later. These are all mild symptoms of the diseases themselves and the children are not infectious either to other children or to adults. Very occasionally children may have a more serious reaction to the MMR injection, and about one child in a thousand has a convulsion. This is, however, less than the number of children who would suffer convulsions if they actually caught measles.

If your child has a fever, you can give her a dose of paracetamol to bring her temperature down, and carry out the other actions to lower her temperature as described in the next section 'When Your Baby is Ill'. You can always call your doctor if you are worried that your child's reaction is worse than you had been led to expect.

Polio The polio vaccine, given orally, is a live vaccine giving the baby a very mild form of the disease to build up her own immunity. Because it is a live virus, it will be passed into your baby's nappies for up to thirty days after each dose. It is, therefore, especially important at this time to be scrupulously hygienic when changing your baby's nappies, and disposing of the contents. If you know, or suspect, that you or your partner has not been immunized against polio, you can arrange to be immunized at the same time as your baby if you wish.

Any immunization should only be carried out when a baby or child is quite well, with no signs of illness. There are some children who should not automatically be immunized. Reasons you might wish to think twice about having your child immunized include:

When to think twice

- ○ A CHILD WHO DOES NOT SEEM TO BE DEVELOPING AS ONE WOULD EXPECT
- ○ A CHILD WHO SHOWED ANY SIGNS OF BRAIN ABNORMALITY AT BIRTH—EVEN IF THIS IS NOW FULLY CLEARED UP
- ○ A CHILD WHO HAS SUFFERED FITS OR CONVULSIONS, OR ONE WHO HAS CLOSE RELATIVES WITH EPILEPSY
- ○ A CHILD WHO HAS A SERIOUS DISEASE
- ○ A CHILD WHO IS TAKING ANY KINDS OF DRUGS (PARTICULARLY STEROIDS)
- ○ A CHILD WHO HAS SOME FORM OF ALLERGY, IN PARTICULAR A CHILD WHO HAS HAD A PREVIOUS SEVERE REACTION TO EATING EGGS
- ○ A CHILD WHO HAS PREVIOUSLY HAD A STRONG REACTION TO IMMUNIZATION

If your baby or child falls into any of these categories, you will need to discuss the most appropriate course of action with your doctor, or specialist if appropriate. Ask for a second opinion if you are unhappy with any of the information you are given.

WHEN YOUR BABY IS ILL

Calling the doctor

Mothers are the best judges of whether or not their babies are ill, so, if you feel there is something not quite right with your child, but cannot put your finger on anything specific, go and see your GP. He would rather see a child who is fine than miss seeing a sick child. If you are sufficiently concerned to call your GP out at night, he should always come. There are very few people who call a doctor out at night without being very worried about a child's health. If it is difficult to be objective, which it often is at 2.00 a.m., try to pretend this is someone else's baby, and imagine what you would say to your friend in this situation.

With new babies, it is hard to be sure what will turn out to be normal and what will not. In the very early days, you can ask your midwife when she calls; after that you will have to decide when to visit the doctor.

Symptoms that should always be taken seriously

If your baby shows any of the following signs, it is potentially very serious, and you need to call your doctor or go to the nearest Accident and Emergency Department immediately:

○ IF SHE IS HAVING FITS, IS NOT BREATHING OR IS UNCON-SCIOUS, TURNS BLUE, OR IS VERY PALE

○ IF SHE HAS DIFFICULTY BREATHING OR HER BREATHING IS VERY RAPID, OR IF SHE IS GRUNTING

○ IF SHE HAS ANY UNEXPLAINED BLEEDING FROM ANY PART OF HER BODY

○ IF SHE HAS A HIGH TEMPERATURE THAT DOES NOT COME DOWN AFTER YOU HAVE TAKEN MEASURES TO BRING IT DOWN (SEE BELOW)

○ IF SHE IS EXCEPTIONALLY HARD TO WAKE, UNUSUALLY DROWSY, OR DOES NOT SEEM TO KNOW YOU

Symptoms that may be serious

Other signs of illness, which are less urgent but might make you think about visiting or calling the doctor, are:

○ IF SHE HAS AN UNUSUALLY HOT OR COLD FOREHEAD

○ IF SHE IS OFF HER FOOD FOR MORE THAN ONE FEED

○ IF SHE HAS VOMITING AND DIARRHOEA (TINY BABIES QUICKLY BECOME DEHYDRATED)

○ IF HER CRYING SOUNDS UNUSUAL, OR IF SHE IS CRYING CONTINUOUSLY OR SCREAMING

○ IF SHE APPEARS LISTLESS AND DOES NOT SHOW THE USUAL SOCIAL RESPONSES TO YOU

○ IF SHE HAS ANY UNUSUAL WEIGHT LOSS

Even if you have consulted your GP, but your baby is not improving, tell him again the same day.

RECOGNIZING MENINGITIS The Hib immunization will protect your baby against the Hib form of meningitis, but not against the other forms of meningitis—meningococcal, pneumococcal, or viral. Recognizing meningitis early on, before the infection takes a hold on a young child, is extremely important, and it is worth being aware of some of the signs which often accompany meningitis. The early symptoms look much like flu, but the illness can develop very rapidly, and you should call your doctor if you are at all worried about your child's symptoms. Apart from the potential serious signs described above, you also need to look out for the following in young babies:

- ○ **GENERAL FRETFULNESS**
- ○ **REFUSING FEEDS**
- ○ **A HIGH-PITCHED, MOANING CRY**
- ○ **PALE OR BLOTCHY SKIN COLOUR**

An older child might also complain of the following:

- ○ **HEADACHE**
- ○ **STIFF NECK**
- ○ **PAINS IN THE JOINTS**
- ○ **INTOLERANCE TO BRIGHT LIGHTS**
- ○ **RASH OF REDDISH PURPLE SPOTS OR BRUISES**

As with all worrying illnesses in a baby or child, if you feel your doctor is not treating the problem seriously, trust to your own instincts and keep asking for help.

Lowering a baby's temperature

If your baby will not stay still long enough for you to take her temperature with a clinical thermometer, you can test her temperature by putting your lips to her forehead, or by using a strip thermometer (available from chemists).

If your baby has a fever, you need to lower her temperature, which will make her feel more comfortable and will reduce the risk of febrile convulsions. Convulsions may not be serious, but are extremely frightening. If your child has a convulsion, call your doctor then start to cool her down.

- ○ **REMOVE CLOTHES EXCEPT FOR A VEST AND NAPPY AND COVER HER WITH NOTHING BUT A SHEET.**
- ○ **LET THE ROOM TEMPERATURE DROP TO 65 °F IF IT IS HIGHER, BUT WITHOUT MAKING IT TOO DRAUGHTY FOR YOUR BABY.**

○ BREASTFEED HER TO KEEP UP HER FLUID INTAKE (OFFER WATER IF YOU ARE BOTTLEFEEDING AND IT IS NOT TIME FOR A FEED).

○ TRY GIVING HER PARACETAMOL SYRUP IF HER TEMPERATURE IS STILL HIGH AFTER ABOUT TWENTY MINUTES. ASK YOUR CHEMIST FOR A SPECIAL NON-SPILL SPOON OR DROPPER FOR GIVING MEDICINE TO SMALL BABIES. TRY TO AIM FOR THE BACK OF THE MOUTH OR YOU WILL HAVE A STICKY MESS ON THE BABY, ON YOU, AND ON THE FLOOR OR BED. CHILDREN SHOULD NOT BE GIVEN ASPIRIN IN ANY FORM.

○ SPONGE HER WITH TEPID WATER. USE WARM WATER AND SPONGE HER ALL OVER HER BODY, LEAVING THE WATER TO DRY OFF NATURALLY.

Emergency action

While waiting for a doctor or ambulance to arrive:

BABY NOT BREATHING

○ STIMULATE BABY BY FLICKING THE SOLES OF HER FEET OR PICKING HER UP. IF NO RESPONSE, BEGIN RESUSCITATION THROUGH HER MOUTH AND NOSE.

○ PLACE BABY ON HER BACK ON A TABLE OR OTHER FIRM SURFACE.

○ SUCK THE BABY'S NOSE CLEAR.

If baby does not gasp or breathe:

○ SUPPORT THE BACK OF HER NECK, TILT HER HEAD BACK-WARDS, AND HOLD HER CHIN UPWARDS.

○ OPEN YOUR MOUTH WIDE AND BREATHE IN.

○ SEAL YOUR LIPS AROUND HER MOUTH AND NOSE.

○ BREATHE GENTLY INTO HER LUNGS, USING ONLY THE BREATH YOU HOLD IN YOUR CHEEKS, UNTIL HER CHEST RISES.

○ REMOVE YOUR MOUTH TO ALLOW THE AIR TO COME OUT, AND LET HER CHEST FALL.

○ REPEAT GENTLE INFLATIONS, A LITTLE FASTER THAN YOUR NORMAL BREATHING RATE, REMOVING YOUR MOUTH AFTER EACH BREATH.

The baby should begin to breathe within a minute or so.

FITS OR CONVULSIONS

○ LAY BABY ON HER TUMMY WITH HER HEAD LOW AND TURNED TO ONE SIDE.

○ CLEAR HER MOUTH AND NOSE OF ANY SICK OR FROTH.
○ IF SHE IS HOT, COOL AS DESCRIBED ABOVE.

Burns or scalds

○ PUT THE BURNT OR SCALDED PART IMMEDIATELY IN COLD WATER; HOLD IT THERE FOR AS LONG AS POSSIBLE.
○ LIGHTLY COVER WITH A VERY CLEAN CLOTH OR STERILE DRESSING.
○ DO NOT APPLY OINTMENTS; DO NOT PRICK ANY BLISTERS.

In the event of an accident

○ IF YOU KNOW HOW, GIVE FIRST AID.
○ IF YOUR BABY HAS SWALLOWED PILLS, MEDICINES, OR HOUSEHOLD LIQUIDS, TAKE THE BOTTLE TO THE HOSPITAL AS WELL.

First Aid

It may be that you feel rather ignorant, and concerned that you might be helpless should an emergency arise. What about going on a First Aid course run by the Red Cross or St. John Ambulance? In some areas, too, the NHS paramedic teams will come out and run basic resuscitation courses for groups. Could you organize this through your local toddler group, school, or playschool, or through your local NCT branch? Even if you never have the need to use your skills, at least you will feel confident that you would know what to do in an emergency.

When you see the doctor

When you are worried about your baby, it can be hard to think what you need to know from your GP, or remember exactly what was said. If you find you have forgotten what was said at the surgery once you get home, do ring up your GP — he would rather you got it right than muddled through.

Ask your GP:

○ WHAT HE THINKS IS WRONG
○ WHAT THE TREATMENT IS
○ HOW LONG THE ILLNESS SHOULD LAST
○ HOW LONG THE TREATMENT SHOULD LAST
○ HOW LONG THE CHILD WILL BE INFECTIOUS, IF RELEVANT
○ WHAT WOULD INDICATE THAT THE CHILD IS GETTING WORSE
○ WHEN YOU SHOULD COME BACK TO SEE THE GP
○ IF ANY TREATMENT MIGHT CAUSE OTHER PROBLEMS, SUCH AS ANTIBIOTICS POSSIBLY CAUSING THRUSH

Preventing problems

If you have a baby who often seems to be catching colds or other infections, perhaps you could think about the amount she is exposed to infection. Do you have other children who bring infections home from school? Do you meet lots of other children at toddler groups or coffees who could be passing things on? Would it be worth keeping the baby away from other children (not your own of course) for a little while?

Is your house centrally heated, and so warm that bugs do not get killed off so easily in cold weather? Some fresh air in the house every day, even in the coldest weather, is a good idea, as is going out for walks. Fresh air is good for a healthy baby, but avoid draughts and make sure you keep her well wrapped up in cold weather, with a pram hood up if it is especially cold or windy. Keep her warm and out of draughts if she does have a cold or cough. If it is very hot, do not forget to use a sun-shade on the pram or push-chair.

If you are breastfeeding, is your own diet sufficiently full of the necessary vitamins and other nutrients to ensure good health for both of you?

Safety in the home

Tiny babies do not get into too much trouble, but they are often more mobile than you expect. They can roll off beds or changing areas easily; if you have to leave a baby somewhere, the safest place is usually the floor.

If you have a toddler who is rather unpredictable in his or her behaviour, it is wisest not to leave the two alone together in a room, even if it does mean you all have to go to the lavatory together.

If your baby sleeps in a Moses basket, or sits in a bouncing cradle, do not leave it up on a work surface; babies wriggle and can move their seats, or you might accidentally knock it off when passing.

Once your baby is older and more mobile, there will inevitably be lots of changes you will need to make to your home to make it safe. The trick is to stay one step ahead of your baby all the time; get down to her level and look for any potential objects of interest or danger. Use your imagination. It may help to invite a friend plus her slightly older baby or toddler to get some idea of what your baby will be into and up to next.

You may need to move everything she might get at:

- O **HOUSEHOLD CLEANERS**
- O **COSMETICS**
- O **MEDICINES**
- O **BREAKABLE ITEMS**
- O **ANYTHING YOU CARE ABOUT**
- O **POISONOUS HOUSEPLANTS**

○ **KETTLES**
○ **ELECTRICAL LEADS AND WIRES**
○ **HOT MUGS OF TEA**
○ **SAUCEPAN HANDLES**
○ **PETS' FOOD AND WATER BOWLS**
○ **CATS' LITTER TRAYS**

If necessary, shut doors or use gates and fire-guards to keep her away from stairs, steps, fires, garden pond, the road, etc. You can fix a cooker-top guard, and it is wise to turn saucepan handles sideways, and use back rings and burners on your cooker whenever possible.

COT DEATH

Cot death—or sudden infant death syndrome (SIDS), as it is also known—is a leading cause of death in babies aged between one month and one year. The vast majority of cot deaths occur between the first and sixth months. The term cot death is applied to any baby's death which is sudden and unexpected, and where no cause for the death can be found at the post-mortem examination.

Many parents are understandably fearful that, having come safely through pregnancy and birth with a healthy baby, they might then lose this baby for no apparent reason and with no warning. The very unexpected nature of a cot death, along with the fact that no clear reason may be found, can heighten parents' distress. For parents who have tragically suffered a cot death, this distress may also be increased by the fact that the police and coroner will have to be involved as the death is unexpected and sudden. However sympathetic and sensitive the various authorities may be, this is still an extra burden of formality for parents to cope with at an already difficult time.

The publicity given to this topic over the past few years has had a considerable effect in helping to raise awareness of the problem, and has also helped to lower the number of cot deaths occurring in the United Kingdom. Although no advice can guarantee protection from cot death, there are measures you can take to reduce the risk for your baby. There may well be more than one factor involved in many of the cot deaths, and experts suspect that in many cases several factors interact to put certain babies at risk. What you can do is to try and reduce as many of the known individual risk factors as possible.

○ **DO NOT SMOKE AND AVOID SMOKY ATMOSPHERES.**
○ **PLACE YOUR BABY ON HER BACK OR SIDE TO SLEEP.**
○ **DO NOT LET YOUR BABY GET TOO HOT.**
○ **IF YOU THINK YOUR BABY IS UNWELL, CONTACT YOUR DOCTOR.**
○ **BREASTFEED YOUR BABY.**

Reducing the risk

SMOKING   A mother who smokes during her pregnancy greatly increases the risk of her baby suffering a cot death. This is true not only for babies who have a low birth-weight because their mothers have smoked, but also for those who have a normal birth-weight. Babies whose parents smoke during the postnatal period are also at increased risk of cot death, so it makes sense not to subject your baby to any form of passive smoking.   If you do not smoke yourselves, but have friends or family who do, your new baby's health and safety may be an excellent reason for making your home a smoke-free zone.

SLEEPING   Sleeping positions for a tiny baby have already been discussed earlier in this chapter, but are worth repeating given the success of the 'Back to Sleep' campaign in reducing the cot-death figures. Babies placed on their backs or sides to sleep are far less likely to suffer a cot death than babies laid on their tummies. The reason for this has not been clearly established as yet, but whatever the reason, the evidence shows that it is safer for babies to sleep on their backs.

There has recently been some controversial research linking the use of fire-retardant chemicals in mattresses with cot death. This link appeared only when parents were using second-hand mattresses. The suggestion was that gases might be given off once a new baby's warmth caused a reaction between these chemicals and any moulds lingering in the mattress which had been stored. The results of this piece of research have not so far been duplicated and are dismissed by many medical authorities.   This dismissal has not necessarily reassured all parents intending to use a mattress more than once, however.   If you are at all worried, you can make sure any mattress you use is as clean and well aired as possible, and that you take care to reduce any other risk factors.   Laying your baby on her back to sleep and making sure she cannot overheat will lessen the chances of her being affected by anything in the mattress.

OVERHEATING   Babies who become overheated by being overwrapped or in a room with an excessively high room temperature are also at greater risk of cot death.   Overheating alone may well prove not to be a cause of cot death, but, in conjunction with other factors such as smoking, sleeping position, or infection, high temperatures can put a baby at extra risk because these may reduce her ability to lose excess heat.

Common sense is a useful guide here.   Babies do not need lots of layers of clothing plus duvets or blankets in centrally heated houses. They do not need the same amount of clothing and bedding inside as outside. Babies sleeping on their fronts with their faces buried cannot lose heat as effectively.   A fever will also reduce a baby's ability to lose heat, as will bedclothes covering her head, or simply too much clothing, too tightly wrapped. Of course, your baby does need to be protected from cold, but not to the extent of becoming overheated.

The Department of Health now recommends that you do not use pillows, duvets, or cot bumpers for babies under one year, and that you put your baby to sleep well down the cot or pram so that she has further to wriggle up her bed before her head becomes pressed against the sides.

ILLNESS As discussed earlier in this chapter, it is important to contact your doctor if you suspect your baby may be unwell. Most cot-death babies were apparently perfectly healthy before they died, and there is no suggestion that illness on its own is a risk factor in cot deaths. Some cot-death babies, however, have been found to have signs of minor infections or illnesses. It is worthwhile checking with your doctor if your baby shows any signs or symptoms of illness as described in the section, 'When Your Baby is Ill'. Simply being alert for any unusual behaviour or signs in your baby will mean one potential risk factor reduced.

BREASTFEEDING Although studies are as yet inconclusive about the value of breastfeeding as a specific risk reduction factor in cot death, there are so many benefits of breastfeeding that it is a useful addition to this list. Apart from the fact that breastfed babies are less likely to suffer infections anyway, breastfeeding encourages a speedier recovery after infection. Above all, it is a positive step you can take towards caring for your baby, and will help you feel that you are taking all possible preventative measures.

As with all tragedies, parents whose baby has died suddenly and unexpectedly will inevitably ask themselves, 'What if . . .'. At least by taking as many of these preventative measures as possible, you will be doing your best to take sensible avoiding action.

Looking after a baby is very hard work; there is more to think about and take into consideration than ever before. If this is your first baby, you may find it all very strange in the beginning. With a second or subsequent baby you may feel unbelievably tired looking after an energetic toddler or child, as well as a new baby. Gradually, you will get used to it; babies do learn to do things for themselves little by little, and, if it is hard in the early weeks, think about what you can leave undone while you do the essentials of caring for yourself and your baby.

The things that seemed so difficult in the beginning, when you felt all fingers and thumbs, or were constantly worried by what every cry, every change in your baby's normal pattern, might mean, will soon become second nature, until you are able to sit back and enjoy every minute with her, confident in your handling of her.

- *I found it quite frightening actually. There I was, responsible for this tiny baby and I hadn't the faintest idea what was the 'proper' way to do it!*

- *I kept worrying that she was too warm, too cold; sleeping too long, feeding too often; I was picking her up too much, letting her cry too long, etc. Eventually I relaxed and stopped being obsessed and did what felt about right.*

- *Beforehand we had thought we would fall into a routine after a few days. That was our first misconception. It took something like four months before any sort of pattern or routine showed itself.*

- *It was unbelievable. Every time I put a decent set of clothes on myself or the baby, either she was sick on both of us, or my breasts leaked within ten minutes.*

- *My mother kept telling me to put him in his pram in the garden straight after his feed and change. Well, I didn't take any notice — we used to cuddle up on the sofa after a breastfeed. He would lie on my chest and we'd have a doze together. After a while, I gave up worrying about my mother's disapproval, and she gave up telling me I was doing it all wrong.*

Looking After Yourself

27

These early weeks with a new baby are immensely exciting and challenging, but the inevitable change in your life means that this will be a stressful time too. Any change in life, however positive, takes a lot of energy during the period of adjustment. Once you have a new baby you are adapting to the added responsibility of your new roles as parents; to the fact of having a new person in your family; to a different financial situation; you are coping with any changes in your own relationship and relationships with other family members, and all this on top of disturbed, sleepless nights! For you as a new mother, at home with your new baby, busy juggling the needs of your baby, your partner, and your other children as well as looking after your home, it can be very easy to forget yourself.

STRESS

If you are finding life with your baby particularly difficult or stressful, finding that there are more 'lows' than 'highs' in your day, it can help to know something about stress and how you can deal with it.

Stress can be described as an imbalance between the demands being made on you and your perceived ability to cope with these demands. There are many factors which will influence how you respond to certain situations, such as your personality, your past experience, or lack of it, the information you do or do not have about the situation, and any additional demands on you at this time. Some of these factors can be changed; others cannot.

STRESS RESPONSE The body's stress response is geared to coping with situations of real danger, so it causes a change in the nervous and hormonal systems which make our bodies deal with the danger. This is known as the 'fight or flight response'. In other situations, however, if we perceive that the demands on us are greater than our ability to cope with them, our bodies may also switch into the stress response. If this response continues over a prolonged period of time, then real health problems may eventually ensue.

Stress response	Relaxation response
raised blood pressure	lowered blood pressure
faster heart rate	slower heart rate
increased breathing rate	slower breathing rate
muscle tension	reduced muscle tension

SIGNS OF STRESS Signs of stress may include:

- O **HEADACHES**
- O **ACHING SHOULDERS OR FACE DUE TO MUSCLE TENSION**
- O **POOR APPETITE**
- O **DISTURBED SLEEP PATTERNS**
- O **DIFFICULTY IN CONCENTRATING**
- O **WORRY**
- O **ANXIETY**
- O **FRUSTRATION**
- O **FREQUENT FEELINGS OF IRRITATION AND ANGER**

It is important to be able to recognize these signs as they are developing and to know what you can do to get things back on to an even keel.

An ABC of managing stress

AWARENESS Identify your own signs of stress, and also those situations which cause you to feel stressed.

BALANCE Discover your own optimum stress level — one which is enough for stimulation and motivation, but does not leave you feeling overloaded; learn to say 'no'.

CONTROL Combining awareness and balance can lead to a feeling of greater self-responsibility and control of your own life, so you feel better all round.

You may find the following suggestions helpful in minimizing stress levels in your life:

- O **TALK IT OUT:**   **SHARE IT WITH SOMEONE.**
- O **WRITE IT OUT:**   **HELP GET THINGS IN PERSPECTIVE.**
- O **BREATHE IT AWAY:** **USE YOUR RELAXATION AND BREATHING TECHNIQUES.**
- O **SORT IT OUT:**   **MAKE LISTS OF YOUR PRIORITIES AND PRACTICAL OPTIONS.**
- O **WORK IT OFF:**   **DO SOMETHING ENERGETIC AND PHYSICAL.**

○ **LAUGH IT OFF:**	**TRY TO LIGHTEN THE SITUATION; SINGING CAN HELP.**	
○ **DISTANCE IT:**	**TRY TO IMAGINE THINGS SOME MONTHS OR YEARS FROM NOW.**	
○ **BALANCE IT:**	**TRY THINKING OF SOME POSITIVE ASPECTS.**	
○ **HOLD IT:**	**STOP, PAUSE, THINK, AND TAKE A FRESH LOOK.**	
○ **WIN THROUGH:**	**IMAGINE YOURSELF BEING SUCCESSFUL, COMING THROUGH THE OTHER SIDE!**	

It is unrealistic to expect yourself to be able to cope with all the things you used to do around the house as well as look after a baby, plus managing with less sleep than you have had in years. If you and your partner can work out some plan of action, you may be able to relax a little about any chores that are not getting done. Many people believe now that fatigue and feelings of inadequacy are major contributory factors towards postnatal depression, so recognizing your capabilities and limitations early on may be very important to you and your baby's well-being. Try to find even a few minutes each day to do something you enjoy that is just for you and that you know will make you feel better.

DIET

A healthy, balanced diet is essential for all new mothers, whether they are breastfeeding or bottlefeeding. Even if you are short of time, you should not skimp your own meals. This can add to your feelings of tiredness and depression so should really be avoided. Eating regularly every two or three hours during the day will help to keep your blood-sugar level more constant, and this in turn may keep depression at bay, leaving you better able to cope with whatever crops up. Sugary snacks, however tempting, are best avoided, because they raise blood-sugar levels too rapidly and cause a subsequent dip in levels, worse than before. Fresh fruit (particularly bananas), dried fruit, a wholemeal cheese sandwich, or a glass of milk and some crackers are all more beneficial in the long run, though there is no reason why you should not enjoy the occasional sweet snack as well. It may not be as healthy and nutritionally valuable, but the odd slice of a chocolate bar or cake is not the end of the world. See Chapter 6, Looking After Yourself, for details of a healthy, balanced diet.

REST AND RELAXATION

Both partners may be finding it hard to cope if nights are very disturbed. If you were working in a job which required you to be awake at night, you would probably sleep during the day to make up for the lost sleep, but many parents who are losing sleep at nights, maybe for many months, expect to be able to carry on as before during the day. You need to work out a solution that suits you both. This may involve mum coping with the baby at nights during the week, and dad taking the baby and any other children out at the weekend leaving mum time to catch up on lost sleep. You may find you both need to bring your usual bedtime forward an hour or two for a while. It is also important that a new mother finds some time during the day to rest, and is realistic about what she can achieve in a day. Relaxation techniques that you learned antenatally can be a great help in keeping muscle tension at bay, and a quick relaxation is particularly restorative and restful postnatally. With practice, you will soon learn to relax anywhere — driving, feeding the baby, washing-up, watching television, and when trying to get back to sleep after being disturbed.

Babies excel at picking up signals from their parents. If you are feeling tense, the chances are that your baby will pick up those feelings and may be more fretful as a result; but if you practise relaxation with her, you can pass on those positive messages to her.

YOUR POSTNATAL CHECK

About six weeks after the birth of your baby you will need to visit your GP or the hospital for a postnatal check-up. This is to ensure that your body is returning to normal following the many changes of pregnancy and birth, so that any problems may be dealt with.

If you have had a Caesarean section, if yours was a particularly difficult delivery, or if your baby was stillborn, then you will probably have to see the consultant or registrar at the hospital.

This appointment should be an opportunity for you and your partner to ask any questions that may still be concerning you about your delivery. You may not be entirely clear as to the reason for your Caesarean or instrumental delivery, and it is helpful to discuss it with the people who were involved with the decision at the time.

If your baby died, it is important that you have an opportunity to talk through your feelings about the labour and how you are coping with your loss as well as having your general health checked.

DISCUSSION Whether you see your GP or the consultant, the postnatal check should include an opportunity to discuss how your labour progressed, how your baby is settling into the family, and how her feeding is going. Some GPs will include the baby's six-week check at the same time.

You will probably be asked if your periods have resumed yet; if you have thought about the various methods of contraception; if you still have any discharge from the vagina; if any stitches you had, or your Caesarean-section wound, are fully healed. You should also be asked if you have any particular problems you would like to discuss. It is useful to have thought about what you would like to discuss with the doctor and perhaps make a note of everything in case you forget.

PHYSICAL CHECK There will also be a general examination, including blood pressure, a urine test, an internal examination, and possibly a cervical smear test if you have not recently had one. Some doctors do include a check of your abdominal and pelvic-floor muscles, but not all do this, and this might be something you would like to ask for. You should certainly discuss with the doctor any problems such as stress incontinence, or if you feel your abdominal muscles are not coming together as they should. Now is a good time to sort out any problems or difficulties, however shy or embarrassed you may feel talking about 'difficult' topics.

SEX AFTER CHILDBIRTH

Resuming sex

There are many physical and emotional factors which govern how men and women feel about sex after childbirth, which can only be touched upon here. The sense of having shared the making of this baby as a couple can be very powerful, and many couples do find this feeling of sharing and closeness continues throughout parenthood. Others, however, find that the baby becomes the focus of so much attention that it is difficult to find time for themselves. The very closeness with the baby can also lead to a couple finding sufficient sensual fulfilment in feeding and handling the baby, so that their normal sexual relationship returns only gradually. What matters is that you should both feel happy about the relationship you are enjoying, and not feel pressurized into anything which does not feel quite right for you. Whatever you decide to do, make sure you talk to each other about your feelings, and try to make time to nourish your own relationship as partners while you are finding out about your new relationship as parents.

Traditionally, women have expected to wait until the 'all-clear' from their doctors at the six-week postnatal check before resuming love-making. You may, however, find that you feel ready for sex very soon after the birth, well before the six weeks are up. This is fine, though you will need to give some thought to the matter of contraception.

SORENESS Making love after childbirth can be pretty uncomfortable and you may feel reluctant to make any attempts for several weeks. You may feel that your body needs time to recover, especially if you have had stitches or piles which have been causing soreness and pain. If you are still feeling hesitant, or if you find that your vagina feels rather sore and tight, it may help to use a lubricant such as K-Y jelly or contraceptive cream both in the vagina and smoothed on to your partner's penis before penetration. The hormonal changes which occur during breastfeeding may well mean that you are not producing the same amount of vaginal lubrication as usual, and you may need to continue using extra lubrication for many weeks and months. It also helps to make sure that you are fully aroused before penetration takes place, and it is important to find the most comfortable angle of entry which does not rub any sore spots.

CAESAREAN SCARS If you have had a Caesarean section, the scar may be tender for quite some time, so you will need to find positions which avoid any pressure on it. Some of the suggestions for sex during pregnancy may also be useful (see Chapter 8, Sex in Pregnancy). You may be anxious that your scar has made you less attractive than before; this is something you need to discuss with your partner, rather than keeping your worries to yourself.

THE PELVIC FLOOR You or your partner may be concerned that your vagina will have been irrevocably stretched during birth, resulting in less pleasurable sex for both of you. The vaginal walls actually return to their normal size very soon after the delivery, but the pelvic-floor muscles may be weakened. Doing your pelvic-floor exercises will strengthen your muscles and encourage them to return to their pre-pregnant state.

BREASTFEEDING You may find the physical and emotional aspects of breastfeeding totally satisfying and have little desire for sex. The hormonal changes involved in breastfeeding are responsible for this, though some women do say they feel drained by breastfeeding, and have no energy left for sex. Either of you may feel that the breasts somehow 'belong to the baby' and that they are no longer sexual. This usually stops once the baby has been weaned or is no longer so dependent on breastfeeding for her nourishment.

You may find that breastfeeding enhances your sense of yourself as a sexual person and that you wish to make love more than you had expected. You will find further discussion of the effects of breastfeeding on sex, and vice versa, in Chapter 24, Feeding your Baby.

The effects on sex of being a parent

The demands of being a parent can be quite overwhelming at times, so much so that an extra half-hour's sleep, or some time to yourself, can come to seem infinitely preferable to making love. Feeling simply too tired to make love is a normal and understandable reaction in these early days with your new baby. The more both partners can share in the ordinary household chores and the care of the baby, the more time you will both have for yourselves and each other, and the more sex will begin to seem like a pleasurable option.

Some babies seem determined to wake up every time one of you even thinks about sex, so that you have either to try to make love in unaccustomed silence or to give up your attempts in order to pacify your screaming baby. Some babies choose to wait until orgasm is approaching before waking up, which is equally frustrating.

If your baby is sharing your room, you may decide to make love elsewhere for a few months, or choose instead to move the baby. Trying to find occasions for love-making when your baby is not likely to be needing a feed, and is probably going to sleep for some while, may become a rather fraught exercise, especially if your baby is one who enjoys her wakeful time during the evening, as so many do.

If your baby will sleep on regardless, you might move her or yourselves, or you may decide to stay in the same room or bed; do whatever feels comfortable for you.

You may well find that the experience of becoming parents offers you a golden opportunity to explore different ways and means of making love, in the same way that pregnancy can. The important thing is to tell each other what works and what does not, to talk over any problems, and to try different approaches. If you can both be open to change, can allow plenty of time for adjustment to your new roles, and are prepared to explain your needs and feelings to each other, your sexual relationship can be stronger and more exciting as a result of your baby's birth.

Contraception

It is worth considering the form of contraception you wish to use before the birth, as there may be too much else to think about once your baby has arrived. There is no really ideal form of contraception available, so you will have to make the most of those choices that are on offer.

It is possible to become pregnant again very soon after giving birth, which may not be in your scheme of things. Breastfeeding on an unrestricted basis certainly reduces the likelihood of a pregnancy occurring, but you may prefer not to rely on this. Women vary as to when their periods start again; some will menstruate before the six-week check, while others may not menstruate until they stop breastfeeding or until the baby starts solid foods. If this is your first baby, you will not know what your body's pattern is. Ovulation may occur either before or after the first period, and, unless you have clear indications from your body that you are ovulating, you will not know which comes first for you.

THE PILL The Pill is a reliable form of contraception, but you may prefer not to take it while breastfeeding. Low-dose progestogen-only pills have the least effect on milk supply, but may nevertheless affect the quality of milk you produce, and can make you feel depressed. The combined Pill can affect both quality and quantity.

It is not yet known what effect taking the Pill whilst breastfeeding might have on the long-term health of the baby.

INTRA-UTERINE DEVICE An intra-uterine device (IUD or coil) cannot be fitted until at least eight weeks after the birth, and many doctors prefer to wait until three months. If you wish to have an IUD fitted, you will need to think about some other form of contraception in the meantime.

CAP A cap can normally be fitted at about six weeks, and most women need a different size from the one they were using before the pregnancy. As your body and your weight may continue to change for some months after the birth, you should remember to have the cap checked within a few months.

CONDOMS Many couples find condoms a useful form of contraception, if only for a short while after having a baby.

NATURAL METHODS If you are interested in using a natural form of contraception, involving an observation of your body's rhythms, it is a good idea to contact someone who can teach you precisely how to use this method most effectively (see Chapter 1, Beginning a Pregnancy, for information on natural methods for achieving or avoiding pregnancy). Your local Family Planning Service should be able to give you details on this and on all methods of contraception.

POSTNATAL EXERCISES

The child-bearing years are a time when many women find themselves more in tune with their bodies than they have ever been previously. It can be a time of discovering how good exercise can be for both physical and emotional well-being. If your baby has been born in hospital, you may be advised by the physiotherapist about which exercises you need to help regain the strength in your weakened pelvic-floor and abdominal muscles. It is important to do these exercises regularly before joining any exercise class. Your baby will probably lie on a blanket on the floor beside you, watching you while you exercise, and, as she gets older, there are exercises you can do with her.

The hormonal changes which affect your joints and ligaments during pregnancy will last for three or five months following the birth of your baby. Because of this, you will need to remember the following when exercising:

○ **START APPROPRIATE EXERCISES AS SOON AS POSSIBLE AFTER THE BIRTH AND REPEAT THEM OFTEN.**

○ **WORK AT YOUR OWN PACE AND NOT TO THE POINT OF
   EXHAUSTION; LISTEN TO YOUR BODY.**

○ **DO NOT EXERCISE WHEN YOU ARE TIRED OR ILL.**

○ **CHECK YOUR POSTURE, ESPECIALLY WHEN EXERCISING,
   LIFTING, CARRYING, FEEDING YOUR BABY, AND PERFORM-
   ING EVERYDAY TASKS.**

○ **NEVER TRY TO STRENGTHEN YOUR ABDOMINAL MUSCLES
   BY LYING FLAT ON YOUR BACK WITH YOUR FEET HELD
   DOWN DOING SIT-UPS, AS THIS WILL CAUSE YOUR
   HIP FLEXOR MUSCLES TO WORK AND CAN CAUSE STRAIN
   ON THE BACK IF YOUR ABDOMINAL MUSCLES ARE VERY
   WEAK.**

○ **NEVER LIE FLAT ON YOUR BACK AND LIFT BOTH LEGS IN
   THE AIR. THIS IS NOT STRICTLY AN ABDOMINAL EXERCISE
   AND CAN BE POTENTIALLY DANGEROUS FOR A RECENTLY
   DELIVERED MOTHER WHOSE LIGAMENTS AND MUSCLES ARE
   STILL LAX AND WEAK.**

THE FIRST SIX WEEKS

CHECKING YOUR ABDOMINAL MUSCLES You will need to check that
your abdominal muscles which stretched and separated as your
pregnancy advanced (see p. 71) are returning to normal a few days
after the birth and to keep checking them until you are sure they
have returned to normal. To check this, you must make the muscles
work strongly. You will need to do exercises to strengthen the
muscles.

*The
abdominal
muscles*

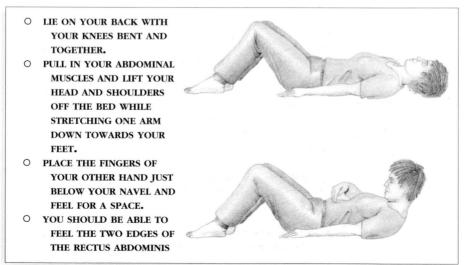

○ **LIE ON YOUR BACK WITH
   YOUR KNEES BENT AND
   TOGETHER.**

○ **PULL IN YOUR ABDOMINAL
   MUSCLES AND LIFT YOUR
   HEAD AND SHOULDERS
   OFF THE BED WHILE
   STRETCHING ONE ARM
   DOWN TOWARDS YOUR
   FEET.**

○ **PLACE THE FINGERS OF
   YOUR OTHER HAND JUST
   BELOW YOUR NAVEL AND
   FEEL FOR A SPACE.**

○ **YOU SHOULD BE ABLE TO
   FEEL THE TWO EDGES OF
   THE RECTUS ABDOMINIS**

MUSCLES AS FIRM RIDGES ON EITHER SIDE OF YOUR
NAVEL, AND HAVE A SPACE AT LEAST TWO FINGERS
WIDE BETWEEN THEM. (SOME PEOPLE MAY HAVE A GAP
OF ABOUT 4–5 FINGERS WIDE INITIALLY.)
O   AS YOUR MUSCLES IMPROVE IN STRENGTH, THE GAP
SHOULD NARROW UNTIL IT IS SO SMALL THAT IT IS
ONLY ABOUT THE WIDTH OF THE TIP OF ONE OF YOUR
FINGERS.

LEG SLIDING

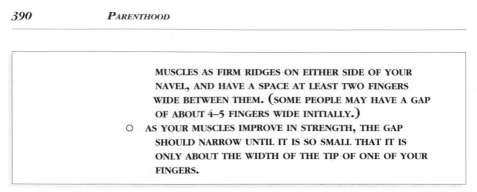

O   LIE WITH YOUR KNEES
BENT AND TOGETHER.
O   AS YOU DID FOR PELVIC
ROCKING, BREATHE
OUT, PULL IN YOUR
ABDOMINAL MUSCLES,
AND PRESS THE SMALL
OF YOUR BACK
AGAINST THE BED.
O   HOLD YOUR BACK ON
THE BED AND SLIDE
YOUR LEGS AWAY
FROM YOU AS FAR AS
YOU CAN.
O   AS SOON AS YOUR BACK STARTS TO ARCH OFF THE BED,
RETURN TO THE STARTING POSITION, BREATHE IN, AND
REPEAT AGAIN.

Initially, when your muscles are very weak, you will not be able to
slide the legs very far without your back coming off the bed.

O   REPEAT SIX TIMES, GRADUALLY INCREASING TO FIFTEEN.

CURL-UPS

O   LIE ON YOUR BACK WITH YOUR KNEES BENT.
O   BREATHE IN, AND, AS YOU BREATHE OUT, PULL IN YOUR
ABDOMINAL MUSCLES.

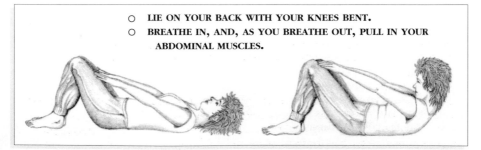

○ **TUCK YOUR CHIN ON TO YOUR CHEST, AND, SLIDING YOUR HANDS UP YOUR THIGHS TOWARDS YOUR KNEES, LIFT YOUR HEAD AND SHOULDERS AS HIGH AS YOU CAN OFF THE BED.**
○ **HOLD FOR A COUNT OF FOUR AND THEN SLOWLY LOWER.**
○ **REPEAT SIX TIMES, GRADUALLY INCREASING TO FIFTEEN.**

The pelvic floor

You will need to go back and re-read the section on pelvic-floor exercises in Chapter 6, Looking After Yourself, to refresh your memory about their importance and how to do them.

Many women feel unsure about how to do the pelvic-floor exercises correctly, and may be afraid of doing damage if that area is already bruised, swollen, and painful following delivery because of an episiotomy or tear. Starting the exercises as soon as possible after delivery will not only improve the circulation so that the healing processes are speeded up but will make the whole area feel more comfortable. Do these exercises little and often throughout the day. If, when you get home, you find it difficult to remember to do them, linking them with regular activities during the day, as before, is helpful. Some people find it helpful to place those little coloured-dot stickers you buy from a stationer's in strategic places around the house, or even on their watch face, as a constant reminder. You do not have to tell anyone else why you have got green dots on the fridge, the telephone, or the bathroom mirror — unless, of course, you want to!

As well as checking you are using the right muscles by stopping your flow of urine mid-stream, you can enlist your partner's help when you are making love. Squeeze your vagina tightly round his penis, and then ask if he can feel that. If he says, 'Feel what?' you have some more work to do!

Stress incontinence If, in common with many women, you find you are 'leaky' after giving birth, this is a problem which can nearly always be cleared up by exercise, without the need for an operation. It is essential to tighten your pelvic-floor muscles regularly, particularly before lifting anything, and before doing any exercises, especially running and jumping.

Once you feel you have control over your pelvic floor when you are sitting down or standing still, you can learn to have control when you are on the move. Vigorous breast-stroke swimming helps to strengthen your pelvic-floor muscles too.

If you suspect you may have any problems with your bladder or your pelvic floor, do go to see your GP. The problem will not go away of its own accord.

Back care and posture

Your posture, which is largely controlled by reflexes, can also be affected by other factors — for example, depression and tiredness, weight change, and weakened muscles. During pregnancy, the changes which occurred to your posture were gradual; the increasing weight of the baby and uterus gradually altered your centre of gravity. The changes following your baby's birth tend to be more rapid. Your body has some re-adjusting to do as you get used to your new weight, an altered centre of gravity, weakened and stretched muscles, and enlarged breasts. It can, in the first few days, seem as if you are inhabiting someone else's body as it all feels so unfamiliar. Correcting your posture at this time is as important as strengthening muscles and protecting joints. Muscles and joints can remain in incorrect alignment causing discomfort and possibly long-term joint changes if you do not.

Backache is one of the most common problems encountered in the early months following the birth. The joint laxity due to hormonal changes makes you very vulnerable to strain, so it is important that you protect your back during everyday activities and exercise the back and abdominal muscles so that they return to full strength. Carrying the baby and sitting in a poor position to feed her can also cause fatigue and discomfort in the muscles of the lower back and thoracic region (upper chest). Mothers who have had an epidural anaesthetic during labour may experience back problems and will need to take extra care.

PELVIC ROCKING Pelvic rocking (see p. 77) is a very useful exercise with which you will be familiar from your antenatal preparation. It can help ease backache and the discomfort of post-Caesarean wind problems as well as being important in maintaining good posture.

LOWER BACK AND BUTTOCKS EXERCISE

○ LIE ON YOUR FRONT ON THE FLOOR, HEAD RESTING ON YOUR HANDS.

○ PLACE TWO PILLOWS, ONE UNDER YOUR WAIST, ONE UNDER YOUR HEAD, WITH A GAP FOR YOUR BREASTS IF THEY ARE TENDER.

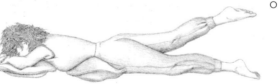

○ LIFT ONE LEG, KEEPING IT STRAIGHT, KEEPING YOUR HIPS ON THE FLOOR AND WITHOUT ALLOWING THE PELVIS TO TWIST SIDEWAYS.

○ BREATHE OUT AS YOU LIFT.

○ HOLD FOR A COUNT OF FOUR AND LOWER TO THE FLOOR.

○ REPEAT WITH THE OTHER LEG.

○ IF THIS CAUSES DISCOMFORT IN THE LOWER BACK, TRY PUTTING ANOTHER PILLOW UNDER YOUR WAIST.

○ TRY THIS SIX TIMES WITH EACH LEG, PROGRESSING TO TWELVE, ALWAYS ALTERNATING LEGS. (DO NOT LIFT

BOTH LEGS TOGETHER AT THIS STAGE, AS IT IS PROBABLY
TOO STRENUOUS.)

SIDE BENDS

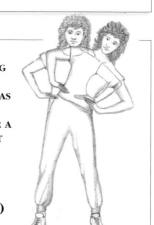

○ STAND WITH YOUR FEET APART, HANDS ON HIPS.
○ SLOWLY AND SMOOTHLY BEND TO THE LEFT, KEEPING
YOUR HIPS STEADY AND FACING FORWARDS WITH
YOUR FEET FLAT ON THE FLOOR, BREATHING OUT AS
YOU BEND SIDEWAYS.
○ MOVE AS FAR AS YOU COMFORTABLY CAN, HOLD FOR A
FEW SECONDS, AND THEN RETURN TO THE UPRIGHT
POSITION, BREATHING IN.
○ REPEAT ON THE OTHER SIDE.
○ DO NOT BOUNCE TO INCREASE THE MOVEMENT AND
DO NOT BEND FORWARDS OR BACKWARDS. (THIS
EXERCISE CAN ALSO BE DONE SITTING ON A CHAIR.)
○ DO THIS 6–12 TIMES EACH SIDE.

TRUNK, KNEE, AND HIP BENDS

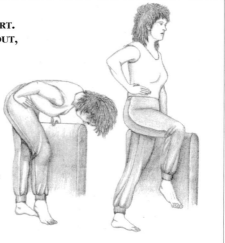

○ STAND TALL, FEET ABOUT 18" APART.
○ PLACE HANDS ON A CHAIR FOR SUPPORT.
○ BREATHE IN, AND, AS YOU BREATHE OUT,
CURL YOUR HEAD DOWN, CURVING
THE SPINE SO THAT THE HEAD IS
LOW.
○ RAISE ONE KNEE TOWARDS YOUR
HEAD.
○ RETURN TO THE START POSITION
AND REPEAT WITH THE OTHER LEG.
THE SUPPORTING LEG SHOULD NOT
BE HELD STIFFLY AND THE MOVE-
MENT SHOULD BE SMOOTH AND NOT
JERKY. DO NOT BRING THE KNEE
TOO HIGH, AS THIS LIMITS THE
MOVEMENT IN THE BACK.
○ DO 6–12 BENDS.

HEAD, TRUNK, AND ARMS ROTATING

○ SIT ON A STOOL WITH HANDS AND ARMS REACHING
DIRECTLY FORWARD AT SHOULDER HEIGHT.
○ KEEP YOUR SHOULDERS RELAXED AND NOT HUNCHED UP TO
YOUR EARS.
○ TURN YOUR HEAD, ARMS, AND SHOULDERS AROUND TO

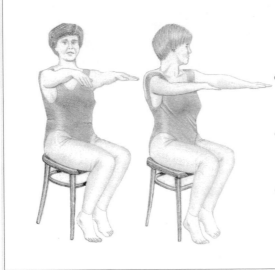

ONE SIDE, BENDING THE
FRONT ARM ACROSS YOUR
CHEST. YOUR HIPS
SHOULD FACE FORWARD
AND SHOULD NOT TWIST.

o HOLD THIS FOR A FEW
   SECONDS, RETURN TO THE
   MIDDLE, AND REPEAT ON
   THE OTHER SIDE.

o YOU SHOULD BREATHE OUT
   AS YOU ROTATE, AND
   BREATHE IN AS YOU
   RETURN TO THE CENTRE.

o DO THIS 6–12 TIMES TO
   EACH SIDE.

SIX WEEKS TO THREE MONTHS

You will probably find that you are able to make more time for
your exercises now, as you get to know your baby and her
sleeping and feeding patterns better. It is important to progress
your exercises as you grow stronger. This is done by increasing
the load on the muscles:

O BY INCREASING THE NUMBER OF TIMES YOU PERFORM A
   CERTAIN EXERCISE.
O BY INCREASING THE FREQUENCY WITH WHICH YOU
   PERFORM THE EXERCISE DURING THE WEEK.
O BY INCREASING THE INTENSITY OF THE EXERCISE, E.G.
   BY CHANGING THE WAY YOU DO THE EXERCISE TO
   INCREASE THE RESISTANCE AND MAKE THE MUSCLES
   WORK HARDER.

Additional
abdominal
exercises

Continue to use the back exercises like side bends, hip, knee,
and trunk bends, and arm, shoulder, and back rotating as a
warm-up before doing the other exercises. Your pelvic-floor
exercises should be continued on a daily basis too, even if there
is no apparent problem. The ultimate check for pelvic-floor-
muscle strength is to jump up in the air and cough with a slightly
full bladder and see whether your pants stay dry. If they do not,
you need to be doing your pelvic-floor exercises more often, but
do check first that you are doing them correctly (see p. 79).

CURL-UPS

Do your curl-ups to about 45 ° off the floor, as on p. 390, but with arms folded across your chest instead of stretched out in front of you. Be careful not to jerk to get up. If you cannot perform the movement smoothly, it is probably still too strong an exercise for you, so go back to the original curl-ups. Do this exercise six to fifteen times.

DIAGONAL CURL-UPS

- ○ LIE ON THE FLOOR, WITH KNEES BENT AND ARMS BY YOUR SIDE.
- ○ PULL IN YOUR ABDOMINAL MUSCLES FIRMLY AS YOU BREATHE OUT, TUCK YOUR CHIN ON TO YOUR CHEST, AND REACH ACROSS WITH YOUR RIGHT HAND TO TOUCH YOUR LEFT KNEE.
- ○ HOLD FOR A COUNT OF FOUR AND LOWER, THEN REPEAT ON THE OTHER SIDE.
- ○ REPEAT SIX TIMES TO EACH SIDE, PROGRESSING TO FIFTEEN.

CURL-DOWNS

- ○ SIT UP STRAIGHT WITH KNEES BENT AND ARMS STRETCHED OUT IN FRONT OF YOU.
- ○ LET YOUR BACK ROUND AS YOU PULL IN YOUR ABDOMINAL MUSCLES, TIP THE PUBIC BONE UP TOWARDS YOUR NAVEL, AND SLOWLY CURL DOWN TOWARDS THE FLOOR AS YOU BREATHE OUT.
- ○ IT IS VERY IMPORTANT NOT TO HAVE YOUR BACK HELD STRAIGHT — IT REALLY IS A **CURL-DOWN.**
- ○ WHEN YOU REACH HALF-WAY, HOLD IT FOR A COUNT OF FOUR AND THEN SLOWLY RETURN TO THE UPRIGHT POSITION. YOUR MUSCLES SHOULD NOT BE SHAKING WHEN YOU HOLD FOR THE COUNT OF FOUR.
- ○ DO THIS 6–15 TIMES.

ARM-, SHOULDER-, AND CHEST-STRENGTHENING EXERCISES

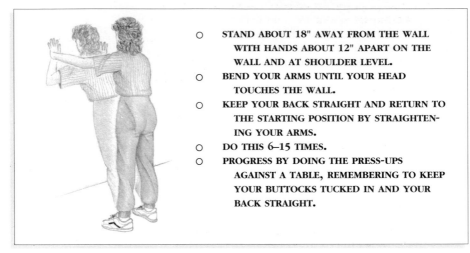

- ○ STAND ABOUT 18" AWAY FROM THE WALL WITH HANDS ABOUT 12" APART ON THE WALL AND AT SHOULDER LEVEL.
- ○ BEND YOUR ARMS UNTIL YOUR HEAD TOUCHES THE WALL.
- ○ KEEP YOUR BACK STRAIGHT AND RETURN TO THE STARTING POSITION BY STRAIGHTENING YOUR ARMS.
- ○ DO THIS 6–15 TIMES.
- ○ PROGRESS BY DOING THE PRESS-UPS AGAINST A TABLE, REMEMBERING TO KEEP YOUR BUTTOCKS TUCKED IN AND YOUR BACK STRAIGHT.

LEG-STRENGTHENING EXERCISES

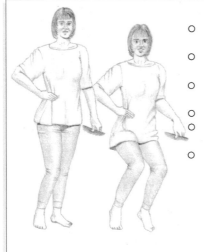

- ○ STAND TALL, FEET HIP-WIDTH APART, AND WITH ONE HAND RESTING ON A CHAIR.
- ○ GO UP ON YOUR TOES AND THEN BEND YOUR KNEES TO A SEMI-SQUAT.
- ○ STRAIGHTEN YOUR KNEES AND RETURN YOUR HEELS TO THE FLOOR.
- ○ DO THIS 6–15 TIMES.
- ○ PROGRESS BY REMOVING THE SUPPORT OF THE CHAIR.
- ○ YOU COULD ALSO DO THIS EXERCISE WITH YOUR BABY IN YOUR ARMS TO ADD RESISTANCE, BUT USE A WALL BEHIND YOUR BACK FOR SUPPORT.

BACK AND BUTTOCK EXERCISES

- ○ KNEEL ON ALL-FOURS.
- ○ BRING YOUR RIGHT KNEE TOWARDS YOUR HEAD, PULLING YOUR ABDOMINAL MUSCLES IN AT THE SAME TIME.
- ○ THEN STRETCH THAT LEG STRAIGHT OUT BEHIND YOU, FEELING YOUR BUTTOCKS TIGHTEN AS YOU DO SO.

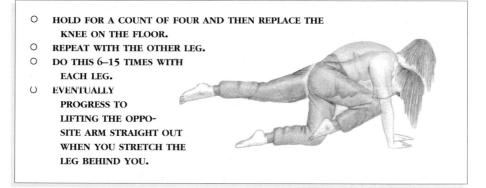

- HOLD FOR A COUNT OF FOUR AND THEN REPLACE THE KNEE ON THE FLOOR.
- REPEAT WITH THE OTHER LEG.
- DO THIS 6–15 TIMES WITH EACH LEG.
- EVENTUALLY PROGRESS TO LIFTING THE OPPO-SITE ARM STRAIGHT OUT WHEN YOU STRETCH THE LEG BEHIND YOU.

HIP-HITCHING

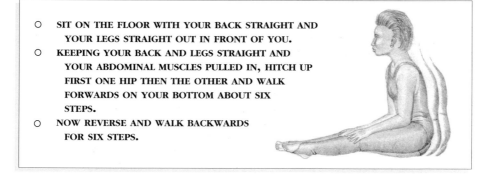

- SIT ON THE FLOOR WITH YOUR BACK STRAIGHT AND YOUR LEGS STRAIGHT OUT IN FRONT OF YOU.
- KEEPING YOUR BACK AND LEGS STRAIGHT AND YOUR ABDOMINAL MUSCLES PULLED IN, HITCH UP FIRST ONE HIP THEN THE OTHER AND WALK FORWARDS ON YOUR BOTTOM ABOUT SIX STEPS.
- NOW REVERSE AND WALK BACKWARDS FOR SIX STEPS.

Moving on

When you feel confident that you can take these early exercises in your stride, you will probably feel ready to join an exercise class with others. Many leisure centres run crèches where your baby can be safely left while you swim, play badminton, dance, or whatever you have chosen. If there are no facilities near you, you could get together with a group of other mothers and arrange your own informal crèche arrangements, taking turns to look after the babies. Some NCT branches also run postnatal exercise classes, where you can combine exercises with group discussion sessions on a variety of postnatal topics.

POSTNATAL SUPPORT

Many women settle into their new role as a mother at home with a new baby better than they imagined they would. They may be surrounded by friends and family, welcome the release from their previous employment, and enjoy the opportunity to take up many of the home-based activities which they may not have had time for up till now. Others may feel lonely and isolated, far from friends and family, and missing the contact they previously enjoyed with their workmates.

NCT postnatal support

An NCT postnatal support group offers contact with other new mothers in your area and a chance to talk through and share the many new experiences that life with a young baby brings. It is amazing how reassuring it can be to discover that other mothers are having some of the same experiences as you, and can perhaps share with you some of the solutions to particular problems, just as you, in your turn, can offer support and suggestions to other new mums.

These groups often meet in mothers' homes on a weekly, fortnightly or monthly basis, and many branches organize other activities too, such as baby-sitting rotas. You may have heard about these activities if you attended your local NCT antenatal classes, but these meetings are normally open to any new mothers in the area, so, even if you have not been to NCT classes, do contact the local branch secretary and find out what is available near you. You will probably find the telephone number in the local directory, or you can contact NCT Headquarters.

NEWSLETTER Most branches produce a newsletter, which will be full of all sorts of local information as well as details of the NCT meetings; it will also contain interesting articles on all sorts of topics.

SPECIALIST GROUPS Some branches have specialist groups of people who have experience of particular situations, such as miscarriage, Caesarean section, single parenthood, working mothers, etc., and these groups meet to provide mutual support in their special circumstances.

EXPERIENCES REGISTER Branches will also hold Experiences Registers giving details of people with whom you can be put in contact on a one-to-one basis if you or your baby has a particular problem or handicap.

POSTNATAL SUPPORTERS Most branches operate a postnatal support scheme whereby mothers who have been to NCT antenatal classes are put in touch with another local mother; this may be on a one-to-one basis, or a supporter may be allocated to a particular class. This support will be separate from the group meetings mentioned earlier. It offers an opportunity for the class members to meet another mother who has recently experienced all the changes that come with introducing a new baby into the family. Sharing experiences and having someone to ring when you are feeling low can be a real lifeline to a lonely new mother. These supporters often provide help in the form of shopping or baby-minding, especially

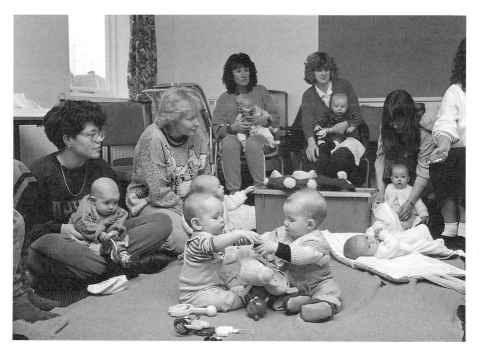

in a crisis, for example if you are ill, but it is important for each mother and her supporter to work out between them what help is most needed and what the supporter can realistically provide, given the constraints of her own family commitments. If you feel a bit shy about meeting lots of new people at once, you could go along to a local coffee together, as a spot of mutual support. In some branches, support groups for the fathers are also provided.

In the early weeks you may find it difficult to get yourself organized in time to be at the local coffee meeting, but, once you have made the effort, you will probably realize that it was well worth it; many new friends have been made at NCT coffees all over the country. If you are moving house it is also a wonderful way of meeting people in your new area.

Meeting new people with whom you have things in common is an important part of looking after yourself and, providing you enjoy it, should be seen as an important part of your life with your new baby, and not as a trivial activity, only to be squeezed in if you have the time. You need adult company, too, and your partner may not be able to fulfil all the companionship roles you need now you no longer have work colleagues to talk with each day. Apart from any other consideration, your baby will also enjoy meeting new friends before many months have passed, and this is an excellent way to begin her social life as well!

‘ Having those few minutes to myself every day kept me sane. ’

‘ I didn't mind the extra weight, but I hated feeling flabby, so I started exercising pretty quickly. I also went swimming once a week, leaving Helen in the crèche, which was a good morale-booster too. ’

‘ Days when I was extra tired were difficult because I was irritable with the children, and everything got on top of me more quickly. If I do have a bad night now, I try to make sure we have a fairly quiet day, and I give up on any housework. ’

‘ They said I'd be tired, but I didn't expect to be this tired. ’

‘ I was told I'd be exhausted all the time and I was expecting the worst. It's not that bad though, much more fun than I thought. ’

POSTNATAL DEPRESSION   28

Postnatal depression has, in recent years, become well known as a risk for women within the first year after having a baby. The term is used to refer to a wide spectrum of feelings and experiences which differ in many important ways. The research literature — as well as the number of media accounts by women themselves — is rapidly growing, but the result has been the identification of many possible causes, and many possible ways of being helped. This chapter will try to unravel for you some of the key themes which are emerging from what is known both by the professionals and by women themselves.

BABY BLUES

The baby blues has already been discussed in Chapter 22, Early Days, and though, as a new mother, you may feel very weepy and highly emotional for a day or two, this common occurrence cannot properly be classified as postnatal depression. You need only feel concerned if this period does not pass as quickly as it arrived. You may find that your emotions are unreliable until your hormones have settled into a non-pregnant pattern again; this will not be until you have had two consecutive normal menstrual cycles.

MILD DEPRESSION

Signs and symptoms

During the early months of motherhood, you may find yourself feeling somewhat tired and listless. You may begin to doubt your own competence, and to be a bit more easily upset or irritated than usual. You may not feel completely fulfilled and joyous in your new role, and may not find your baby as wholly rewarding as you think you should. You may even suspect, somewhat guiltily, that other women are coping better, and that all this is due to some personal shortcoming on your part. All these feelings could be described as mild depression.

Many women would regard feelings like these as relatively normal, but why should women experience these feelings, and are they really depression?

Reasons for depression

In a way, the label 'depression' is not very helpful. What is perhaps more important is to think about what often happens to the mother of any new baby, whether it is her first or her fifth, and what might help her to cope better.

BIRTH EXPERIENCE Some women may find that if their birth experience failed to match up to their expectations, the ensuing grief and resentment causes depression to set in. This may be particularly true for women who have had a Caesarean section, but any woman who feels that her own role in the birth process was undermined or taken away by the medical management, may become depressed following the baby's birth.

DEMANDS OF A BABY On a practical level, new babies are hard work, and usually mean a significant loss of normal uninterrupted sleep. Hard work and poor sleep patterns generally make people feel noticeably under par. The hard work of a new baby is emotionally, physically, and intellectually demanding. Looking after a baby is virtually a full-time job in itself, often leaving little time or energy for looking after a home and any others in the family. Tired people with too much to do tend to become irritable.

Under other circumstances, tired people who face heavy demands tend to get sympathy and support from others to see them through. Mothers of new babies, however, may well find that all the attention which was focused on them during pregnancy is suddenly transferred to the new baby, just at the time when they could most do with it themselves.

IMAGES OF MOTHERHOOD At the same time, the popular images of motherhood suggest that mothers should be radiant, beautiful, slim, and energetic, living in immaculate houses with ever-supportive and supported partners. Mothers themselves will often present themselves to the outside world as if this were the reality. This tends to perpetuate the myth of motherhood, and might make you imagine you are the only one who is not coping. Experienced mothers, whose children are well past the baby stage, or even grown up, will often have forgotten what these early months were like, so even they may find it hard to understand why you appear not to be coping.

CHANGE OF LIFE-STYLE An additional factor may be that, although you have gained a much-wanted baby, you have also lost your previous life-style — irrevocably. This applies whether you were a mother of older children who was coping well, or a person with a successful job or career. Your partner, too, will have both gains and losses, and the nature of your relationship will have changed. Coping with any major change in your life-style, however much it was wanted and however much it is valued, involves working through the losses so that you can adjust to and appreciate the change as a gain, and so that what is happening now can be fully enjoyed by both of you.

You are likely to find the early months of motherhood easier if you are able to talk frankly about how you feel and make friends with people who are understanding and sympathetic, rather than passing judgements. You are also more likely to find quite a number of other women who have been feeling much the same, but have felt too inhibited or guilty to say so.

Talking to others

    For outsiders, whether partners, relatives, friends, or professionals, a very important contribution is to create conditions under which a new mother can talk about how things really are, when she can feel safe to speak freely about her emotions. On the whole, this means listening and supporting rather than judging and advising. Recent research has shown how very helpful these supportive relationships can be, in both preventing and alleviating depressive feelings and experiences.

Practical help can also be invaluable in preventing or relieving these feelings. A friend who calls round with a casserole to put in the oven, or wearing old clothes and offering to clean the bathroom, will be much more welcome in the long run than the one who sits around all afternoon, leaving behind her a stack of dirty coffee cups and plates. Genuine offers of baby-sitting so that you as a couple can leave both the house and the baby, are also useful. It helps, too, if your partner manages not to ask what might be perceived as disparaging questions about what on earth you have been doing all day! Above all, it helps if your partner and others take notice of you as a person in your own right, rather than just a necessary appendage to the baby.

Practical help

SEVERE DEPRESSION

Severe depression, of the sort which would be clinically recognized by a psychiatrist or psychologist, will usually be experienced as a much stronger version of what has just been described here as mild depression. Typically, early morning waking and loss of appetite (or, in some women, over-eating) are combined with strong feelings of inadequacy, guilt, and worthlessness. Sometimes emotions will be generally very flat, but there may also be feelings of anxiety, irritability, tension, or agitation. At times, feelings of anger or rage may surface unexpectedly. Some women may feel neutral or even very negative towards their babies, which can in itself be an added concern. At times they may be frightened that they will neglect or harm their babies. Many depressed women may actually give

Signs and symptoms

excessive physical care to their babies, but without offering either love or eye contact. The responsibilities of looking after a young baby are likely to feel enormous if a mother is depressed in this way, but the depression will mean that it will seem impossible to meet them. This in turn is likely to worsen any feelings of guilt and inadequacy. These feelings may also make a mother want to hide her true feelings from friends and relatives through shame or fear of their reactions. She can often develop very effective ways of doing this, which unfortunately deprive her of just the help and support which could be of greatest value.

Causes

HORMONAL There is considerable debate amongst professionals about the causes of this sort of depression. Some have suggested that hormonal difficulties may be part of the cause, believing that some women are particularly vulnerable to the drop in natural steroids occurring after a baby is born. Certainly the hormonal changes after birth and during lactation are massive, but it is not clear why only some women should experience severe depression as a result. Research into biological explanations of this sort of depression is still under way.

SOCIAL AND PSYCHOLOGICAL An alternative theory is concerned with social and individual psychological explanations. Again, it is possible to identify social and personal factors which may make women more vulnerable to severe depression during the first year of motherhood. Some of these are similar to those factors which would make a woman vulnerable to depression in any case, but particularly following major life events, of which the birth of a child is one.

Both researchers who emphasize the biological factor and those who favour social and personal factors have found that women in general are more vulnerable to depression and other psychological difficulties than men, even without the additional events of pregnancy, childbirth, and motherhood. Some professionals believe that it is a combination of causes which is the most likely explanation.

Getting help

As with milder depression, it is known that severe depression can be prevented and helped, at least to some extent, by strongly supportive networks of friends and relatives. Again, this sort of support needs to include both practical help and the creation of conditions where a woman can talk freely without feeling she is being judged, and possibly found wanting. Part of her problem is that she is already judging herself and being severely self-critical.

LAY SUPPORT GROUPS There are national groups with some local branches which put women in touch with others who have had similar experiences, and the local NCT postnatal support organizer will have a list of these, along with information on how to contact them. Your local postnatal support organizer may also be able to put you in touch with someone local from her confidential Experiences Register, who has had similar problems.

There are a growing number of readable books giving women's own stories which may help you to feel less as though you were the only one who had ever felt like this, and the NCT publishes a useful leaflet.

ALTERNATIVE THERAPIES Some women have sought help through alternative medicine (e.g. aromatherapy, reflexology, and others). Formal research evidence is virtually non-existent, but individual accounts clearly illustrate the great care with which many alternative therapists address the woman as an individual, giving her space and support to talk in her own way about her problems and difficulties. Research on more conventional psychotherapies supports the idea that this sort of helping relationship can be very valuable. Besides this, most alternative forms of therapy are rather pleasant and many women feel that they have a more equal relationship with their alternative therapist than they suspect may be the case with more conventional doctors. They may also feel there is less stigma attached to seeking help from alternative medicine than from conventional forms. You will usually have to pay for alternative therapies, though some complementary therapies, such as homoeopathy, are available on the NHS.

COUNSELLING AND PSYCHOTHERAPY Counselling and psychotherapy are both available on the NHS, sometimes by direct self-referral and sometimes through the GP. Availability varies considerably, however, and in some areas of the country resources are very scarce indeed. These forms of help generally involve seeing a therapist, alone or in a small group, at a regular time each week over an agreed period of time. Although there are a number of different approaches, what they all offer is the opportunity for a woman to gain a clearer understanding of herself, her feelings, and thoughts, and ways in which it would be useful for her to change.

Some therapists have medical training, others have trained primarily as therapists. The professionals may include counsellors, clinical psychologists, psychotherapists, psychiatrists, and community psychiatric nurses. Occasionally local authority social workers are able to offer similar help.

There are a growing number of private counsellors and therapists, particularly in the major cities. There is no universal system of licensing or registration, so, where possible, it is worth checking credentials, or going on personal recommendation. Costs vary but tend to be pricey. Some volunteer and charitable groups use professional people, whilst others use trained volunteers, and fees are often based on a person's ability to pay.

Medical help

Severe depression, however, does usually call for outside professional or expert help. There are a number of routes to getting this help. If you are suffering from this condition, health visitors and GPs should be your first ports of call. It is important to understand that neither your health visitor nor your GP is likely to be shocked or to be dismissive of a woman who describes any of the feelings or experiences mentioned here. If your GP is dismissive or initially unhelpful, it will be worth persisting, perhaps taking your partner or a friend with you on the next occasion you visit so that you can be sure you are explaining your problems fully. In some areas there are drop-in centres which offer counselling or other help with emotional or psychological difficulties.

MEDICATION Medical practitioners, either GPs or psychiatrists, may wish to prescribe medication for depression. Sometimes this will be the major form of help offered; sometimes it will be in conjunction with therapy. Most forms of anti-depressant medication take a week or two to have any significant effect, and instructions need to be carefully followed. If you are breastfeeding, you should make sure your doctor knows this, so that he can prescribe appropriate drugs. It is important to find out what view is being taken of your depression and what sort of treatment is being proposed.

You will need to know what effect you can expect the medication to have; how long you will need to be taking it; what side effects there may be, and what long-term help is envisaged.

Given the wide range of views on the causes and treatments of postnatal depression currently held by the professionals, there may be various options available to you. If you feel unhappy about what's actually being offered, you may like to ask for a second opinion. The views of consumer organizations will also vary, but the self-help groups can give you the range of consumer experiences to different approaches to treatment and help.

HOSPITALIZATION Very occasionally, a mother may be admitted to hospital for a short period. This will generally be because it is felt that more intensive help is necessary and that the mother would benefit from being relieved of her ordinary domestic and family responsibilities. It is generally felt better that women should be with their babies in hospital, and should be responsible for their care. There are a number, still very few, of mother-and-baby units for women experiencing some form of postnatal depression. Sadly, these tend to be over-subscribed and often some considerable distance from home. Their main advantages are that the staff have both considerable expertise and interest in helping women with these problems, and that all the patients are likely to have things in common, so can be supportive to each other.

If it is recommended that you should be admitted to hospital for a while, then you will need to talk it over very carefully with your partner and your medical carers, so that you can discuss at length the advantages and disadvantages it might offer to all members of the family, especially to you, and how this treatment compares with the alternatives on offer. Your partner may also need to bear in mind that a woman suffering from postnatal depression may be unlikely to be able to look at her problem and the solutions with the same rational perspective as usual.

Whatever you decide to do should be based on a careful assessment of your individual circumstances and experiences, so that you receive the help that is most appropriate for you.

Offering personal support

Although friendship and personal support can be extremely important for a mother experiencing some degree of depression, and in many cases this can make a significant difference, the mother may not accept it readily, or it may be that her needs are greater than can be met by supportive friendship alone. It is important for friends and relatives to recognize this and to encourage the mother to seek outside help if it is needed. Sometimes she may be unwilling to do so, or may be too depressed to do anything about it. It is possible to contact the health visitor or GP in confidence if you are worried about a friend or relative and have not got anywhere by discussing it with the person involved. Above all, you may need to accept that even friendship and family relationships have their limitations and that you should not try to take the whole responsibility on yourself. You too may need support if you are trying to help and especially if you feel you are not succeeding. Equally, if the mother has hidden her problems from you, you may need reassurance to help you with any guilt you may be feeling as a result.

POSTNATAL (OR PUERPERAL) PSYCHOSIS

Very rarely indeed, a mother may develop a serious mental illness after the birth of a baby. This can be frightening for both the mother and those close to her, and definitely requires professional help from skilled and experienced people.

Symptoms

The onset may be sudden or gradual and the symptoms are variable. They may include severe withdrawal from everyday life into a world of her own, or intense over-activity. She may experience hallucinations or delusions, including feelings of persecution or seeing strange images. She may feel impelled to do bizarre or dangerous things to herself or others, including her baby. Sometimes the mother will be able to express her fears and feelings, but she may neither recognize, nor be able to express, what is happening to her.

Getting help

She should be strongly urged to get help from her GP, who should be involved as soon as possible, even if the mother is reluctant. The GP will probably involve a psychiatrist with specialist knowledge and experience in these sorts of problems. Treatment is liable to involve a combination of medication and other therapy and may need to continue for some months with close monitoring. She may be strongly advised to accept treatment in hospital, at least during the initial acute phase.

Support for the family

Support for partners and the rest of the family from friends and relatives is very helpful, as they may be feeling bewildered, maybe even in some way responsible.

As the mother begins to recover and resume her ordinary life, help and friendly support to welcome her back can be invaluable. Some people are afraid of mental illness and, because of their fears and uncertainty over what to say or do, may avoid someone who has had these problems. Equally, the anticipated reactions of others can be a serious worry to someone recovering from mental illness. Expressions of friendship and acceptance, plus a willingness to listen and talk about what has happened, can make the process of readjustment much easier for the mother, and also for those around her. Eventually, too, a mother who has experienced such a mental illness will be glad to be able to join groups of other mothers and enjoy being an ordinary mother herself.

Although postnatal psychosis is as serious and as much in need of good professional help as any other mental illness, it is rare. Even though loving and supportive friendship will not be able to cure it on their own, they will be invaluable in helping both a mother and her family during and after an illness of this kind.

- *The most overwhelming feeling was one of total failure. I felt inadequate as a mother — I had been a competent teacher, yet I couldn't even cope with one baby. But at the same time I felt so totally responsible for James that I was frightened to leave him even for a couple of hours.*

- *My stomach was in a permanent knot, and my temples ached and pressed so much I felt my head would burst open. I couldn't relax, and found it impossible to sleep without sleeping tablets.*

- *It wasn't until about nine months after the birth that I began to notice I wasn't well at all. The main thing was a dreadful sore throat which just went on and on. At the same time I had dizzy spells and nausea.* ❜

❛ *I found out why I was depressed — which to me was the beginning of the "cure". It wasn't quick or easy; there is no wonder drug to cure it, but it's more a question of self-cure. Gradually you realize that you are beginning to relax and enjoy the children. The edginess you felt every time a decision had to be reached disappears.* ❜

29 BABIES IN SPECIAL CARE

Although this chapter is primarily concerned with those babies who require special care, for whatever reasons, much of the information, particularly that on maintaining a supply of breast milk under difficult conditions, will also apply to parents of babies in other situations. Such situations might include:

- ○ **PRE-TERM BABIES**
- ○ **SMALL-FOR-DATES BABIES**
- ○ **ILL BABIES, OR THOSE RECOVERING FROM OPERATIONS**
- ○ **BABIES REQUIRING HOSPITALIZATION**
- ○ **BABIES WITH JAUNDICE WHO NEED PHOTOTHERAPY**
- ○ **BABIES WITH PHYSICAL PROBLEMS, E.G. CLEFT PALATE**

Discovering that you are not alone in facing your problem is a great help for many anxious parents. You may well be feeling disappointed, bewildered, worried, and distressed for yourselves and your baby, and it may be especially difficult if you have to be on a postnatal ward amongst other mothers and fathers with their healthy, full-term infants. Understanding what is happening to your baby and why, finding out how best you can care for her, and recognizing that other parents have been through similar experiences can help you to feel less isolated and confused, whilst providing some of the support and reassurance you will need.

THE SPECIAL CARE BABY UNIT

Reasons for admission

(Opposite) Your new baby may seem quite overwhelmed by the equipment in Special Care

Not all babies in the Special Care Baby Unit (SCBU) are pre-term, but this is the main reason for babies to be admitted. Babies born with birth-weights below 2 kg. (4 lb.), or those born earlier than 34 weeks, are usually admitted. This is because these babies do not have the same capacity for survival as larger, more mature babies. Some babies go into the SCBU because there have been problems surrounding their birth, or because they are unwell. Seriously ill babies will normally be admitted to the most suitable specialist unit for their condition, which may well not be local, and may add to the difficulties for the parents who will have to travel.

The majority of babies in Special Care are normal, healthy babies

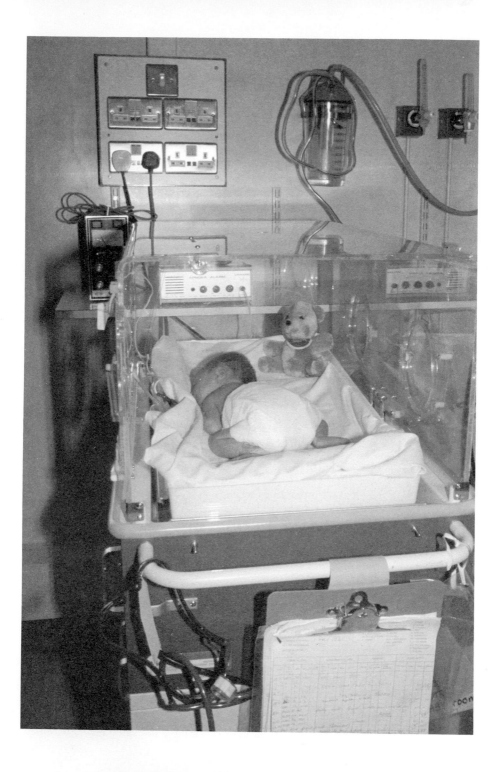

who need to have their environment and feeding conditions regulated. Very small or pre-term babies will need constant, careful monitoring to check their heart rate, respiratory rate, blood pressure, and temperature.

Most babies born prematurely are over 30 weeks, but some are younger even than this and very tiny indeed. These babies require even more intensive nursing and will seem particularly frail. Modern technology has made it possible for babies as young as 23 or 24 weeks to be kept alive, but this is uncommon, and there are often complications arising from their extreme immaturity. There may be developmental problems and weaknesses which cause difficulties in later years for these smaller, sicker babies. If your baby is over 30 weeks, however, the chances for her are generally good.

Your baby in Special Care

Seeing your baby nursed in an incubator can be extremely distressing. It looks rather like a spaceship, but is, in fact, only an open cot with plastic sides and top. This means that nurses can observe your baby at all times to detect any slight change in her colour or breathing. If she were covered up in blankets in a cot, the nurses would have to be disturbing her frequently to monitor her condition. With your baby in an incubator, you will be able to put your hands through the portholes to touch and talk to her. Even if you are not able to do this, you will be able to watch her as she moves, and will feel closer to her by being able to see her more clearly.

You may feel rather afraid of touching your baby for fear of disturbing all the wires to the monitors. Many parents have said that it has been hard to see their baby in the incubator, as she is surrounded by so much equipment both in and around the cot. You may feel sorry for your little child who has had to experience unpleasant procedures so early in life, and want her to understand that it will not always be like this. You may feel it is all your fault that she is subjected to this —your feeling may be illogical, but that will not necessarily prevent you feeling it.

Staff on the SCBU will listen to your concerns, and will help you find practical ways of establishing contact with your child.

Problems for the pre-term baby

A baby who is pre-term may, because of the prematurity, have specific problems.

BREATHING The baby's immature lungs may need help in the form of oxygen or a ventilator. Tiny babies breathe irregularly and sometimes simply stop breathing, although they are quite healthy. They are therefore laid on an 'apnoea' mattress ('apnoea' means 'no breathing'), which will alert staff by sounding an alarm if the baby stops breathing.

TEMPERATURE Small babies do not have the same layers of subcutaneous fat as full-term infants, so need the warmth of an incubator to maintain a steady temperature.

FEEDING A pre-term baby has only weak sucking and swallowing responses, and will be unable to suck on a nipple (either yours or a bottle's). Some form of alternative feeding is therefore necessary. Her delicate, immature gut is also highly susceptible to infection. Your baby may be fed via a nasal tube to her stomach (naso-gastric tube), or she may need to be fed intravenously. This involves feeding the baby via a drip into a vein for immediate absorption into the bloodstream.

Appearance

If your baby has been born pre-term, it is possible that she may not look all that much like your idea of a baby. She may be unbelievably small, yet appear rather wizened. She may be covered in hair, her skin will be very red, and she may be incredibly skinny. Mothers have sometimes described their pre-term babies as resembling rats or skinned rabbits.

Communicating with hospital staff

When things are not going smoothly, it is more important than ever to build up a strong line of communication between yourselves and the staff. It is sensible to share any feelings and worries you may have with your partner or husband at all times, then together you can discuss these feelings and worries with the staff in the unit. They are there to help and inform you. If there is anything you do not understand in your baby's treatment, or regarding the machines, do keep asking until you are confident you understand. You will naturally be worried and may not easily be able to take in information on first hearing. Staff should be used to this and be happy to explain as often as you need. You can also ask for an appointment with your baby's paediatrician who can give you a clear, full run-down of the treatment and the prognosis for your baby. Staff are usually very open about the likely outcome for your baby, which can be helpful if you are experiencing wild swings from optimism to utter despair.

FEELING INVOLVED Parents are as much a part of the caring team as the unit staff are, and in most units parents are encouraged to become involved, are welcomed, and are cared for sensitively. You need not feel it is silly to keep asking questions or to have regular discussions with the paediatricians; it is your baby, and eventually you will be the carers. The more involved you can be from the beginning, the easier it will be to establish a good relationship once you are all together at home.

One of the biggest problems mentioned by parents whose babies have been in the SCBU is the feeling that their baby does not really belong to them, but to the hospital staff. Most staff will help you by encouraging you to care for your baby while she is in the SCBU, explaining the unit routines to you, and making you feel part of the team. Others, unfortunately, may still regard parents as some sort of interlopers into their private domain. If you do experience this sort of insensitivity, try to find someone sympathetic on the unit and explain your feelings to him or her, so that a more encouraging attitude can be adopted both now and in the future.

Making contact with your baby

Try to visit your baby as often as possible; touch her and talk to her, so she will get to know what you feel, smell, and sound like, and you will begin to get to know her. Many women with babies in Special Care say they did not feel as if the baby knew they were any different from all the nurses, so they could not really feel like the baby's mother. The more contact you have with your baby, the more you will feel like her mother, and the more likely she will be to respond especially to you. Even very tiny, sick babies show a response, by a slight change in heart rate or movement, when their mothers touch them, which they do not have for anyone else. You are no stranger to your baby after all the months she has spent inside your body!

If you find out what times are best to be with your baby in Special Care, you can avoid feeling 'in the way'. You can also make sure you do not miss your own mealtimes or medication on the postnatal ward. If your mealtime does coincide with your baby's feed-time, ask the ward sister if she would keep your meal back for you. Most wards now have microwave ovens so that you can heat it up when you get back.

BREASTFEEDING YOUR BABY

Many mothers find it comforting to provide breast milk for their baby in Special Care, as it is the one thing only a mother can do for her baby when everyone else is caring for her. Even if your baby is seriously ill, you will feel you are doing something worthwhile and positive for her if you express your milk. This is a very personal choice, and you should be happy with whatever you decide to do. If you decide not to continue with breastfeeding for whatever reasons, you can still feel assured that even a small amount of breast milk will have benefited your baby enormously.

Benefits of breast milk for pre-term babies

Breast milk is the best food for new-born babies. It is especially suitable for your pre-term baby, because of her immature digestive system, and because her size and early arrival make her more vulnerable to infection. Breast milk contains protective factors which help to protect your baby from infection and allergy. Recent research shows that breast milk from mothers of pre-term babies is higher in protein than breast milk from mothers of full-term babies.

This extra protein will help your baby's growth and development. If your baby is particularly tiny (1.5 kg. or less), the paediatrician will usually recommend supplements to your breast milk to ensure your baby is receiving the best possible nutrition for her needs.

Although you may have been able to have a brief cuddle and quiet talk with your baby immediately after delivery, you may feel disappointed that she was not able to feed after her birth. The reasons why she could not suckle may be perfectly understandable, but you might still feel somewhat cheated. You can send a message straightaway to the sister in charge of the SCBU that you wish to breastfeed your baby and, if possible, would like her only to have expressed breast milk.

Tell the sister on your postnatal ward too that you intend to breastfeed, and she will help you to hand-express your milk, or will show you how to use either a hand pump or, more likely, an electric one. You can start expressing very soon after delivery, providing your medical condition allows. Severe high blood pressure or a Caesarean section may delay starting, but neither condition means you cannot feed eventually. If you are having problems breastfeeding, you can contact your local NCT breastfeeding counsellor for help and support.

Your expressed milk will be given to your baby through a naso-gastric tube. The tube is left in place between feeds, being regularly replaced with a clean one. Sometimes the milk is given as a continuous feed with the aid of a small electric pump. Feeding in this way enables your baby to get her food without using up any energy, so that all her food can go into her growth.

Try to arrange to express your milk every three hours, so that you are expressing *at least* four times a day — more whenever possible. This way your breasts will be stimulated to produce enough milk. It is a good idea to get into some sort of routine as soon as you can:

Expressing milk

- ○ WHEN YOU WAKE UP
- ○ 10 A.M., OR MID-MORNING
- ○ 1 P.M., OR LUNCH-TIME
- ○ 4 P.M., OR TEA-TIME
- ○ 7 P.M., OR SUPPER-TIME
- ○ 10 P.M., OR BEFORE YOU SETTLE FOR THE NIGHT

Your milk should be given direct, without any treatment, to your baby. Some hospitals, however, do prefer to treat the milk before giving it to the baby. Ask particularly that *your* milk should be kept for *your* baby.

If you are not initially supplying sufficient milk for your baby's needs, it will be mixed with expressed breast milk from the hospital milk bank, or with formula milk. If your hospital cannot provide expressed breast milk, and few hospitals have milk banks now, it may be possible for the local branch of the NCT to do so. Small babies do need relatively more food than full-term, average-weight ones, so you need not feel depressed if you are not producing enough in the beginning.

Using an electric pump

You should have a fair amount of help using an electric pump while you are still in hospital, but if you have to go home before your baby, the following suggestions may help:

○ MAKE SURE YOU FOLLOW THE INSTRUCTIONS THAT COME WITH THE PUMP AND THAT YOU ARE CAREFUL TO WASH YOUR HANDS WELL BEFORE BEGINNING TO EXPRESS.

○ RELAX AS MUCH AS YOU CAN. PERHAPS A PHOTO OF YOUR BABY MIGHT HELP YOU TO RELAX AND THE MILK TO FLOW. SOME MOTHERS IMAGINE THEY ARE ACTUALLY FEEDING THE BABY. THERE IS NO REASON WHY YOU SHOULD NOT RELAX BY READING OR WATCHING TELEVISION, OF COURSE.

○ PUMPING FOR FIVE MINUTES A SIDE EVERY THREE HOURS WILL PRODUCE MORE MILK THAN PUMPING FOR FIFTEEN MINUTES EVERY FOUR HOURS.

○ A HOT BATH OR WARM FLANNEL ON YOUR BREASTS MAY ENCOURAGE YOUR LET-DOWN REFLEX.

○ TRY TO EXPRESS AT WHAT YOU KNOW ARE YOUR BABY'S FEED-TIMES — IT WILL HELP YOU FEEL CLOSER.

○ SAVE ANY SPILLS ON YOUR CLOTHES BY COVERING YOURSELF WITH TOWELS.

○ WHEN YOU ARE AT HOME IT IS NICE TO HAVE SOMEONE AROUND WHO WILL SORT OUT ALL THE PUMP EQUIPMENT AT THE END OF A FEED, AND WASH AND STERILIZE IT FOR YOU. YOU WILL HAVE ENOUGH TO DO YOURSELF WITHOUT THE EXTRA WORKLOAD PUMPING WILL ENTAIL.

○ MAKE SURE YOU ARE GETTING ENOUGH REST AND FOOD YOURSELF JUST LIKE ANY OTHER NEW MOTHER BEGINNING TO BREASTFEED HER BABY.

Moving from tube to breast

When your baby is well enough to come out of the incubator for a short time, you may be able to put her to the breast. When you hold her for the first time, do not attempt to feed her, just have a cuddle and talk to her. Though it may be difficult, try not to be too nervous handling your baby. She is a tough little thing really, though she looks frail, and she will be sensitive to your moods.

At the first feed, try not to expect too much as she will have to learn how to suck and will tire easily. If she has been having bottlefeeds, she has to relearn how to suckle from the breast. Use what you know of positioning a baby at the breast to help you recognize when she is well latched on, and, if you feel unsure, ask staff to sit with you for the first few feeds. It is a good idea to continue your pumping routine even when she is on the breast and sucking well, as her stimulation alone might not be enough to keep up your supply. Feed your baby first when your breasts will be full and, after the feed, express as usual. The expressed milk can be given to your baby by tube or bottle when you are not there.

When you are discharged, you will probably only manage to visit the hospital for one or two feeds a day, so you will need to continue expressing your milk at home and bringing it in each day. You will find the information about storing breast milk in Chapter 24 (p. 329–31). Your community midwife or health visitor will also be able to help you with this.

As you approach the day when your baby will be able to come home with you, try to arrange a full day at the hospital when you can breastfeed every feed without any 'topping-up'. Some hospitals have a system where mothers can stay in for a few days before their baby goes home, so it may be worth finding out if your hospital will allow this. You might also like to ask if she can wear her own clothes in hospital before coming home, if she is not already wearing them, so that you get more used to the fact that soon this baby really will be part of your family at home.

Preparing to bring your baby home

Remember to continue using the pump for a while until breastfeeding is established; any surplus can be kept in your fridge or freezer in case you need it once you get home. Your baby may not be as 'old' as a full-term baby even now, and may need shorter, more frequent feeding for a time as her stomach capacity will be small. Most pre-term babies are prescribed iron medicine, as they have been born before having time to lay down stores of iron in their livers.

There are several little tricks you can use to help your baby suck:

Encouraging a reluctant baby to suck

○ HAND-EXPRESSING A LITTLE MILK CAN HELP THE NIPPLE TO STAND OUT AND MAKE IT EASIER FOR THE BABY TO FIX ON.

○ EXPRESSING IS ALSO HELPFUL IF YOUR BREASTS ARE FULL OR YOU HAVE A SLOW LET-DOWN REFLEX.

○ WARM COMPRESSES CAN HELP THE LET-DOWN REFLEX.

○ AN ORTHODONTIC BOTTLE TEAT HAS A MORE 'NATURAL' SHAPE AND CAN BE USED WITH BOTTLES OF EXPRESSED BREAST MILK.

○ STIMULATING HER LIPS TO SUCKLE BY STROKING THEM VERY GENTLY FROM THE MIDDLE TOWARDS THE OUTSIDE OF HER MOUTH WITH YOUR LITTLE FINGER OR A VERY SOFT BRUSH.

FAMILY RELATIONSHIPS AND SUPPORT

If you are discharged before your baby, it can be difficult to fit in hospital visits, using the breast pump, making time for other children and your partner, not to mention getting adequate food and rest. Try not to let all of this weigh you down: take opportunities to get out of the house, meet friends, and have the odd evening out with your husband or partner.

Partners may feel very left out when so much of your energy is directed at feeding and visiting your baby, so making time for talking to each other every day, when you can develop the emotional support you need from each other, is important. Many couples feel disorientated having a premature baby, and often need to discuss their feelings with each other or with friends and relatives.

Many mothers feel very emotional after they have given birth, and, with the added strain of being separated from your baby, you are almost bound to feel miserable or depressed at times. Crying is a good safety valve for letting out worry, frustration, and tension — men are as liable as women to feel emotional and will need to cry as well. This is entirely natural, and a normal emotional response — far better than bottling up all your negative feelings.

It may be hard for you to accept a baby with whom you have had so little physical contact. She may seem more like an object in a glass case than a real person, while her physical appearance may make it difficult for you to find her attractive. It is quite normal not to have any particularly motherly or fatherly feelings just yet — they usually develop once you can really hold and feel your baby and she becomes more responsive.

Siblings Your other children may feel resentful towards this new baby, who is getting so much of your time and attention. Try to let them visit the hospital and see their baby brother or sister. If you can arrange it with the sister on the SCBU, let them touch their baby if possible. Your children might like to buy a present such as a cuddly toy for the new baby which can then be hung up in or near the incubator. Explain gently to them why their new baby has to stay in hospital and keep them as well informed as you feel is appropriate for their ages and comprehension. Small children will take in as much as they want to or can understand, so it is better to give information than not. It can be very confusing and frightening for children when adults talk of serious matters of which they cannot quite grasp the implications. Children are sensitive to atmosphere and tension and hate being left out. If they are included and helped to accept the new baby, you will be minimizing the amount of resentment which might otherwise build up.

Some mothers and fathers feel they ought not to become too involved with a sick or premature baby in case the baby should die. If you feel like this, it might help to consider that, difficult as it may be to cope with at the time, any involvement now will help you to cope better in the years to come, whatever the outcome for your baby. Sometimes a mother will be very involved with the baby, while the father chooses to remain aloof; this can build up resentment between the couple and needs to be talked through. As a mother you may prefer your partner to share your involvement and feel that sharing the experiences will be more supportive for the whole family during this difficult time. Trying to remain supposedly 'strong' and detached may not be the most helpful way of supporting others. Different people have different needs and ways of expressing their needs — talking about your needs and feelings will help to keep your relationship strong and healthy.

Being involved

Some parents need support from others who have been through a similar experience. Many hospitals now run groups, with parents whose babies have left the hospital having been in Special Care talking with those who are still going through it all. Most SCBUs have photographs of their previous babies as toddlers, so that parents can see that their tiny, pre-term baby will eventually become a healthy, well-developed child.

Support outside the family

There are also two national organizations, Baby Life Support Systems (BLISS) and Nippers, which offer support to parents of babies in Special Care. You will find their addresses listed at the back of this book.

• *The staff were wonderful — they were completely professional, yet always kind and understanding. Whenever I felt weepy or anxious, there was someone to talk things over with, who could reassure me.* •

• *No one ever talked down to us, or pretended that it was better than it really was. I appreciated that honesty — it made me feel human, and a part of the caring team.* •

• *Trekking off to the hospital every day after I'd gone home without Nicholas was dreadful. It was exhausting and demoralizing. When I was at home I couldn't imagine I had a baby, and when I was in the hospital I found it hard to imagine we would ever all be at home together.* •

30 TWINS AND SUPERTWINS: LIFE AFTER BIRTH

The normal tiredness experienced by most new mothers is inevitably compounded when more than one baby is involved. This is due partly to the extra demands made by extra babies, and partly to a backlog from the pregnancy and birth. The last weeks or months of a twin (or more) pregnancy will have put an added strain on your body; you may have felt tired and uncomfortable yet unable to enjoy a good night's sleep. When you add to that the trauma of the birth, which may have happened prematurely, and which may have been a highly supervised technological process, it is not surprising if you feel that what you could really do with right now is a relaxing period of convalescence!

Instead of this, of course, you have a new and awesomely responsible job on your hands: that of nourishing and caring for two or more tiny human beings. If this is your first birth, this will be a totally new challenge for you, and one with which you may feel ill-equipped to cope. If, however, you have the benefit of previous experience and are parents already, you will be juggling the pressing needs of the new babies with those of a young toddler or other children. Many mothers of twins or triplets stress that tiredness, sometimes to the point of exhaustion, was a marked feature of their lives during the first weeks after the birth.

If you have twins or more babies, there is a greater possibility of one of them being in Special Care for a while, and this may add to your anxiety for your babies, and also to the demands on your time and energy.

ADJUSTING AND BONDING

The process of growing to love a new baby happens in different ways and at different rates for different parents. It does tend to be more complex for parents of two or more babies for a variety of reasons, not the least of these being the fact that you are adjusting to loving two or more new people as equally as possible. The relationship cannot be the same with each baby, and many factors may influence the way you react to your babies. You may, for instance, feel a more instant bond with your first-born twin or triplet. For some mothers it is the most vulnerable one for whom they feel most strongly at first; for others, the

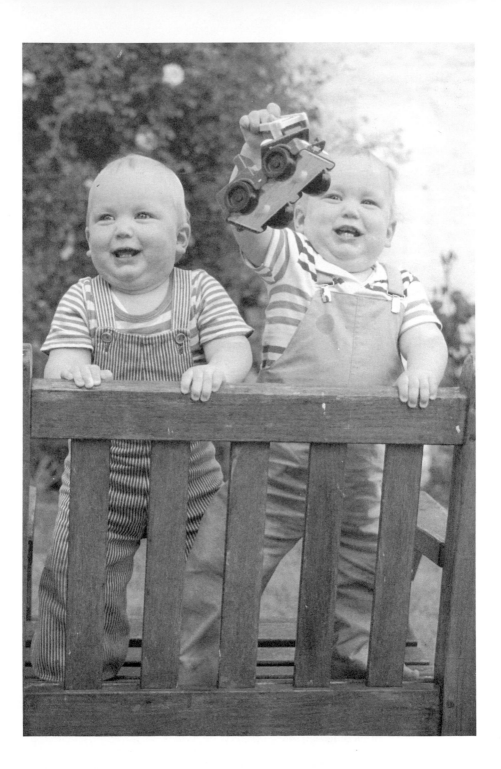

biggest, strongest one. For some, it will be the baby who is least demanding and easiest to care for; for others, the one who demands most attention and time. In the end it will not matter that one baby gained your special attention a little sooner than another, but you may nevertheless feel somewhat guilty or uncomfortable initially. Occasionally, with twins, one of them will become more attached to the father, and one to the mother, at a fairly early stage, and this can work to everyone's advantage; unfortunately, such a helpful arrangement cannot be ordered in advance!

BREASTFEEDING

It is perfectly possible to breastfeed twins or triplets totally, as your body will produce sufficient nourishment for all the babies. It is possible to breastfeed quads too, but in this case the time element could be rather daunting. There is an extra reason for breastfeeding twins or triplets: the antibodies in breast milk will be particularly valuable if they are tiny or born pre-term, and therefore more vulnerable to illnesses. The pre-term baby's immature gut will also have more trouble attempting to digest formula milk.

If you have decided to breastfeed, it is important to understand the supply-and-demand system which produces the milk: the more your babies suckle at your breast, the more milk your breasts will produce for them. Understanding how breastfeeding works will help you have the confidence in your ability to breastfeed. You will find this information in Chapter 24, Feeding your Baby: Breastfeeding and Bottlefeeding.

Support

You will need plenty of support from those around you who believe, as firmly as you do, that breastfeeding is the best option for your babies and that you do indeed have plenty of milk for them. Nothing shakes a new mother's confidence more than a relative tut-tutting about the size of one of the babies, and implying that she is not as big as someone else's baby, or her own sibling, because of the decision to breastfeed! It is well worth trying to ensure that your mother, your partner, your in-laws, and others around you do understand the benefits of breastfeeding and the way it works, and will be prepared to offer you practical and emotional support. If you are keen to breastfeed and want more information, or help in overcoming problems, do contact your local NCT breastfeeding counsellor for both support and information. Contacting another mother locally who has breastfed twins success-fully may also be helpful. You can do this through the NCT or the Twins and Multiple Births Association (TAMBA).

Establishing breastfeeding

Breastfeeding more than one baby is not always plain sailing, and you will probably need help when you are establishing a successful pattern of feeding.

There are several reasons why it may be more difficult than breastfeeding one baby:

○ IF THE BABIES ARE SMALL, THEY WILL TAKE LONGER TO FEED.

○ IF YOU FEED THE BABIES SEPARATELY, THE SECOND MAY BE CRYING WITH HUNGER WHILE YOU FEED THE FIRST.

○ IF YOU FEED THEM SIMULTANEOUSLY, THE LATCHING-ON HAS TO BE EXACTLY RIGHT, AS YOU HAVE NO SPARE HAND TO READJUST A BABY WHO IS UNCOMFORTABLY POSITIONED.

○ ONE BABY MAY NEED WINDING WHILE YOU ARE STILL FEEDING THE OTHER.

○ IF THE BABIES ARE OF VERY DIFFERENT BIRTH-WEIGHTS AND RATES OF DEVELOPMENT, YOU MAY HAVE TWO (OR MORE) DIFFERENT FEEDING PATTERNS TO COPE WITH.

There are many combinations and variations possible when breastfeeding twins or triplets. You might decide to feed them separately, attending first to the one who wakes first, and then waking the second (and third) baby once the first has finished. By arranging the feeds evenly like this you have perhaps more chance of getting them into a routine. It may be that the second (and third) baby is not sleeping during the feeding of the first, and then you could prop her (or them) up beside you to talk to and play with while the first is busy sucking. They then swap places.

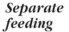
Separate feeding

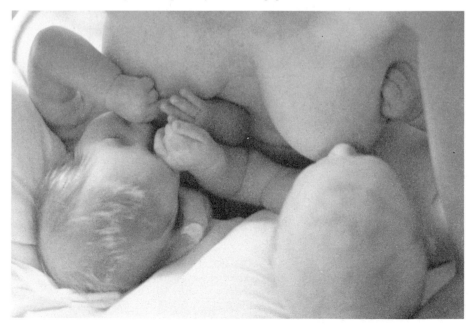

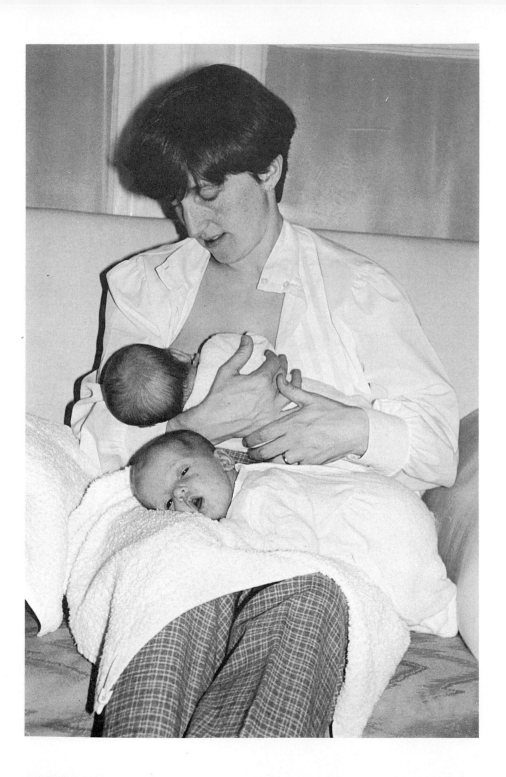

The pattern of breastfeeding the babies separately does take more time, but it also enables you to have a quiet, close time with each baby individually, when you can get to know them. It does give you more freedom to practise good latching-on techniques as well, which may be extremely useful, at least in the early days.

If you try feeding your twins simultaneously, it is important to make yourself comfortable, ensuring that your back is well supported, perhaps with a special V-shaped pillow to begin with. Once you have the babies latched on, there will be little scope for rearranging yourself. Although at first you may feel you have to handle each baby with great care, mothers of twins and triplets do become adept at scooping them up with one hand. This usually becomes easier as the babies' muscles grow stronger, and they are no longer so floppy. One baby can be propped up on your shoulder, or laid face down across your lap, to be winded, while the other carries on feeding.

Simultaneous breastfeeding

For the first few times you breastfeed two babies simultaneously, you will need someone to sit with you to help you — if only to hold one baby while you get the other one latched on, and to hand the second one gently to you so that the first is not dislodged from her position. If one comes off the breast, you will certainly need someone to help position her again. It may be a good idea to try simultaneous feeding when your midwife or breastfeeding counsellor is there to help you latch the babies on.

POSITIONS There are various ways of positioning your two babies at the breast:

- ○ **YOU MIGHT HAVE THEIR HEADS TOGETHER ON A PILLOW ON YOUR LAP, WITH THEIR BODIES OUT EITHER SIDE OF YOU, RESTING ON MORE PILLOWS (OR ON ONE V-SHAPED PILLOW).**
- ○ **YOU MIGHT HAVE ONE BABY IN THE TRADITIONAL POSITION, HER HEAD IN THE CROOK OF YOUR ARM, WITH THE OTHER BABY LYING PARALLEL, HER BOTTOM IN THE CROOK OF YOUR ARM AND YOUR HAND SUPPORTING HER HEAD.**
- ○ **ALTERNATIVELY, EACH BABY CAN BE IN THE TRADITIONAL POSITION, WITH BOTH LYING IN YOUR LAP, ONE IMMEDIATELY BEHIND THE OTHER.**

You may sometimes wish to feed simultaneously — at night, for instance, so that feeding takes less time — but normally prefer to feed separately, particularly if you have a toddler who also wants a cuddle at feed-times, or an older child who is willing to amuse whichever baby is not being fed.

(Opposite) Some mothers find it easier to feed one twin at a time

Boosting your milk supply

If you do have problems with your milk supply and want to produce more, feeding simultaneously will help to stimulate the let-down reflex and the supply, so you could try it for a few days while boosting your supply, even if you do not want to use this method all the time. Frequent feeding will also stimulate your supply. In any case, you will probably find that twins need feeding at least every three hours.

Different feeding patterns

Parents are often surprised by the many differences between their babies, and it is quite normal for one to be a far stronger sucker than the other, to grow more quickly, and possibly to settle more easily. This can throw any feeding routine you had envisaged completely off balance. You may find that you are having to give the smaller baby shorter and more frequent feeds initially, but this inequality often levels off after a couple of months, making it possible for you to plan your days a little.

Twins often have their own preferred breast and will more readily latch on to that one. They will receive sufficient milk from just the one breast, if that is how you decide to feed them. If, however, you do have babies whose weights and growth rates are very different, it may be worth getting them to swap breasts occasionally, so that the bigger baby with the stronger suck will stimulate a greater milk supply to the smaller one's breast. With each keeping to her own side, each breast will be stimulated differently and produce differing amounts of milk. You may even become slightly lop-sided, though this will probably be visible only to you.

If your babies are more even in their demands and weight gain, it is possible that you may prefer to go for a system of modified demand feeding, rather than aiming to be available whenever either baby wants feeding. With a modified system, the aim is to get the babies feeding either both at the same time, or with one directly following the other.

Perhaps for triplets, exclusively breastfeeding all three may seem too much to aim for and you may choose to compromise, so that two are breastfed and one bottlefed at each feed, each taking it in turns with the bottle. But, if you are determined, exclusive breastfeeding is an attainable goal.

Your diet

(Opposite) A useful position in the early days till the babies get too big

It is not surprising that a mother breastfeeding two or even three babies needs a greater intake of food and drink than a mother of one baby, and eats much more than she did in her pre-pregnant state. You will possibly always feel hungry, but rarely have time to cook — a frustrating situation. It is worth having plenty of nutritious snack foods permanently available. You may even find that you have to take in some sort of meal as well as a drink when you are feeding the babies during the night. Never refuse an offer of a meal from someone else — relative, friend, or neighbour. Your health

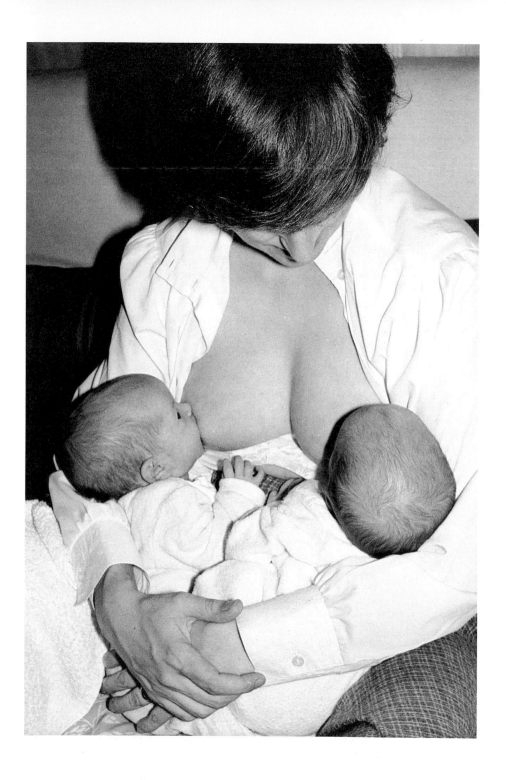

and well-being is a top priority at this time, both for your sake and that of your babies. Make it a conscious aim to look after yourself well as part of your everyday life.

> *I quickly fell into a pattern of feeding one baby off one side and the next off the other and the third off both sides. I tried a few times to feed a baby on each side at the same time . . . but for me this proved uncomfortable and unsatisfactory.*

> *I'm glad that I was very determined to breastfeed because it was much harder than I thought it was going to be. John, the bigger twin, was much more difficult to feed and was very slow to gain weight. But it was worthwhile in the end. Health-care professionals were all too keen to say give it up and bottlefeed; it will be easier for you. But really, once established, it was very easy, particularly with a V-shaped pillow so that I could feed both babies simultaneously, heads towards the middle, and a body tucked under each of my arms. Another V-shaped pillow behind me would have made it more comfortable for me in the early days.*

THE EARLY MONTHS

Practical help

Almost all mothers of twins or more find the first three months after the birth a very difficult period, when they seem to be feeding and changing babies perpetually, while the rest of their life is in a state of chaos all round them. At this stage, having some extra help on a daily basis is tremendously valuable, and, if there is any way you can afford it, it is a worthwhile investment for preserving your health and sanity. You may be fortunate enough to have relatives or friends who can provide regular help. Most people are prepared to do a bit of clearing up, ironing, or vacuuming for you; or to take the babies off your hands completely while you have a much-needed rest, or go out on your own for an hour or so.

Gradually your days will take on a more predictable pattern and you will begin to feel more in control of your life. Most parents of twins or triplets find it important to establish some sort of routine to the day, and to become reasonably well organized.

> *Good organization paid dividends. We used both paid and unpaid help, as two people were needed day and night (one of our babies was very sickly). The parents have to be in a routine, even if the babies aren't! Planning and preparation included always having the bottles ready, and having the change of clothes right on hand. Always try to anticipate the next need — not so easy when you are already fully occupied — and make a special effort to involve and not neglect your older child.*

Getting out of the house with two or more small babies seems a mammoth effort. If it takes half an hour to organize an outing with one baby, how does one ever make it with two? It is, however, worth all the effort, even for a short outing, as it is so easy to feel trapped in the house otherwise. Outings are a particular strain when the babies both (or all) want you within their sight at all times, and you simply have to leave one (or two) safely in one place while you transport the other from house to car, or vice versa. There may be some distress and crying, but this is usually balanced by the stimulation of other company or simply being in the fresh air. Supermarket shopping, on the other hand, is almost impossible with two babies. If you do attempt it, you will probably end up having to use two trolleys — not the easiest means of supermarket travel at the best of times!

Getting out

When it comes to acquiring equipment for the babies, it is well worth buying second-hand or borrowing. If there is a Twins' Club or a branch of TAMBA in your area, there is probably an informal network for the passing around of double buggies, twin prams, extra car seats, etc., as they are needed.

Equipment

You may wonder what your twins will do for sleeping arrangements; will they share or have separate cots and carry-cots? As they grow bigger, they will probably need separate accommodation, but in the early days they can share, and, in fact, some parents have found that putting a crying baby in the same cot as her sleeping twin does wonders in settling her down.

Sleeping

There is almost bound to be more crying in a household with two or more babies, simply because virtually all babies cry some of the time, and this amount will be multiplied by the number of babies you have. Moreover, you will not always have your hands free to comfort a crying baby. All parents find it difficult to cope with a baby's crying, and you will need to use all your relaxation skills to prevent yourself becoming tense and anxious whenever one of your babies screams. Since you have at least two babies to deal with, you cannot possibly be instantly available to each of them. If you accept this, and relax a little, you will feel less exhausted and better able to cope. They will learn to wait, and many mothers of twins say that by six months or so the babies are more independent and able to amuse each other.

Crying

Parents sometimes remark that twins have a pattern for crying and seem to take turns. If one is particularly upset or ill, the other will be quiet and undemanding, as though there were some understanding of each other's needs. When both (or all) of the babies do cry together in the early months, the scene may well be completed by the mother collapsing in tears as well. It is quite an achievement to learn to live with the multiple pressure of your babies' demands at a time when you are getting far less sleep than you were used to.

Fathers' involvement

Rearing twins, triplets, or more is more work than one pair of hands and one person's stamina can reasonably cope with. Fathers find themselves far more heavily involved in day-to-day care than with a single baby, and are surprised at just how much there is to do. Fathers, too, may experience the exhaustion of life after birth.

It can also be quite a strain on a marriage. This is partly because it is so unrelenting a task, and therefore neither parent has the energy to take a fresh, objective view of problems as they crop up. There is the anxiety that the extra responsibility brings, both physical and emotional, not forgetting the added financial burden. There is also the lack of time and attention that husband and wife are able to give each other in these early months. On the other hand, bringing up twins is a source of great satisfaction and pride.

Involvement with each other

Many parents notice a sympathy at work between their babies from a very early age — in their crying and in their sleeping patterns, for example — but it is at about nine months that they really start to play with each other. Besides the immense fascination for the parents in watching this happen, there are practical benefits too. The babies may be happy to amuse each other on waking in the morning, not crying to be lifted out of their cots, so that some of that sleep deficit might be restored! On the other hand, it can also mean double trouble, as they will be more independent and adventurous together than a single baby would be. They enjoy exploring together once they become mobile.

DEVELOPMENTAL DIFFERENCES

Because multiple babies often start life at different weights and in different states of health, they cannot be expected to develop at the same rates. Although a more active, stronger twin is sometimes a stimulus to the smaller one, extra time will have to be allowed for the weaker baby. One may need solid food weeks before her sibling(s), and a smaller baby may benefit from being breastfed for longer, so you should be prepared for the babies to have very different needs. When they move on to solid foods and begin to handle spoons, they may find it easier to spoon-feed each other than themselves. You may find that less food ends up in ears and hair and on the floor this way!

The differences between twins and triplets often take parents by surprise. There is an assumption in society, and perhaps in the parents during pregnancy, that all babies born as a 'batch' will be identical in personality, and will respond in the same ways towards life. But the babies, genetically identical or not, develop separate identities, and as time goes on there is no way that parents can treat them the same, or expect the same from them. It is helpful to think of yourselves as coping with two single babies: a couple, not a unit.

At some point the babies themselves might need help in separating their identities from each other — just as a single baby has to make the step of regarding herself as a separate being from her mother. Parents can help by treating them as individuals, perhaps dressing them differently for day-to-day wear, and not giving them names which sound too similar. Parents need to help others to see them as separate people, too. Making them look exactly alike and do the same things can be confusing to outsiders, so that they are just referred to as 'Twins' instead of each by her own name. This problem is obviously lessened with twins who are clearly non-identical, but even they may need some help in establishing their own individual personalities.

Separate people

It is important, too, to find some time alone with each baby or child, so that each can make her own special relationship with her parents. This will also help you to enjoy each individual's growth and companionship over the years.

* *Having twins is hard work! But because I've had to be more involved helping with them, I feel much closer to them somehow. After having just one child, we didn't realize just how easy life was in comparison. For instance, Pauline, my wife, was the main one who cared for our first child: bathing, changing nappies, feeding, etc. My job didn't change much. I still went to work, and when I came home, had a cuddle with the baby if I was lucky. But twins are a different matter entirely. It's like having two jobs — one when you go out to work all day, the other when you get home, helping with the twins all evening and night.*

* *Many days you are drained of all energy. You tend to be short-tempered with your partner and not able even to think of his needs. At the same time you expect the impossible of him — to do a full day's work, to take over the babies from you when he comes home, sometimes to cook an evening meal and then to get up to two screaming babies at 3.00 a.m.*

* *At nine months the twins are starting to enjoy playing with each other. Each twin loves to see the other twin enjoy himself. As parents, our love for them seems to grow all the time. We feel so proud of every little achievement.*

31 PARENTING IN SPECIAL CIRCUMSTANCES

Being a parent is never easy, requiring as it does vast amounts of time, energy, and commitment each day for many years. There are situations, however, which can make the task a good deal less straightforward than normal, and this chapter looks at ways in which parents can cope with their own particular circumstances. Because the scope of this book is inevitably limited, only those matters which other parents have found to be especially useful or important for them have been included. Most of the areas covered have a reasonably good range of literature available, either in book form or from the appropriate self-help organizations. You should be able to find more detailed information about your situation from these sources. You will find book titles, and names and addresses of some of the relevant organizations, listed at the back of this book.

Whatever your circumstances, you will find yourself experiencing many of the same pleasures, worries, and fears as any other parent, though it may be difficult to judge whether a particular problem is in fact totally normal or a product of your situation. Meeting other parents at mother and baby/toddler groups, talking with friends and relatives, and discussing your problems with members of your NCT postnatal support group can all help you to differentiate between what is normal and to be expected of babies and their families, and what is heightened by your own circumstances. Sharing experiences and feelings is something which helps most mothers and fathers put problems into context, and it can be a huge morale-booster to discover that what you may have assumed was a problem for you alone is shared by many. Knowing what seems to be normal can also help you to pay extra attention to those areas which seem to be different or unusual.

Most parents in difficult situations do find it useful to meet other parents in similar circumstances to pool problem-solving, benefit from others' experience, and to help them feel less isolated. It is, however, also useful to maintain contact with other parents who do not share your particular problems in order to enjoy simply being another parent; ordinary rather than 'special'.

ADOPTING A BABY

The first few days

It is difficult to generalize about adopted babies, as, like all babies, they are individuals who will respond to life in their own ways.

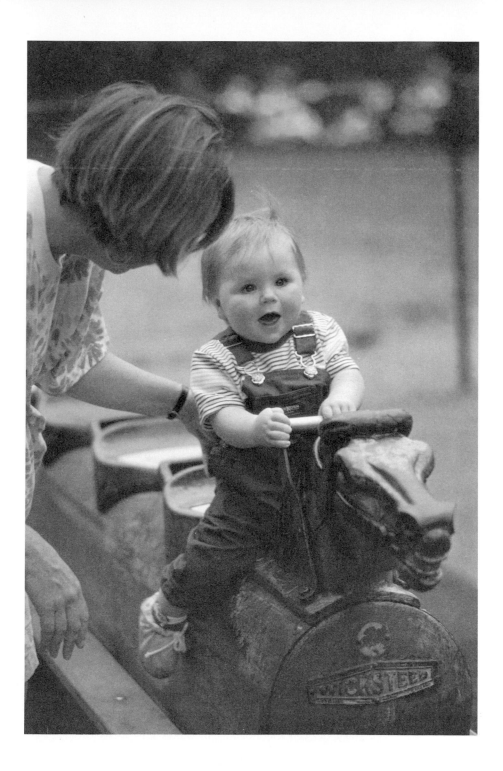

Many may have had a rather different start to life from the majority, coming to their adoptive parents after a period in hospital and sometimes weeks or months with foster parents. A baby is extremely sensitive to her environment from birth, and may well show signs of distress once she arrives at your home. She will have come to depend on hospital staff or her foster parents for comfort and reassurance, and will be accustomed to everyday sights and sounds in another place. It is not surprising, therefore, that many adopted babies are restless and distressed when they first settle into their new homes. Natural parents often experience similar upsets when they bring their babies home from hospital, or when staying in another house or on holiday.

If this is your first baby, you may be feeling very anxious, in common with all first-time parents, though you will have the added anxiety of legal procedures to cope with. Although you will not actually be recovering from the birth as a natural mother is, you will still become exhausted by your new baby's demands and the emotional adjustments to a new way of life. It is as important for you to rest and relax and enjoy your new baby as for any new mother, and to remember to put your own and your baby's needs before worrying about the housework.

The arrival of your long-awaited baby may come as rather a shock. You may be taking this small stranger into your family after the briefest of introductions, and without the benefits of a nine-month pregnancy to prepare you. However certain you may feel that you are going to make a wonderful mother or father, with boundless love to offer your child, the actual arrival may release feelings of total panic rather than the expected love and parental pride. The sense of having let yourself in for more than you can handle is something experienced by many natural parents despite the months of preparation. However much you have wanted your baby, ambivalent feelings towards this small person can be very strong indeed once you have the responsibility.

It can be helpful if adoptive parents are able to visit their new baby a couple of times at the foster parents' home beforehand, so that they have an opportunity to slip more gradually into their new roles. Partners may be feeling as unsure as each other, wondering if they will really be able to love another person's child as well as they would their own, and may welcome any chance to get to know the baby before she comes into the family. Your social worker can be contacted to ask if you can arrange a preliminary visit or two.

Once your baby has been with you for a few weeks and you have grown accustomed to each other, become bound up in each other's lives, you will find your love will grow, even if this is a very gradual, slow process. Many parents find that they take many weeks and months before loving their babies, so there is no need to feel worried or guilty, or even abnormal, if this is how it happens for you.

Some adoptive mothers want to enjoy the close, loving relationship which breastfeeding offers. It is quite possible to breastfeed an adopted baby, even if you have never been pregnant or had a child. You will find information on breastfeeding an adopted baby in Chapter 24, Feeding your Baby: Breastfeeding and Bottlefeeding.

Breastfeeding an adopted baby

If you decide not to breastfeed, you can still enjoy a close bond between the two of you. Holding your baby very close when you bottlefeed, not at arm's length; making sure you have plenty of skin-to-skin contact through bathing together or just enjoying a stroke or massage; simply cuddling up together; all these can help to form a loving relationship that you will both enjoy. After all, most fathers find ways of being physically and emotionally close to their babies without the experience of breastfeeding.

If you are adopting an older baby or toddler, breastfeeding may not be one of your considerations, but it will still be important for you to develop a close, loving relationship. The new child may be rather wary of you initially and may seem to want to reject you at precisely those times when you are offering love and comfort. If you can try to be patient and respect her feelings, allow her to test you and your love, she will soon come to feel she can trust you. Having come this far, though, she may then be anxious not to lose you. She may panic when you go out of the room or leave her, however briefly, and may be unusually clinging when others are present or you are out together. It is easy to imagine that these feelings and reactions are peculiar to your child because she is adopted, but, if you watch other children with their parents, you will notice that they too go through clinging, anxious, timid stages at various times. Discussing your experiences with others may help to put things into perspective for you.

The older baby

As with the arrival of any new baby into a family, existing children can have ambivalent reactions. Excited and proud as they may be when the baby arrives, they may also become extra demanding and 'difficult', rather than the loving, helpful siblings you had been hoping for. This behaviour is certainly not exclusive to children with an adopted brother or sister, but, if you have had less time to prepare, this may make it more extreme in the early stages.

Your other children

If they are old enough, they may well be aware to some degree of the adoption process, and will probably ask lots of tricky questions. It is a good idea to make sure your children do understand that the adoption is not permanent until all the legal procedures have been finalized, or they will feel confused and distressed if the baby has to return to her natural mother. They may feel worried that their own place in the family is not secure if they had understood the baby would be staying and she does not.

How much of your baby's previous history you decide to reveal is of course up to you, but it may be worth bearing in mind that what you tell your children may soon be very common knowledge! You may find there is a difficult balance to be struck between your desire for openness within the family — family secrets are notoriously troublesome — and a natural desire to protect the baby from learning the facts about her birth from your other children in a possibly garbled and incorrect form.

Information for the child

There is obviously no need to give your child too much detailed information all at once, but it might be sensible to write down any actual information you have about her background immediately. In the ensuing months and years you may soon forget what was told to you by the social worker, and what you deduced from the information given to you. Eventually, details of her background will become an important part of your child's understanding of herself, her memories, and her world as it is now, and you can then give her any information you have as and when you feel it appropriate for her age and understanding.

SINGLE PARENTS

Although, clearly, not all single parents are mothers, in these early months and years it is more often the mother who is the parent responsible for a child, which is why it is the mother who is concentrated on here. Single fathers will have to forgive the use of the female form.

Whether your situation as a single parent has been chosen or has been thrust upon you, the effect is the same: you are one person attempting to perform all parental roles in your baby's life for much of the time. Even a baby who is in regular contact with her father or who visits grandparents or friends will still spend most of her time with only one parent. This will bring inevitable difficulties, both practical and emotional, and you may well have found it frustrating that the emphasis in this book has been on the couple and their involvement in the pregnancy, the birth, and the new baby, ignoring the problems of the single parent without any full-time support.

Antenatal classes

Many single mothers find attending antenatal classes geared towards the couple rather than just the mother rather difficult. The closeness and the sharing which so many couples obviously enjoy at this stage of their lives may leave you feeling isolated and even angry. If you suspect that being in a group with couples might upset or irritate you, it may be worth trying to see if there are any 'mothers-only' classes in your area.

NCT teachers often run a mixture of mothers' and couples' classes, and, if you explain your position when you book for classes, it may be possible to find an appropriate class for you. If there are no mothers' classes, you can still feel reassured that your NCT teacher will be sensitive to your needs as an individual within the group. There may well be more than one mother in any class who is on her own, either full-time, or during the classes, which will help you to feel less 'different'.

Some NHS classes run 'Solo' groups of antenatal classes aimed at single mothers; these are, however, often geared to the young single mother, and, if you are in your thirties and the other members of the group are in their teens, you may find that you have little in common besides the pregnancy.

Joining an antenatal course may require an extra burst of courage on your part, but you will have the friendship and support of several other women, which will help you to feel supported during the last weeks of pregnancy and the postnatal period. Joining an NCT class will also introduce you to the local NCT's postnatal support network, which could prove to be a lifeline for you if there is no one else supporting you on a regular basis.

Attitudes

You may already have found that some people are critical of single parents, regardless of their individual circumstances; some friends will be supportive and helpful, others will take the attitude that you should be left to get on with it, whether the initial decision was yours or not. This may be extremely hard to cope with at a time when you are feeling more vulnerable than usual. Some single mothers have remarked that, whereas some people seem to find it hard to be openly supportive of a single pregnant woman, they find a single mother and her baby much easier to relate to. Perhaps a pregnancy is a more obvious indication of sexual activity than a baby!

MEDICAL PROFESSIONALS Some medical personnel are not as sensitive towards single parents as they might be. It is tempting to take these sort of attitudes personally, but often they are the result of an unfortunate manner, or sheer ignorance, rather than deliberate unkindness, although the effect on you may be the same, whatever the motive. If hospital staff have treated you unsympathetically, it may be a good idea to write a letter to a senior member of the relevant department; this can help you get things off your chest, will alert the management to areas which need looking into, and may improve the situation for mothers in the future.

Support

IN LABOUR If your baby's father does not wish to be with you during labour and the birth (or, indeed, if you do not wish him to be there), then you may like to think about whom else you will choose for your labour companion.

There may be someone very obvious such as a close friend, sister, or mother, who could stay with you and act as your labour partner. The majority of hospitals are happy to have someone other than the baby's father accompanying a labouring woman, understanding the need for most women to have with them someone they know well and can trust.

If you already know and like your midwife and have built up a good rapport with her, this may be enough for you, and some women do not feel the need of any other companion. If you have chosen someone else to go in with you, however, it is a good idea to attend antenatal classes together, so that the two of you can prepare for your labour and can discuss beforehand how your partner can most effectively support you in labour.

AFTER THE BIRTH If it is possible to arrange for some help when you first come home with your new baby, then this is a sensible idea. You may have a mother, friend, or sister who can come to stay or will be able to pop in regularly to give practical help and emotional support. It may be that you have friends or relatives who would be willing to stay, but you feel you would prefer to live alone while getting to know your new baby. If you already have other children, this may be an especially difficult time, trying to juggle everyone's needs whilst coping with your new baby and your postnatal self. Whenever any help is offered, accept it thankfully; see if there is someone who would shop for you occasionally, or take the children to school, so that you can concentrate on yourself and your baby. You may find a friend or neighbour who is willing to take the baby out for the odd hour or so, while you rest or do something for yourself — have a leisurely bath, cook a meal, visit the hairdresser. All new mothers need this time for themselves, but, if you have no support living in, it is even more important that you care for yourself properly. This includes making sure you are eating well and resting when the baby does, as well as finding time for the things you enjoy doing which help to recharge your batteries. All mothers need this time, but it may be a lot harder for you to work out how to get it.

You may find that looking after your baby day to day is less easy than for supported mothers, because you have no one with whom to share it. There is no one you can rely on being there at certain times of the day or week to help you with your baby when you could do with a break. If the baby has been whingeing all day and you have had enough, there is no one else to take over; nor is there anyone to share the first smile, the early cooings and gurgles, the night-time wakings. Grandparents and friends may take an active interest, may love her, but will not have the same depth of interest or commitment that you might expect from another parent, and you may find yourself missing this. If you can build a network of physical support around you and your baby, this will help you cope with the emotional demands of motherhood. It is worth trying to get out as much as possible to meet friends, and other mothers too, both to avoid some of the loneliness of being on your own with a tiny baby and to break up the days, which may otherwise come to seem very monotonous, with nothing to make a distinction between day and evening, or between one day and another.

On the plus side, you may find your life has a degree of flexibility about it not enjoyed by women who have others to consider besides themselves, and you may be better able to fit your time round your own and your baby's needs.

There may well be occasions when you feel the need of some support and reassurance from others outside any immediate support network. Use whatever is available: breastfeeding counsellor, friends, relatives, neighbours, other mothers, health visitor, post-natal supporter. Above all, do not feel afraid to ask for help if you need it.

Financial implications

You may be worried about your financial situation with the extra expense of a baby. Whether or not the baby's father is supporting you financially, do make sure you are getting all the benefits and allowances you are entitled to. You will be able to get full details and forms from your local Department of Social Security, whose address will be in your phone book or at your Post Office. If you are on your own, things always seem easier if you are financially secure. You may find the booklet 'Money for Mothers and Babies' published by the Maternity Alliance comes in extremely useful too; you will find the address listed at the back of this book.

If you think you will need to go back to work, perhaps to help make ends meet, see Chapter 32, Returning to Work, which provides information to help you make the right decision, and on the various forms of child care available.

Other relationships

Many single mothers make special efforts to make sure their children have plenty of access to other close friends and relations so that the mother–baby relationship does not become too all-consuming.

Grandparents, aunts and uncles, good friends, with or without children of their own, can all help to build up a strong network of close friends for your child, to take some of the pressure off you. If her father will be keeping in touch with his baby, this is another relationship which can grow and develop over the years for the child's benefit, though it may be painful for you at times.

No one parent can possibly be everything to a child; nor can any two parents, of course, but you may find you are expecting more of yourself than is either reasonable or physically and emotionally feasible. Do whatever you can, encourage your child to enjoy close relationships with a variety of others around you, and try to provide plenty of outside contacts; but, above all, enjoy being her parent.

❛ *The nights are particularly hard work with no one to help take the load off me.* ❜

• *I often wished things were a bit different, that there were two of us to enjoy being her parents together instead of doing it separately, without any contact between us.* •

• *I have honestly never felt either Joe or I was missing out by not having a second parent around. It was entirely my decision to have a baby minus a partner and I don't have any regrets.* •

• *It did take me a while before I dared ask people to help with babysitting while I went out alone, but, once I'd plucked up the courage and realized people weren't condemning me for being a single mother, I felt much better in myself, and started to feel self-confident again.* •

BEING A STEP-PARENT

It is becoming increasingly common for couples who are starting a family together to have stepchildren from previous relationships. This may make everyday life more complicated, as domestic arrangements and circumstances may alter frequently, and there will be the feelings of several other people to be taken into account. The whole subject of step-parenting is vast, but, if you are preparing for a new baby's arrival, some suggestions from other parents who have been in this situation may help.

There is a multiplicity of possible step-parent permutations: either one or both of you may have children already; you may have stepchildren living with you or only visiting on a regular basis; you may have a combination of these — some living with you, others visiting; the children may be grown-up already, even with children of their own. Whatever the circumstances, keeping the children informed and involved in what is going on will be important. Nobody likes to feel excluded from family events, so the more the children are included from the beginning, the less likely they are to feel rejected or insecure. If the children are older, it can be all too easy to assume they have heard the news, which may lead to some difficult moments when you realize no one had actually thought to tell them. Even if you think they already know, most people prefer to be told any news by their own parents than by a third party.

Although many of the problems of step-parenting will be those of practical logistics (who will be staying with whom, and when, and for how long?), many of the other potential problems can be avoided by being tactful, aware, and sensitive to the needs of others — your partner and your (or his) ex-partner, as well as any existing children. It may take a bit of extra effort to sort out the needs of the whole family when so many different relationships are involved.

The new parent

If one parent has children already, whilst this is the first baby for the other, several issues may crop up.

It may be that, as a new mother, you feel less 'special' than other first-time mothers, because your partner has been through it before, and no longer views the birth of a baby as quite so extraordinary. He may find it hard to remember that you have not done all this before and need your confidence building up, just as he did the first time round.

Any parent who already has children needs to be especially sensitive to a partner enjoying a first baby and feeling his or her way into mother- or fatherhood. It is easy to criticize someone, however gently, for not doing things the way you want them done; easy to belittle a partner's early attempts at caring for, or playing with, his or her new baby; you may have to be particularly aware of the danger of making him (or her) feel clumsy, inexperienced, and, ultimately, resentful. You cannot ignore the fact that someone has had a chance to adjust to the role of being a parent before, but making allowances for inexperience, and talking about anything you find especially difficult, will help you both learn together as you work towards becoming the sort of parents you would like to be with this new family.

If your partner's other children were born and brought up several years ago, he (or she) may find it hard adapting to newer and different ideas of child care. The new mother or father who has not had children previously, or whose children are much younger, may have to tread lightly in order not to seem dismissive of ideas which seem out of date or inappropriate. Previous experience is invaluable in many instances, and can be a reassuringly sane voice in times of stress, but it can also create problems if people find it difficult to be flexible or find newer ideas less acceptable.

A mother whose partner has children may also feel that her partner is less interested in this baby than in his talkative, active, older children, with whom he already has a relationship. A father may be so anxious that his other children should not feel rejected by the baby's arrival that he treats them with extra special attention, leaving his new partner feeling that he is favouring them to the disadvantage of her new baby. On the other hand, he may be so fascinated by this new baby with his new partner, may so enjoy building up a new relationship, with all the opportunities it offers, that his other children seem much less interesting. As with any other difficulty in family relationships, these need talking about and airing so that neither partner nor any child is left feeling excluded or unhappy.

Other children

Most children are reasonably pleased at the prospect of a new brother or sister, though they may feel wary of what changes this will bring at the same time. The child may have serious reservations about this baby:

○ WILL THE BABY PUSH ME OUT?
○ WILL MY PARENT/STEP-PARENT HAVE LESS TIME FOR ME?
○ WILL DADDY OR MUMMY LOVE ME LESS ONCE THERE IS SOMEONE ELSE TO SHARE WITH?
○ WILL THEY LOVE THE BABY MORE THAN ME?

You may find it helpful to talk over any concerns you have with other parents who have more than one child — not necessarily step-parents. It can come as a relief to find that children in any family have negative feelings and responses alongside the positive. Most children see a new baby as something of a threat, though a child whose parents have separated may still be feeling vulnerable, and a new baby can highlight any sense of rejection or insecurity. Many of the things you would normally do to smooth over any difficult patches will be exactly the same as in any family situation when a new baby arrives, though you may have to use a little extra sensitivity and forward planning, particularly if you are still unsure of your relationship with your stepchildren.

Helping older children

○ TRY TO INVOLVE THE CHILDREN AS MUCH AS POSSIBLE — IN THE PLANNING, THE EXCITEMENT, THE CARE OF THE BABY. EXPLAIN WHAT NEEDS TO BE DONE AND WHY, AND ALLOW THEM TO SHARE AS MUCH AS YOU CAN.
○ ENCOURAGE THE CHILDREN TO TALK OPENLY TO YOU OR YOUR PARTNER ABOUT THEIR FEELINGS, THEIR WORRIES, AND THEIR FEARS. TRY NOT TO BELITTLE THESE FEELINGS; THEY ARE IMPORTANT TO THEM.
○ TRY NOT TO WORRY IF OLDER CHILDREN DO NOT LOVE THE BABY. THEY DO NOT HAVE TO; IT IS JUST NICER FOR YOU ALL IF THEY DO.
○ TRY TO SET ASIDE SOME SPECIAL TIME FOR YOU AND YOUR CHILDREN, PERHAPS WITHOUT THE BABY — EASIER FOR A FATHER TO ACHIEVE!
○ TRY TO EMPHASIZE THEIR SPECIALNESS TO YOU AND ALL THAT THEY MEAN TO YOU FOR THEMSELVES.
○ TRY NOT TO SHOW ANY FAVOURITISM. THIS MAY BE DIFFICULT, ESPECIALLY IF THE CHILD IS NOT YOURS, BUT IT IS IMPORTANT TO TRY TO BE FAIR. CHILDREN ARE STRONG ON WHAT IS JUST AND WHAT IS NOT, AND ARE QUICK TO NOTICE ANY UNFAIRNESS, ALBEIT IMAGINARY, EVEN WHEN YOU THOUGHT YOU WERE BEING SCRUPULOUSLY FAIR!
○ TRY TO ANSWER ANY QUESTIONS OPENLY AND HONESTLY.

> OLDER CHILDREN MAY TRY TO PUSH YOU BY ASKING ALL
> SORTS OF AWKWARD QUESTIONS. THEY MAY BE AP-
> PROACHING PUBERTY AND FINDING IT EMBARRASSING
> THAT YOU ARE SO OBVIOUSLY HAVING A SEXUAL RELA-
> TIONSHIP. WHAT CLEARER EVIDENCE COULD THERE BE
> THAT YOU ARE 'DOING IT'? THIS IS A COMMON REACTION
> OF MANY TEENAGERS WHEN A PREGNANCY IS ANNOUNCED
> AND IS NOT CONFINED TO STEPCHILDREN; BUT HANDLING
> THESE AWKWARD QUESTIONS MAY BE DIFFICULT FOR A
> STEP-PARENT, WHO MAY HAVE LITTLE EXPERIENCE WITH
> OLDER CHILDREN AND ADOLESCENTS.

Practical arrangements

On a practical level, there may be changes to be made in the usual domestic arrangements. Explain this to the children and keep them in touch with what is going on.

If you have children who come for regular visits, perhaps for weekends, you may need to alter these for a week or two while you get used to the baby. You could try taking them out somewhere special to replace the usual visit once or twice while the new mother has some time alone. They will almost certainly want to see their new brother or sister, but you may prefer to keep the visits brief at first until you are ready to settle into a new pattern.

If the baby is ill, and the children cannot visit, do remember to keep in touch by phone; not only will they be sorry to have missed a visit, but they may be concerned for the baby's health as well. You will also need to alter arrangements if the children are ill. This is all made much easier if you are on good terms with the ex-partners, of course.

As the baby grows a little older, visiting children may bring rather unsuitable toys and games, or may not understand what is and is not dangerous. Children living in a household quickly discover what is acceptable or safe, but those visiting are at a disadvantage; you will have to explain things very carefully to them, without hurting their feelings.

It is very hard work trying to make a cohesive unit of a family who do not all have the same two parents in common. It may take longer to work out all the relationships satisfactorily, may take longer to find a way of life which suits all of you; you may all have to make more compromises than more straightforward families. But the end result may be far richer and, with luck, a lot more fun as well.

❛ I had to be careful not to hurt James's feelings whenever he wanted to do something one way, just as he'd done it before, but which now seemed old-fashioned or not really appropriate for us. ❜

The older children were great with the baby when they came to visit, but I found their visits rather wearing in the early months, while I was still getting used to being a mother.

PARENTS WITH DISABILITIES

People who have disabilities are increasingly taking the decision to become parents, but they are still facing enormous difficulties in getting hold of all the information they need to help them through pregnancy, birth, and the postnatal period. Mothers and mothers-to-be with disabilities often have very restricted access both to the maternity services, and to useful, accurate information. There is, sadly, little literature available from the disability organizations which deals specifically with pregnancy and parenthood. This section of the book does not have the scope to offer particular information on the wide range of disabilities, but it can point you in the right direction so that you can find the information you need.

Where to find help

PARENTABILITY ParentAbility is an NCT network which supports disabled people through pregnancy, birth, and parenthood. On a general level, it plays a significant role in challenging prejudice, improving access to services and information, and raising awareness amongst maternity services personnel. ParentAbility can help you get access to good, clear information by providing:

○ A CONTACT REGISTER AND REGULAR NEWSLETTER ENABLING DISABLED PARENTS TO TALK TO OTHER MOTHERS AND FATHERS WITH SIMILAR CONDITIONS OR DISABILITIES. GETTING IN TOUCH DURING PREGNANCY, OR EVEN WHEN CONSIDERING HAVING A BABY, GIVES PEOPLE THE CHANCE TO GET TO KNOW OTHERS AND FIND THE NECESSARY INFORMATION.
○ A RESOURCE LIST AND OTHER PUBLICATIONS, PROVIDING EASIER ACCESS TO INFORMATION ON PREGNANCY, PARENTHOOD, AND DISABILITY.
○ A PRACTICAL EQUIPMENT HELPLINE, GIVING INFORMATION ON HOW TO GET APPROPRIATE BABYCARE AND NURSERY EQUIPMENT
○ REPORTS ON ACCESS TO MATERNITY UNITS AND COMMUNITY-BASED ANTENATAL CLINICS TO HELP IMPROVE THE FACILITIES, CARE AND INFORMATION OFFERED.

DURING PREGNANCY If you are disabled you need information not only about your pregnancy and birth, but also about how it could affect your condition or impairment:

○ HOW WILL PREGNANCY AFFECT YOUR CONDITION?
○ HOW WILL YOUR CONDITION AFFECT THE PREGNANCY AND BIRTH?

○ **WHAT EQUIPMENT, ADAPTATIONS, AND ADDITIONAL SUPPORT WILL BE HELPFUL TO YOU IN CARING FOR YOUR BABY?**

If your midwife or doctor has limited knowledge of the effects of your disability on the pregnancy and birth, or if your specialist has little experience of mothers with your disability, encourage them to make contact with each other. It may be important to write about this in your birth plan, and to keep a copy yourself in case it is not available at the right times. You might like to take your partner, a friend, or advocate with you to the antenatal clinic when you visit. The Maternity Alliance has published a very useful Charter: 'Listen to us for a Change'. It was written by parents with disabilities working with health professionals and disability organizations. This may help if you find it difficult to explain your point of view, or to get the kind of information and support you want.

You can make contact with other mothers who have experienced similar situations by contacting the relevant self-help organization and NCT ParentAbility.

The maternity services should be sensitive to people wanting ordinary care, not 'special care'—which can make people feel isolated and 'labelled'. You may prefer your midwife to come to your home for your antenatal checks. You may choose to go to the antenatal clinic sometimes, even if it is more complicated, because this may offer you the opportunity to get to know other women in your community who are having babies, to pick up leaflets and information, and to find out about parents' support networks of all sorts.

You and your midwife need time to get to know each other, to talk over where you want to give birth, and to plan for any special needs you may have during labour or after the birth to be met. She can link you in with other services: accessible antenatal/parentcraft classes, sign interpreters if necessary, help in getting useful information about facilities and equipment in the maternity unit and at home. She can also ensure that the maternity unit is ready to meet your needs.

Access to information

All parents need access to accurate, useful information to help them make their choices about their maternity care, and this is even more important for anyone who has special and particular needs. No parent need be fobbed off with less than the best care throughout the maternity or postnatal period simply because his or her needs are not quite straightforward.

NCT ParentAbility's resource list provides a wide range of literature available in different formats. If you have a visual impairment, you can contact the RNIB for a list of books and leaflets available in Braille and on tape. Many NCT publications are available in Braille and on tape, including this book: details are given in the current Maternity Sales Publications List. NCT's quarterly magazine 'New Generation' is also available on tape.

The Maternity Services Charter and any information leaflets produced by your local maternity services should be available in a format you can use; you can ask your midwife to help you get hold of the most appropriate ones for you.

Antenatal classes are an ideal opportunity to gain information as well as to meet other parents. Do not be put off if you are told the classes are not accessible: try talking to the booking clerk or midwife who organizes them to see if an alternative venue could be arranged. If you are not able to attend classes, there are some excellent video films on relaxation, exercises, and preparation for birth available now. NCT Maternity Sales Ltd. also sell an audio tape on relaxation for pregnancy and childbirth.

Benefits and entitlements

There is no benefit at present specifically for disabled people who care for others whether as parents or relatives. Information about maternity and disability benefits and entitlements is available from the Benefits Enquiry Line on Freephone 01800 666555. You can ask for a letter summarizing the advice given, and information is also available in Braille, large print, and audio tape. Specially trained operators can call you back and fill in the form over the telephone, which is then sent back to you for checking, signing, and posting. If you use a minicom, you can receive advice directly onto your screen using 01800 243355.

Practical help

If you think you will need additional help with child care, special equipment, or funding to buy in such help yourself, contact your local social services to see what community-care support they can offer. Resources vary in different parts of the country. Home-Start and Crossroads are two voluntary organizations which can provide practical help if you have branches in your area.

Some parents with disabilities have found it useful to practise handling a baby beforehand. This will give you some idea in advance about what equipment will be of greatest use to you. It is worth planning any help you will need well in advance so that it is all in place when your baby arrives. Your midwife and/or occupational therapist should be able to help you with all this. There may be more useful equipment around than you currently have, and babycare or nursery equipment may need to be adapted or made to order, which inevitably takes time. The ParentAbility Equipment Helpline can provide further helpful information as well.

AFTER THE BIRTH Some mothers with disabilities who give birth in hospital prefer to have the privacy of a side room, but others find being on a ward with other new mothers means they can share the experiences of caring for a new baby. Watching other mothers handle their babies can be a great help for any new mother, particularly with a first baby.

Some disabled women find that fatigue is even more of a factor for them than for non-disabled mothers, and it is worth bearing this in mind when you are planning how much help you will need around the house after your baby arrives. A real life-saver for some women has been finding a way to guarantee a rest every day, even if they happen to have one of those babies who seems to need very little sleep! Perhaps it will be even more important for you than for other new mothers to accept any offer of help, however tentatively suggested.

Many disabled people feel isolated by an inaccessible environment and inadequate transport system, and this may be particularly true for a new mother. You might find it especially useful to have the contact and friendship of a postnatal support group or local postnatal supporters. Your local branch of the NCT should be able to make its services available to you, but when you make contact, do explain what your special needs are. It may be necessary to make arrangements to allow for people's different requirements.

In some areas, there are local parents' support groups where you can meet and talk with other disabled parents. ParentAbility has a list of these. Local disability groups and organizations can also provide useful contacts and information.

Your health visitor or local NCT will have information about activities for parents and babies in your local community. Some areas publish Under-5s guides which should include information about access. (ParentAbility has also published a survey report on access to these kinds of facilities.)

All babies are unbelievably time-consuming and you may find that everything takes far longer than you had expected, and needs much more careful planning. Try to give yourself as much time as possible, including plenty of time to rest if you need this. *Get into Shape after Childbirth* is a book which gives lots of ideas for exercise and relaxation, including a chapter dealing with the specific needs of disabled mothers; this book is also available on audio tape with a poster. You will find details on this and other books in the section 'Further Reading' at the end of this book, or you can contact NCT Maternity Sales Ltd. for more information.

• *It's very easy to be swayed by other people's prejudice, but any disabled person considering parenthood should definitely go for it. Despite the difficulties and disadvantages, you can be strong, powerful, and, most essentially, happy.* •

• *I'm so proud of my children and, even though it's been hard work, I feel my life is so exciting with them. ParentAbility was really helpful in giving me confidence in my abilities as a mother, because it was through them I heard about other disabled parents' experiences.* •

HAVING A BABY WITH A DISABILITY

***Communicating
with medical
professionals*** If your baby does have some malformation, whatever its nature, medical staff should come and explain the situation to you soon after the delivery. You may find yourselves feeling confused and miserable, unable to enjoy the usual delight of new parents. If your baby has a very minor, treatable problem, you may be feeling a curious mixture of elation at her arrival and distress at the malformation. It may be hard for you to comprehend the reality of the situation, and you may not be able to take in much of what is said to you for the first day or two. Do not be afraid to keep asking for explanations; staff will understand your need to be as fully informed as possible, will be aware of the difficulty of absorbing information at such an emotional time, and should not consider you a nuisance for asking. If you are treated with less sensitivity than you would expect, or have your queries brushed aside, remember that this is your baby, these are your decisions and your feelings, and, if they are important to you, you should be given every opportunity to be as informed as it is possible to be. If you are experiencing problems with a junior member of staff, it may be worth asking to speak to somebody in a more senior position to explain your problems and concerns. If it is the specialist who is reluctant to answer your questions, or is dismissive of your worries, it will take courage, but it may be valuable to tell him exactly how you are feeling. He may not find it particularly easy dealing with distressed parents, but, if you point out to him the added misery his behaviour or attitude causes you, as well as your reasons for needing to ask for information, he may begin to understand what you would find it useful for him to do.

***Getting to
know your
baby*** Whatever your baby's problem, whether it is severe enough for her to be admitted into Special Care or moved to a specialist unit at another hospital, or even if she is not expected to live for very long, you will always be free to go and visit your baby whenever you wish. It may be important for you to get to know your newborn baby, just as any mother gets to know her baby. You have the same needs to find out about and build up a relationship with this baby as with any other. If your baby has a malformation, it may be difficult for you to begin creating a bond with her; you may feel that you do not want to see or touch her, may feel it would be better to remain detached. You may feel disappointed that this was not the baby you had hoped for, that she does not come up to your expectations. You may feel guilty or a failure for not having produced a perfect baby and for not being able to love her as you think you would love a normal baby.

Although these feelings are entirely understandable and very common, you may find later on, once things are clearer in your own mind, that you regret not having visited your child from the beginning, not having offered her the same degree of love and care as all new-born babies would like from their parents. Whatever your initial feelings, you will not usually have to make any decisions immediately; there is normally time to mull over what you want to do, to come to terms with what has happened, and what is expected for the future. Talking to your partner, allowing each other to feel angry or bewildered or resentful, is an important way of coping with your situation, whilst keeping close to each other at a difficult time.

Other children

Your other children, if you have them, will find it very hard to comprehend what is going on; they may not be of an age to understand what such things mean, and explanations will need to be kept simple and appropriate for their comprehension. Children always know when there are problems; they are highly sensitive to atmosphere and to other people's unhappiness, and it is only fair to let them know what is happening. Children may end up feeling rejected, miserable and even guilty themselves, if they are not kept reasonably well informed, and may begin to have behaviour problems if they are feeling left out and distressed. Families where both good and bad news is openly shared and discussed will usually find it easier to pick up the pieces afterwards than when events have been hidden away or denied.

Other people

One of the hardest aspects of having a disabled child is coping with the reactions of other people. Parents are often finding it difficult enough to cope with their own emotions, so having to deal with the less helpful responses of others can be very painful. At first, if you know your baby has a disability, whether physical or mental, you may find simply telling other people a most unpleasant task. You may feel that you will somehow be regarded as a failure for not having produced a perfect baby, in a society which only really values perfect people. You may find their shock, horror, or even their sympathy make it more difficult for you. If you can, and want to, ask relatives or friends to do some of the phoning for you. Some people find it easier to tell everyone at once, others prefer to make phone calls or visits as and when they feel ready for them. It can be difficult making sure you have informed everyone who needs to know, but it is worth checking to save embarrassing moments later on.

Support

If you are feeling angry and hurt at your own friends' inability to be supportive at a time when you are more in need of friendship than ever before, contacting someone who has been through something similar but has come to terms with her own situation can be immensely helpful. Most forms of disability and malformation now have a support group and you should be able to get a contact number from your hospital or Social Services, or through the NCT's Experiences Register. You may need to find a number of close friends who will occasionally look after your baby for you if she has a severe disability and needs a great deal more attention than normal. It will be even more important than usual for you to have some time to yourselves in this sort of situation. It may be hard for you to meet your friends with perfect babies for a while, but this may also be a good source of support and friendship as well as a useful forum for sharing a wide variety of experiences as a parent.

* *Some days I can easily ignore people staring at him; other times it gets my back up or upsets me that they consider him a freak to be gazed at.* *

* *People seem to think that just because we have a handicapped child, we're somehow special or wonderful. Well, we're not — we're just normal parents who happen to have been given this extra responsibility, that's all.* *

CONSIDERATION TOWARDS OTHERS

If you have been reading this chapter as a parent in a fairly straightforward situation, you will have become aware of the frequently voiced complaint of parents in other circumstances, that it is very hard to be accepted as an ordinary parent who happens to have one different aspect to his or her life. Whether one is the parent of a child with a disability, a single father, or a blind mother, there is still a need to be able to enjoy simply being a parent and meeting other parents at that level. Many mothers have said how excluded they have felt from already established groups of mothers, especially if their circumstances did not happen to fit in with the group's. Mothers say that it is usually they who have to make the first moves, and how their one different circumstance can make them feel isolated.

How you can help

If you do know a mother (or father) who may be finding it more difficult than usual to look after a baby, you might like to think about making the first moves yourself:

O   **PHONE TO OFFER ANY HELP YOU CAN.**

O   **PHONE OR VISIT TO SHOW YOU WOULD LIKE TO KEEP IN TOUCH.**

O   **INVITE THE MOTHER (OR FATHER) TO ANY MEETINGS WHERE SHE CAN ENJOY BEING AN ORDINARY PARENT AMONG OTHER PARENTS FOR A WHILE.**

○ ACCEPT HER AS SHE IS; DO NOT BE JUDGEMENTAL.

○ TRY TO BE SENSITIVE IN YOUR TOPICS OF CONVERSATION: AN ADOPTIVE MOTHER MAY BE FEELING SAD AND VULNERABLE ABOUT HER OWN INFERTILITY STILL AND MAY NOT FIND IT EASY TO LISTEN TO EVERYONE ELSE'S ACCOUNTS OF THEIR PREGNANCIES AND BIRTHS; A MOTHER WITH A DISABLED CHILD MAY APPRECIATE LESS THAN MOST DISCUSSIONS ABOUT WHOSE CHILD WALKED/TALKED/WAS DRY AT NIGHT FIRST.

○ LISTEN AND OFFER REASSURANCE AND SUPPORT, IF SHE NEEDS IT.

32 RETURNING TO WORK

Despite rapidly changing patterns of employment for women, deciding whether to return to paid work after having a baby can be difficult, both rationally and emotionally, for each individual woman. Whatever the trends, and whatever the views of friends, relatives, and even former colleagues, it is very much a personal and financial decision for both the woman and her partner, if she has one. You may find it helpful to consider the decision from a number of different perspectives.

MAKING THE DECISION

Financial

It may be financially essential to retain your income, or it may be that, although possible to manage without it, the family finances would be very difficult if you were not working. It may not be a straightforward matter of either earning or not earning money, however. You will have different costs to set against your income once you have a child. Apart from the direct cost of child care, it is worth thinking about the less obvious costs of working — travel, clothes, even the likelihood of feeling inclined to spend more on items like convenience foods or domestic help. It may well be that the net profit from your paid work is much less than at first sight. It will certainly be substantially less than before the baby arrived.

Career

The implications of a career break any longer than maternity leave allows can be worrying, particularly if you have actively sought to develop a career. If your career is in a competitive field, then you may feel that you would be seriously disadvantaged by returning later. Equally, in areas which are developing rapidly, a long break may mean you have a lot of catching up to do.

However, partly because of pressure from women and partly because of changes in the employment market, many employers and professions are beginning to make taking a longer break from work a more viable option. More enlightened employers will give options such as returning to a guaranteed job at the same level after a number of years. Increasing numbers of refresher and up-date courses are becoming available for those returning to work. Part-time or job-share employment is now much more widely available, as well, and could be worth negotiating with your employer.

On the other hand, you may feel that developing your career is important enough to tip the balance in favour of a return to work straight after maternity leave.

Your work may well feel like an important part of your identity. However much you love your baby, you may feel that you do not want to lose that part of yourself which is expressed and seen through your work. *Identity*

For many women their new identity as a mother is very important and fulfilling. It is unfortunate that within society as a whole, it is still an undervalued one and one which does not, on its own, appeal to all women. Some women who have chosen not to return to work for a while find that their time as full-time mothers offers prime opportunities for developing new roles or learning new skills.

These opportunities may include studying — whether adult education classes or the Open University — or local community activities. Local organizations are always looking for new members to give their time, and participation can be extremely rewarding. The NCT, for example, as a self-help organization, provides opportunities for such participation, particularly for its more active local and national members.

The issue of having an identity in your own right is certainly worth considering seriously, but paid work is only one of a number of options once you have had your baby.

The conventional image of motherhood may feel very different from the reality. As you will have gathered from previous chapters, having a baby can be far more challenging than a full-time job. Babies are not always contented and many do not sleep to order. Babies can be emotionally and physically very demanding and extremely disruptive of previous, childless life-styles. Not all women are born mothers: many have to learn, often with difficulty, how to do it. In contrast, however, there are many rewards and the role can be indescribably fulfilling. Whether it is or is not, the way in which you choose to spend your time is a highly individual matter. Before, but especially after, you have had your baby, it is well worth talking with other women who have chosen to stay at home, and with those who have chosen to return to paid work, as well as paying careful attention to your own and your partner's feelings. *Considering full-time motherhood*

There are many examples of women who felt absolutely certain that they would return to work after their maternity leave, but then, to their surprise, changed their minds during the first few months of motherhood. There are probably at least as many examples of women who thought that full-time motherhood would be for them, and then decided to return to work. The most unhappy women are those who made either choice, not on the basis of their own feelings and circumstances, but because it was what seemed to be expected, or the right thing to do.

It is also important to consider your health — planning in advance to return to work soon after the birth can be a mistake — you may simply not feel up to it.

Effects on the baby

There has been a considerable amount of research into the effects on babies and children, of having a working mother, and of different forms of child care. In essence, the research suggests that, both in the early years, and later into childhood and adolescence, there are no significant differences either way between infants and children whose mothers go out to work and those whose mothers do not. Other factors, including stability in the home and the general well-being and mental health of the mother, are much more important. Paradoxically, perhaps, mothers should think of themselves first: if they make the right choice for themselves, the children will be happier and thrive better than if they do not.

Babies and small children need to form stable, secure attachments to adults in order to thrive, but these attachments need not simply be to their parents. Children need to feel secure, to understand what is happening in their lives, but there are many different ways of providing this security and you will need to consider how best you can provide this stability when looking at the child-care options available to you.

Partners' attitudes

Neither the decision to return to paid work, nor the decision to remain at home, can realistically or sensibly be made without discussions with your partner, if you have one. The easiest mistake to make is that of assuming his views, without checking with him. Both full-time mothers and those who go out to work are better off if their partners support their choice, or at least understand it. The transition to parenthood involves major transitions for men as well as for women, and your partner will have to adapt in various ways, whether you become a working mother or a staying-at-home one. Both the practical and the emotional implications for the partnership need to be talked about and talked about again.

If the woman stays at home, a well established way of domestic life is dramatically changed, especially for couples who defer their children for some years, or for whom babies do not arrive as quickly as planned. If, as for many couples, the man has taken an equal share of domestic responsibilities, he may feel that part of his role has been taken away from him, despite the convention that women at home will become housewives as well as mothers. On the other hand, he may expect this shift in responsibilities, whilst the woman may expect him to continue to shoulder a substantial share of domestic duties. She may see her new, unpaid job as motherhood, not housework.

For mothers who go out to work, the demands of children and

domestic duties on top of a job are very stressful indeed. Whatever happened before, they are likely to find they need support from their partners now. Even if a partner has not previously been involved domestically, a woman with both children and work will badly need a more active input from her partner.

Studies have shown that, even when both partners are working equal hours outside the home, it is very rare for men to share the domestic responsibilities equally. If you are concerned that your partner may not realize quite how onerous the household chores can be, it may be worth making lists and negotiating a reasonably fair deal for each of you. Women often complain that it is not only the doing of the chores that is time- and energy-consuming, but the thinking about them, the planning of what needs to be done. Lists are a good way of making sure that you both understand what responsibilities are there to be shared. It is easy for someone not directly carrying out a particular set of household tasks to forget that these things do not happen by themselves. Making sure that you are both aware of what needs to be done, and what you can share, will help to keep resentment at an unfair workload at bay. If either of you is feeling overburdened, discuss your feelings, and take action before a minor irritation turns to real anger.

You may also find that you have to work particularly hard at nurturing your own relationship during these transition periods. If both of you are working as well as having to cope with a child and household jobs, it can be easy to forget to spend time with each other. It may feel as though you no longer have any spare time to spend together. Checking that you can get together for at least a ten-minute chat each day, to catch up on each other's news, and deliberately making time to have longer periods together on a regular basis will help to keep your lines of communication open.

As with all the issues confronting new parents, it is helpful for both partners to have opportunities to talk to other people in a similar situation, and to find out how they have managed to cope with the return to work.

CHILD-CARE OPTIONS

There are a number of excellent publications on the market which describe in some detail the child-care options to be considered. The Working Mothers Association, in particular, offers very helpful guidance on choices, based on members' own experiences as well as the experiences of those offering various forms of care. This section will, therefore, simply outline the main options and give some suggestions about the factors you might need to take into account when making your own decision.

It may be helpful to remember that you are not trying to find someone to be a substitute 'you'. You need to feel sure that your baby will be well cared for in a sensitive, stimulating environment, by someone whose outlook on life roughly resembles your own, without feeling you are looking for a perfect replacement for yourself. Many women have admitted that initially they set their sights unrealistically high when looking at child-care options. Only when they realized that finding a second mother for their babies was attempting the impossible did they find a successful solution.

Nanny

A proper nanny is someone, usually a young woman, who has taken an appropriate qualification at a local or national college after leaving school. These courses include both theoretical and practical work on aspects of child development: safety and first aid; health and welfare of children; nutrition and play. Modern nannies do not have to be starchy and uniformed; they are much more likely to be wearing jeans and to call you by your first name. They can be expected to take full charge of your baby or child in every sense, in your absence. They can be living-in or living-out. They can work out quite expensive, relative to other forms of child care, especially as you are expected to meet their tax and national insurance contributions over and above the net wage they will be getting. Although a few nannies may be expecting to lead jet-setting life-styles with their families, many more enjoy working with ordinary families in ordinary homes. Nannies are not only for the rich and famous!

Some nannies are not qualified, but have acquired experience in child care since leaving school. The qualification alone is no guarantee of the quality of child care, and it will be up to you to check whether your prospective nanny is likely to care for your children responsibly and in the way you would wish.

As well as child care, nannies will usually expect to be responsible for keeping the children's areas of the house tidy, dealing with children's laundry and mending, and cooking children's meals, but not for any other areas of work in the home.

NANNY-SHARE A nanny-share is an arrangement whereby two families share the costs of a single nanny. It has considerable financial appeal, but to work well requires clear agreement between the two families and with the nanny about how things will work.

Mother's help

A mother's help is typically a younger person, unqualified, who is employed to do a mixture of child care and housework. Again, she may be live-in or live-out. The great appeal is that wages are usually less than for a nanny. You will, however, need to weigh the relative youth and inexperience against the savings in financial terms.

Au pair

An au pair is a young woman from overseas who lives with a family in this country, with the aim of gaining an insight into British family life and improving her English. She is paid a very small sum of money in return for limited hours of household duties, which might include child care. She usually expects the family to arrange English classes for her. There are strict Home Office regulations about length of stay (for people from non-EEC countries, that is). Hours and conditions of work are also clearly laid down by the more reputable au pair agencies. Employing an au pair is unlikely to be a suitable arrangement for caring full-time for a young baby, but may work well for older children who are at nursery or school. One disadvantage is that au pairs are unlikely to stay for more than six or twelve months.

Your local Social Services office will have a list of registered child-minders in your area. Registration depends on a minder meeting basic requirements of safety, and will specify the numbers and ages of children she may take. Although there has been some bad press about minders, particularly unregistered ones, they can be excellent mother-substitutes. A minder is very often someone with young children of her own, who enjoys child care and has decided to look after additional children in her own home. The advantages are that this form of care is cheaper than a nanny for one child; the minder is likely to be an experienced mother; and your child will meet and get to know other children from the start. The disadvantages include having to take your child to her house and pick her up each day. If your child is ill, then the minder will probably expect (and you would probably want) your child to stay at home. This means time off work for you or your partner. As with any form of child care, her approach to parenting needs to be one with which you agree, and you may wish to visit several child-minders (if there is a choice locally) before deciding which would be best with your baby.

Child-minders

Both public sector and private nurseries are still fairly few in number. Local Authorities tend to reserve their own nursery places in large proportions for families and children with special needs.

Despite recent publicity, workplace crèches are still rather a rarity, though numbers are slowly growing. They can now be subsidized by the employer without being taxed as a perk. They offer the advantage of having your child nearby, and the possibility of popping in at lunch-time. No extra travelling is involved — your child comes to work and goes home with you. If you happen to commute into a major city each day, this may seem more like a disadvantage than a benefit.

The critical issue in nursery-type provision is whether you are satisfied, particularly where babies and very young children are concerned, that staffing is sufficiently high and stable enough that your child will be able to form, and continue, reliable close relationships with relatively few adults. Although all nurseries and crèches have to be Social Services registered, this only assures minimum standards. You will, again, need to do your own thorough checking.

Nurseries and workplace crèches

As with child-minders, you will also need to have contingency plans for those times when your child is ill and cannot attend.

For slightly older children, day nurseries or crèches can be lots of fun and provide plenty of friends and companions, facilities, and activities. They should, however, be regarded with a degree of caution for the very young.

Friends and relatives

Strictly speaking, anyone who looks after someone else's child for money in the carer's own home, must become a registered child-minder. If you have an informal arrangement in mind, then it would be wise for you to ensure that this is complied with, particularly for insurance purposes.

Some parents, however, especially part-timers or job-sharers, arrange to share child care between them, without payment. Some people have mothers or in-laws who are young, fit, and interested enough to take on child-care responsibilities.

Informal arrangements which start off in an amicable but vague way can occasionally run into difficulties, so it is better to have anticipated and discussed how things might be handled in advance, at least to some extent. As with all child care, you will need to clarify and make explicit any definite views you may have about how you would like your child to be brought up. If you do not sort out these matters beforehand, any relationship you already have with the prospective carer risks coming under severe strain should any problems arise.

Role-swapping

For a variety of reasons, there is a small but growing number of couples where the man is taking the major, or a significant, responsibility for child care. Some couples have decided that the mother should be the bread-winner and the father the full-time child-care person. Others have decided to share both roles. Although this is still regarded as unconventional by some, it can work very well indeed. Any issues about whose work is the more rewarding, who earns the most, and who enjoys time at home with the children can be considered. The possible disadvantage follows from the very unconventionality of the situation. Motherhood may be under-valued, but there are strong networks for mothers in most neighbourhoods. Fathers may find it hard to enter into these. It can be difficult for women to re-enter employment after a gap, but at least child care is seen as a fairly legitimate reason for a woman's career break, while at present this is not, unfortunately, the case for men.

Whatever the conventions where you live, it can be important for men to have the opportunity to be a full-time parent, and children can benefit enormously from being presented with much less stereotyped sex-role models.

○ PLACE OF CARE — OWN HOME, ANOTHER HOME, OR NURSERY?

○ EASE OF COPING WITH DISRUPTION (E.G. SICK CHILD, SICK CARER)

○ OPPORTUNITIES FOR CHILD TO FORM SECURE ATTACHMENTS

○ COST

○ HOW WELL YOU GET ON WITH THE CHILD-CARE PERSON

○ COMPATIBILITY OF YOUR AND THEIR CHILD-CARE IDEAS AND ATTITUDES

○ WHETHER YOU WOULD LIKE YOUR CHILD TO BE WITH OTHER CHILDREN

○ DEGREE OF INDIVIDUAL ATTENTION FOR YOUR CHILD

○ FACILITIES IN THE PLACE OF CHILD CARE

○ RELIABILITY OF THE CHILD-CARE PERSON

○ STABILITY OF ARRANGEMENTS (ESPECIALLY FOR LITTLE CHILDREN)

Key considerations in choice of child care

COPING WITH THE RETURN TO WORK

If you have made a firm decision to return, then the return itself is likely to need preparation: for you, your baby, and your partner. The transition to the new arrangements for all of you will probably generate both practical and emotional issues, which all tend to be inter-related but are put under separate headings here for convenience.

Helping your baby

Feeling confident and supported in your decision about the return, and about the arrangements you are making, will itself help your baby, who will be sensitive to both your feelings and your partner's.

In addition, it will help your baby if she has already had some experience of being looked after without you, and has begun to learn that, when you go, you do also come back. It is usually sensible and helpful to introduce the baby and the child-care person to each other in a gradual way during the week or two before you go back to work, phasing yourself out as they grow used to each other. When the time comes to leave your baby, it helps to give a firm, clear 'Goodbye', perhaps in a special way, rather than anxiously prolonging the parting. Some babies will separate fairly easily; others will protest vigorously. It is quite understandable that a baby should protest at the loss of her beloved mother, but most babies will then settle fairly quickly. When you return, you may find that your baby is delighted to see you again, or you may find that there is a brief period of anger, distress, or rejection. Again, all of these reactions are understandable. The more negative ones are likely to diminish quickly after the first few occasions, once your baby becomes familiar with the new carer and your regular departure and arrival.

The important thing is to make sure that you show your baby that you still love her, even if, for a little while, you are not receiving much obvious love in return. Any negative reactions can be looked on as your baby's way of showing a strong attachment to you, which is needing reassurance.

On a practical level, it will help if your new child-care person knows about your baby's normal routine, and her likes and dislikes. It will also help your baby to have some familiar things about her, especially if the arrangement is away from home.

Breastfeeding

Depending on your baby's age and stage of progress towards weaning before you return to work, you may want to continue breastfeeding. It is very easy, and physically perfectly possible, to continue for those parts of the day or night when you are at home. Indeed, nursing your baby can be a lovely way of having some close time together at either end of the day.

If your baby is in a workplace crèche, then you may wish to breastfeed during your breaks from work too. This is perfectly possible. It will help, however, if you and your baby have established some sort of routine beforehand. You will also need to decide what you would like to happen should your baby become hungry or thirsty when you are not there. The options will be either expressed milk or an alternative (another drink or baby food). Staff will need to know what you want, and be willing to support your decision.

If your baby is being looked after near your workplace, it may also be possible to organize your work so that you can slip off to breastfeed in a similar way. If either work demands or distance from your baby make this impossible, you will need to consider whether you would prefer your baby to have expressed milk, or an alternative during your working day. If you choose to express, then you will need to buy or hire a suitable breast pump and ensure that you can have privacy and appropriate storage facilities at work and *en route* home, if necessary. The NCT can help with both pump hire and guidance on expressing and storing milk. Leaflets are available from your local breastfeeding counsellor or from NCT Headquarters. Your local counsellor can be a valuable source of help and support.

Helping your child's carer

It is well worth spending time building up an open relationship with your baby's carer, so that each of you can discuss any problems or concerns and reach satisfactory conclusions about how things should be handled. Inevitably, there will be some differences in the ways you both do things, and it is important to be able to have mutual respect for these differences.

A gradual, phased transition will help both the carer and your baby, providing it is not too protracted. It is essential that your carer is familiar with routines and preferences, and that you are both quite clear about what you expect from each other.

It can be very hard, when it comes to the crunch, to entrust your baby to someone you have not known for very long, but it is important that any anxieties you may have are not expressed so strongly that the new person feels undermined. Equally, doubts and queries are generally best resolved openly and swiftly, rather than left to grow and fester.

You will be dealing both with entrusting your baby to a new carer and with your own return to work, possibly after a gap of nine or ten months.

Your own adjustment

The transition to new child-care arrangements, including actually leaving your baby with the new person on your first day back at work, can be very emotional. Many women who are perfectly satisfied with their decisions and arrangements, and keen to be back at work, still find themselves making the first day's journey with misty eyes, and find their thoughts very much on their babies during the early period at work. It helps a great deal to find other women who have small children, either at your place of work or through local networks, so that you can share experiences and concerns.

The return itself can be rather daunting after some months of nappies and feeding, and even broken nights. Some women pick up where they left off, but others find that they need to work at regaining their self-confidence. It often helps to have remained in at least intermittent contact, and to have visited work a few times before the return proper.

On a practical level, it may take time to develop a good way of handling the often conflicting demands of work, mothering, being a partner, and the domestic chores. Despite the images which sometimes appear in the media, very few people make it into the superwoman league! It can help to make pragmatic decisions about what simply has to go. All of these areas are likely to need some radical rethinking and adjustment.

Some of the issues for partners and for your relationship have already been discussed. Whatever agreements you have reached about how you are planning to organize and share the responsibilities, it is sensible to maintain a degree of flexibility and to review together how things are working out for you both. Theory and practice may often have a yawning gap between them which will need more careful negotiation. Most importantly, remember to discuss anything about which either of you is unhappy.

You and your partner

If you do decide to return to paid work, for whatever reasons, and it is the right decision for you, then it takes some thought and effort to manage the transition. There will always be people who will be critical of what you have done, both at work and at home. The world is not yet well geared to understanding mothers who work, nor to supporting them, either practically or emotionally. The numbers of women who make this choice are growing, however, both out of necessity and out of preference. Both they, their partners, and their children can gain a great deal. For none of these people is it necessarily better or worse than full-time mothering; it is simply different.

I hadn't planned on going back to work for a year or two, but I wasn't ever happy at home just looking after a baby and a house. I feel I'm a much nicer person now I'm back at work.

Both of us working full time makes life fraught at times, and we're very reliant on other people, but there's certainly no lack of stimulation in our household.

I was worried I could get bored or frustrated at home, and there are moments, days even, when I feel like that, but most of the time I love it. I'm not answerable to anyone, and we're free to do what we like when we choose, given the minor restrictions of his sleeping and feeding timetable. If we decide to go to the park one afternoon because the weather's nice, or spend a morning having coffee with his friends and mine, we can.

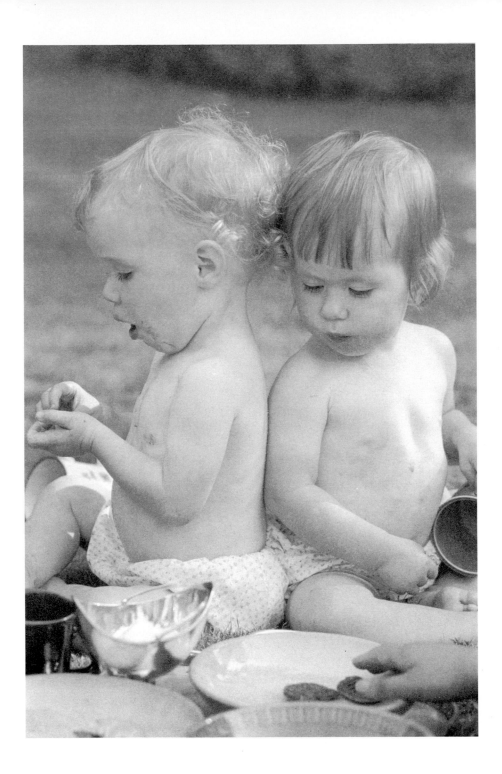

GLOSSARY OF TERMS

abruptio placentae: *see* placental abruption.

acceleration (or augmentation) of labour: process by which labour is artificially speeded up, usually by performing an ARM and using a hormone drip.

alpha-feto-protein (AFP): a protein circulating in the baby's blood before birth, which escapes into the mother's blood and may be used for testing for neural tube defects.

amniocentesis: a test carried out in early pregnancy to detect genetic abnormalities in the fetus; in particular, Down's syndrome.

amniotic fluid (the waters, or the liquor): the clear liquid which cushions and protects the baby throughout pregnancy. It is contained in the amniotic sac.

anaemia: a lack of haemoglobin in the red blood cells, often caused by insufficient iron. Symptoms might include tiredness, breathlessness and lack of energy, because of the inability of the blood to carry oxygen to all the body tissues efficiently. Anaemia can exacerbate postnatal problems of tiredness.

antenatal: before birth.

anterior: front: as in anterior shoulder of the baby, or anterior position of the baby in the pelvis.

augmentation of labour: *see* acceleration.

birth canal: term used to describe the joined uterus and vagina once the cervix is fully dilated, and through which the baby will travel before delivery.

breech birth: delivery of a baby who is born bottom or feet first rather than head first.

Caesarean section: the delivery of a baby via an incision in the mother's abdomen and uterus.

cephalic: the position of a baby who is head down in the uterus.

cervix: the ring of muscle at the neck of the uterus which acts like a drawstring. It remains tightly closed during pregnancy, then dilates during labour to enable the baby to be born.

colostrum: the first food for the baby, produced by the breasts, sustaining and protecting a baby during the first few days of life.

contraction: tightening of the muscle fibres of the uterus during labour. As the fibres tighten, they grow shorter, causing the uterus to become smaller, thus pushing the baby out.

chorionic villus sampling (CVS): an alternative test to amniocentesis, for the detection of certain genetic abnormalities.

Down's syndrome: a genetic disorder causing mental and physical handicaps.

ectopic pregnancy: a pregnancy complication where the fertilized egg implants and begins to grow outside the uterus, most usually in the Fallopian tubes. This necessitates an emergency operation before 10 weeks, as the tubes cannot accommodate the growing fetus.

embryo: a baby or fetus of less than 7 weeks gestation.

engagement (lightening): the descent of the baby's head into the pelvis. This usually happens during the last four weeks of pregnancy with a first baby, but may not occur until the start of labour in a second or subsequent pregnancy.

fetus: a baby in the uterus, from 7 weeks gestation to birth.

fetal movements: the kicks, wriggles, punches, and squirms of a baby in the uterus.

gestation: the time in weeks from the last period to the birth of a baby.

hydatidiform mole: an uncommon form of miscarriage in which the egg fails to develop but the placenta continues to grow.

hormone: chemicals made by the body which enter the blood as 'messengers' to other parts of the body. Many hormones are specifically produced during pregnancy and breastfeeding.

hypertension: medical term for high blood pressure.

induction: a procedure by which labour is artificially started.

incompetent cervix: a rather unpleasant term used to describe a condition in which the cervix opens suddenly during pregnancy, usually occurring after the first trimester (*see* Shirodkhar stitch).

inevitable miscarriage: bleeding from the uterus in early pregnancy, usually coupled with pain, which will definitely end in an actual miscarriage because the fetus has died.

inverted nipple: a condition where one or both nipples are turned inwards instead of sticking out. If the condition does not right itself during pregnancy, a baby with a good strong suck usually will. If not, a midwife or breastfeeding counsellor will be able to help.

ketones: chemicals in the blood which indicate that the body is low in blood sugar and therefore short of energy.

kick chart: a record of fetal movements. It involves counting the number of movements the baby makes each day, so that any change in the baby's pattern, which might call for further investigation, will be noticed.

ligaments: tough, fibrous tissue connecting one bone to another.

lanugo: the downy hair present on some babies' skin.

meconium: the tar-like substance which plugs the baby's bowel before birth.

occiput: the crown of the baby's head.

oedema: swelling due to fluid retention in the tissues. It is one of the three possible signs of pre-eclampsia, though slightly swollen ankles or fingers are not necessarily any particular cause for concern.

oestriol test: a test which may be carried out if doctors are concerned that the placenta may not be functioning properly. The results are not conclusive and are normally used in conjunction with other forms of fetal monitoring.

pelvic floor: the sling of muscle surrounding and supporting the bladder, vagina, and rectum.

perineum: the skin between the back of the vagina and the anus.

placenta (afterbirth): the organ which grows in pregnancy and provides the means whereby the baby receives oxygen, nutrients, and certain protective factors from the mother, and eliminates waste products via the mother's system. One side is attached to the wall of the uterus, at the site where the egg first implanted; the other side is connected to the baby via the umbilical cord.

placental abruption: an emergency situation in which the placenta suddenly separates from the uterine wall. Bleeding from the vagina is a possible symptom. Both mother and baby are at grave risk and urgent action must be taken.

placenta praevia: a complication whereby the placenta grows over the cervix, blocking the baby's exit. If the placenta completely covers the opening, a Caesarean section is necessary.

placental insufficiency: a condition in which the placenta fails to supply adequate nourishment for the growing baby. The baby may be small for its gestational age or become less and less active.

polyhydramnios: a condition where there is more fluid in the amniotic sac than usual.

posterior: back, as in posterior position of the baby in the pelvis, when the back of the baby's head is against the mother's spine.

post-mature: born after 42 weeks. Signs at birth might include dry, peeling skin, long nails, and extreme hunger!

postnatal: the time after the birth.

premature (pre-term): born before 37 weeks.

pre-eclampsia (or pre-eclamptic toxaemia (PET)): a complex condition occurring in about 10% of pregnant women. The causes are unclear and it will disappear soon after birth. There are three indications of pre-eclampsia: oedema, hypertension, protein in the urine. The presence of all three signs may mean that the placenta may not be functioning effectively. In severe cases the baby may have to be delivered by Caesarean section for the sake of her and her mother's health.

proteinuria: protein in the urine.

rubella: German measles.

Shirodkhar stitch: a purse-string stitch in the cervix to stop it opening if there is any sign of an incompetent cervix. The stitch will be loosened with a snip as labour begins or shortly before the expected date of birth.

show: the mucus plug in the cervical opening during pregnancy which will come away during labour, often as the first indication that labour may soon begin.

small for dates: a baby who is considered to be small for her apparent gestational dates.

term: the date at which your baby would be expected.

threatened miscarriage: bleeding in the early weeks of pregnancy which may or may not result in an actual miscarriage.

toxaemia: the old-fashioned term for pre-eclampsia.

trimester: 'a third'. Pregnancy is divided into three sections of roughly equal length: first, second, and third trimesters.

ultrasound (scan): a means of looking at the baby in the uterus using sound waves.

uterus (womb): the muscle which surrounds and holds your baby during pregnancy, growing with her and tightening or contracting to push her out at birth.

vernix: the creamy-white coloured substance which protects the baby's skin before birth.

vulva: a woman's external genitals.

FURTHER READING

There is a wealth of literature available on many topics related to pregnancy, childbirth, and parenthood. Here are some which provide further information on many of the topics covered in this book.

Pregnancy and birth
Ashdown-Sharp, P., *The Single Woman's Guide to Pregnancy and Parenthood* (London, 1975).

Balaskas, J., *New Active Birth* (Cambridge, 1989).

Balaskas, J., and Gordon, Y., *Water Birth* (London, 1990).

Brooks, M., *Caesarean Section* (London, 1989).

Clement, S., *The Caesarean Experience* (London, 1991).

Enkin, M., Keirse, M., Renfrew, M., and Neilson, J., *A Guide to Effective Care in Pregnancy and Childbirth* (Oxford, 1995).

Goldsmith, J., *Childbirth Wisdom* (Brookline, 1990).

Inch, S., *Birthrights* (London, 1994).

Jain Campion, M., *The Baby Challenge* (London, 1990) (for mothers with physical disabilities).

Kitzinger, S., *Freedom and Choice in Childbirth* (London, 1987).

Lewison, H., for NCT, *Your Choice for Pregnancy and Childbirth* (London, (1991).

Oakley, A., *et al.*, *Miscarriage* (London, 1990).

Odent, M., *Birth Reborn* (London, 1984).

Parry, V., *The Antenatal Testing Handbook* (London, 1993).

Phillips, A., *Your Body, your Baby, your Life* (London, 1989).

Pickard, B., *Eating Well for a Healthy Pregnancy* (London, 1984).

Priest, J., *Drugs in Pregnancy and Childbirth* (London, 1990).

Savage, W., and Reader, F., *Coping with Caesareans and Other Difficult Births* (Edinburgh, 1983).

Wesson, N., *Alternative Maternity* (London, 1989).

Postnatal
Atkinson, C., *Step-Parenting* (Wellingborough, 1986).

Brannen, J., and Moss, P., *New Mothers at Work* (London, 1988).

Bryan, E., *Twins in the Family* (London, 1984).

Dunn, J., *Siblings* (London, 1984).

Fletcher, G., for NCT, *Get into Shape after Childbirth* (London, 1991).

Friedrich, E., and Rowland, C., *Twins Handbook* (London, 1983).

Kitzinger, S., *Breastfeeding your Baby* (London, 1989).

—— *The Crying Baby* (London, 1992).

—— *The Year After Childbirth* (Oxford, 1994).

Kremant, J., *How it Feels to be Adopted* (London, 1984).

Leach, P., *Baby and Child* (London, 1988).

Luben, J., *Cot Death* (London, 1989).

Rankin, G., *The First Year* (London, 1988).

Redshaw, M., Rivers, R., and Rosenblatt, D., *Born Too Early* (Oxford, 1989).

Renfrew, M., Fisher, C., and Arms, *Bestfeeding* (California, 1990).

Seel, R., *The Uncertain Father* (Bath, 1987).

Smale, M., *The National Childbirth Book of Breastfeeding* (London, 1992).

Welburn, V., *Postnatal Depression* (London, 1984).

Welford, H., *The A-Z of Feeding in the First Year* (London, 1988).

Working Mothers Association, *Working Mothers' Handbook* (London, 1990).

NCT leaflets

So You're Pregnant—The First Few Months

Healthy Eating for Pregnancy

Sex in Pregnancy and after Birth

Caring for your Pelvic Floor, Before, During, and After Childbirth

Becoming a Father

Miscarriage

A Guide to Labour for Expectant Parents

Induction of Labour

The Third Stage of Labour

Caesarean Birth

Thinking about Breastfeeding?

Breastfeeding after a Caesarean Section

Breastfeeding—a Good Start

Breastfeeding—Avoiding Some of the Problems

Breastfeeding—Making Plenty of Milk for Your Baby

How to Express and Store Breast Milk

Breastfeeding—Too Much Milk?

Breastfeeding if your Baby Needs Special Care

NCT booklets

Accessible Health—A Survey of Physical Access to Primary Health Care Services in the UK

Breastfeeding a Toddler

Breastfeeding—Returning to Work

Emotions and Experiences of Some Disabled Mothers

Giving Birth at Home

Mothers Writing about the Death of a Baby

Postnatal Infection Survey

Rupture of the Membranes in Labour— Survey of Women's Experiences

Some Women's Experiences of Epidurals

The Challenge of Change—Helping Lay Representatives to Work for Change in Childbirth

The Perineum in Childbirth—A Survey of Women's Experiences and Midwives' Practices

What Women Want from Midwives, Obstetricians, GPs and Health Visitors

Useful Addresses

It will be helpful to include a stamped addressed envelope when writing to any of these organizations.

The National Childbirth Trust
Alexandra House
Oldham Terrace
London W3 6NH
0181 992 8637

Action Against Allergy
43 The Downs
London SW20 8HG
0181 947 5082
(Information, advice, leaflets, on allergy problems.)

Active Birth Centre
55 Dartmouth Park Road
London NW5 1SL
0171 561 9006
(Workshops, classes, information for those interested in active birth methods and exercises. Also rent birthing pools.)

Association of Breastfeeding Mothers
10 Herschell Road
London SE23 1EG
0181 778 4769
(Local support groups.)

Association of Crossroads Care Attendance Schemes
10 Regent Place
Rugby
War CV21 4RN
01788 573653
(Help for disabled people.)

Association for Improvement in the Maternity Services (AIMS)
21 Iver Lane
Iver
Bucks SL0 9LH
01753 652781
(Offers information, support, and advice on all aspects of maternity care.)

Association for Postnatal Illness
25 Jerdan Place
London SW6 1BE
0171 386 0868
(Self-help groups offering one-to-one support for mothers.)

Association of Radical Midwives (ARM)
62 Greetby Hill
Ormskirk
Lancs. L39 2DT

Association for Spina Bifida and Hydrocephalus
ASBAH House
42 Park Road
Peterborough
Cambs PE1 2UQ
01735 555988

Baby Life Support Systems (BLISS)
17–21 Emerald Street
London WC1N 3QL
0171 831 9393
(Help and information for parents of babies needing Special Care.)

Benefits Enquiry Line
Freephone:
0800 666555

Birthright
27 Sussex Place
Regent's Park
London NW1 4SP
0171 723 9296
(Raises money for research, and produces leaflets on aspects of maternity care.)

Birthworks
Unit 4E
Brent Mill Trading Estate
South Brent
Devon TQ10 9YT
(Hire of birthing pool for home birth.)

British Diabetic Association
10 Queen Anne Street
London W1M 0BD
0171 323 1531

British Epilepsy Association
Anstey House
40 Hanover Square
Leeds LS3 1BE
01324 639393

British Pregnancy Advisory Service
Austy Manor
Wotton Wawen
Solihull
W. Midlands B95 6BX
01564 793227/5
(Offers pregnancy tests, counselling, abortion, vasectomy, sterilization, and other services.)

Anne Buckley
14 Brookway
Grasscroft
Oldham OL4 4EU
(Supplies nursing supplementer.)

Caesarean Support Network
c/o Mrs Tunstall
2 Hurst Park Drive
Huyton
Merseyside L36 1TF
0151 480 1184

Cleft Lip and Palate Association
1 Eastwood Gardens
Kenton
Newcastle-upon-Tyne NE3 3DQ
0191 285 9396

Compassionate Friends
53 North Street
Bedminster
0117 953 9639
(Support for the bereaved.)

CRY-SIS
BM Cry-sis
London WC1N 3XX
0171 404 5011
(Support for parents of crying babies.)

Down's Syndrome Association
155 Mitcham Road
London SW17 9PG
0181 682 4001

The Disability Information Trust
Mary Marlborough Lodge
Nuffield Orthopaedic Centre
Headington
Oxford OX3 7LD
01865 227592

Exploring Parenthood
Omnibus Workspace
39–41 North Road
London N7 9DP
(Runs workshops on problems and pleasures of parenthood.)

Family Planning Association
27–35 Mortimer Street
London W1N 7RJ
0171 636 7866
(Information and leaflets on all aspects of family planning and contraception.)

Foresight
The Old Vicarage
Church Lane
Whitley
Godalming
Surrey GU8 5PM
(Information, leaflets, and advice on pre-conceptual care.)

Foundation for the Study of Infant Deaths
35 Belgrave Square
London SW1X 8QB
0171 235 0965/1721
(Raises funds for research and offers support to bereaved parents.)

Gingerbread
35 Wellington Street
London WC2E 7BN
0171 240 0953
(Organizes local self-help groups for single parents and their children.)

Home-start
140 New Walk
Leicester LE1 7JL
0116 233 9955

In Touch Trust
10 Norman Road
Sale
Cheshire M33 3DF
0161 962 4441
(Information and contact for all aspects of mental handicap.)

Independent Midwives Association
94 Auckland Road
London SE19 2DB

La Leche League
BM 3424
London WC1V 6XX
0171 242 1278
(Encouragement, information, and support for breastfeeding mothers.)

Maternity Alliance
45 Beech Street
London EC2P 2LX
0171 588 8582
(Campaigns for improvements in maternity care.)

Maternity Alliance Disability Working Group
c/o **Maternity Alliance**

Meet-A-Mum-Association (MAMA)
14 Willis Road
Croydon CR0 2XX
0180 665 0357
(Self-help groups for new mothers.)

Miscarriage Association
c/o Clayton Hospital
Northgate
Wakefield
W. Yorkshire W1 3JS
01924 200799
(Offers information and support during and after miscarriage.)

National Association of Nappy Services
0121 693 4949
(Nappy laundry service: delivery and collection.)

National Association of Parents of Sleepless Children
PO Box 33
Prestwood
Gt. Missenden
Bucks NH16 0SZ
(Responds by letter to individual enquiries; leaflets available.)

National Childminding Association
8 Mason's Hill
Bromley
Kent BR2 9EY
0181 464 6164
(Information on finding a registered child-minder.)

National Council for One-Parent Families
255 Kentish Town Road
London NW5 2LX
0171 267 1361

Natural Family Planning Service
Clitheroe House
1 Blythe Mews
Blythe Road
London W14 0NW
(Information on natural ways to plan and avoid pregnancy.)

NCT Maternity Sales Ltd.
Burnfield Avenue
Glasgow GL6 7TL
0141 633 5552

NIPPERS
Sam Segal Perinatal Research
Unit
St Mary's Hospital
Praed Street
London W2 1NY
0171 725 1487
(Information and practical help
for parents of premature or sick
new-born babies.)

Parentability
c/o NCT
(Help and support for disabled
parents.)

Parentline OPUS
Rayfa House
57 Hart Road
Thundersley
Essex SS7 3PD
01268 757077
(Organization for parents under
stress.)

Parent Network
44–46 Caversham Road
London NW5 2DS
0171 485 8535

Pre-Eclampsia Society (PETS)
Bryn Mor
Carmel
Caernarfon
Gwynedd LL54 7AD
01286 880057/01702 205088
(Encourages research into causes
of PET; offers support, advice
and information.)

**Pre-school Playgroup
Association**
61–63 King's Cross Road
London WC1X 9LL

REMAP
c/o Mr J. Wright
Hazeldene
Ightam
Sevenoaks
Kent TN15 9AD
01732 883818
(Engineering help for disabled
people.)

Royal College of Midwives
15 Mansfield Street
London W1M 0BE
0171 580 6523

Splashdown
17 Wellington Terrace
Harrow-on-the-Hill
Middlesex HA1 3EP
0181 422 9308
(Hire of birthing pool for home
birth.)

**Stillbirth and Neonatal
Death Society (SANDS)**
28 Portland Place
London W1N 4DE
0171 436 5881
(Resource and information
service; encourages greater
awareness of feelings and
needs of parents by health
professionals.)

**Support after Termination
of Fetal Abnormality
(SATFA)**
The Hospital for Women
29–30 Soho Square
London W1N 6JB
0171 631 0285

Spembley Medical
Newbury Road
Andover
Hants. SP10 4DR
(Hire of TENS machines.)

**Twins and Multiple Births
Association (TAMBA)**
Sheilagh Payne
59 Sunnyside
Worksop
North Notts.
Helpline (6pm–11pm and
weekends): 01732 868000
(All aspects of twins.)
TAMBA Administrator (office
hours): 0151 348 0020

**Working Mothers
Association**
77 Holloway Road
London N7 8JZ
0171 700 5771

ACKNOWLEDGEMENTS

The publishers wish to thank the following for supplying photographs for this book:

Page v, Lupe Cunha Photography; page 1, The Hutchison Library/Nancy Durrell McKenna; page 24, Camilla Jessel; page 51, The Hutchison Library/Simon McBride; page 53, Department of Medical Illustration, St Bartholomew's Hospital; page 65, Lupe Cunha Photography; page 68, Lupe Cunha Photography; page 86, Lupe Cunha Photography; page 92, Lupe Cunha Photography; page 112, The Hutchison Library/ Nancy Durrell McKenna; page 126, Camilla Jessel; page 139, Lupe Cunha Photography; page 146, Bubbles/Gena Naccacne; page 147, The Hutchison Library/Nancy Durrell McKenna; page 148, The Hutchison Library/Nancy Durrell McKenna; page 155, The Hutchison Library/Nancy Durrell McKenna; page 161, Lupe Cunha Photography; page 168, Lupe Cunha Photography; page 172, Lupe Cunha Photography; page 175, Lupe Cunha Photography; page 177, Lupe Cunha Photography; page 179, Lupe Cunha Photography; page 190, Science Photo Library/Larry Mulvehill; page 196, The Hutchison Library/Nancy Durrell McKenna; page 205, Lupe Cunha Photography; page 209, Lupe Cunha Photography; page 234, Lupe Cunha Photography; page 237, NCT/ Alan Perkins; page 240, Nancy Durrell McKenna; page 244, Sheila Kitzinger; page 248, Sheila Kitzinger; page 250, Sheila Kitzinger; page 253, Camilla Jessel; page 256, Camilla Jessel; page 262, The Hutchison Library/Nancy Durrell McKenna; page 275, The Hutchison Library/Nancy Durrell McKenna; page 277, Lupe Cunha Photography; page 283, Lupe Cunha Photography; page 291, Camilla Jessel; page 294, The Hutchison Library/Nancy Durrell McKenna; page 297, The Hutchison Library/Nancy Durrell McKenna; page 299, Camilla Jessel; page 301, Lupe Cunha Photography; page 302, Lupe Cunha Photography; page 303, Ann Nursey; page 304, Camilla Jessel; page 309, The Hutchison Library/Nancy Durrell McKenna; page 312, Bubbles/Loisjoy Thurston; page 314, The Hutchison Library/Nancy Durrell McKenna; page 317, NCT/Alan Perkins; page 318, NCT/Hilary English; page 319, NCT/Hilary English; page 320, NCT/ Alan Perkins; page 325, NCT/Hilary English; page 331, The Hutchison Library/Nancy Durrell McKenna; page 338, NCT/Julie Perkins; page 341, The Hutchison Library/ Nancy Durrell McKenna; page 344, Camilla Jessel; page 348, Lupe Cunha Photography; page 350, Camilla Jessel; page 352, Lupe Cunha Photography; page 357, Ann Nursey; page 367, The Hutchison Library; page 399, Camilla Jessel; page 411, The Hutchison Library/Simon McBride; page 421, Camilla Jessel; page 423, The Hutchison Library/Nancy Durrell McKenna; page 424, NCT/Alan Perkins; page 427, NCT/Alan Perkins; page 433, Camilla Jessel; page 463, Camilla Jessel.

INDEX

Index compiled by Frank Pert